CRASH

Nerv
System

SECOND EDITION

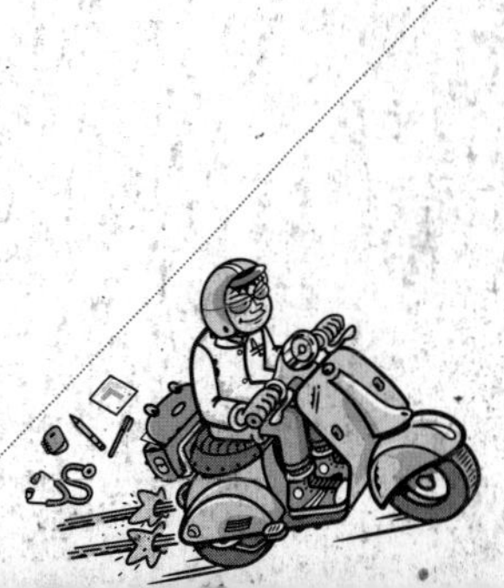

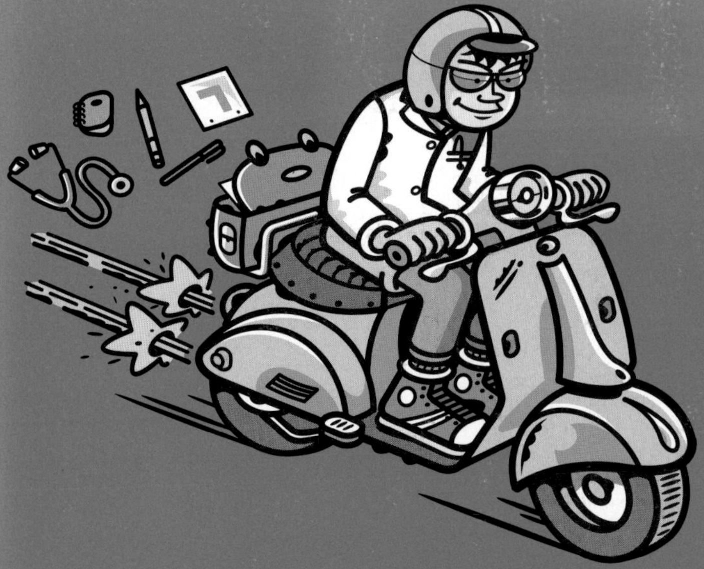

Series editor
Daniel Horton-Szar
BSc (Hons) MBBS (Hons)
GP Registrar
Northgate Medical Practice
Canterbury

Faculty advisor
Professor Anthony Angel
BSc (SpHons) PhD
Department of Biomedical Science
University of Sheffield
Alfred Denny Building
Western Bank
Sheffield

Nervous System

SECOND EDITION

Charlie Briar
BA BM BCh (Oxon)
Green College
University of Oxford

First Edition Authors
Daniel Lasserson, Carolyn Gabriel, Basil Sharrack

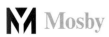

Mosby

London • Edinburgh • New York • Philadelphia • St Louis • Sydney • Toronto 2003

MOSBY
An affiliate of Elsevier Science Limited

Commissioning Editor	**Alex Stibbe**
Project Manager	**Frances Affleck**
Project Development Manager	**Duncan Fraser**
Designer	**Andy Chapman**
Cover Design	**Kevin Faerber**
Illustration Management	**Mick Ruddy**

First edition 1998
Second edition 2003

ISBN 0723432902

British Library Cataloguing in Publication Data
A catalogue record for this book is available from the British Library

Library of Congress Cataloging in Publication Data
A catalog record for this book is available from the Library of Congress

Note
Medical knowledge is constantly changing. As new information becomes available, changes in treatment, procedures, equipment and the use of drugs become necessary. The author, editors and the publisher have taken care to ensure that the information given in this text is accurate and up to date. However, readers are strongly advised to confirm that the information, especially with regard to drug usage, complies with the latest legislation and standards of practice.

Typeset by Kolam, Pondicherry, India
Printed in Spain by Graphycems

The publisher's policy is to use **paper manufactured from sustainable forests**

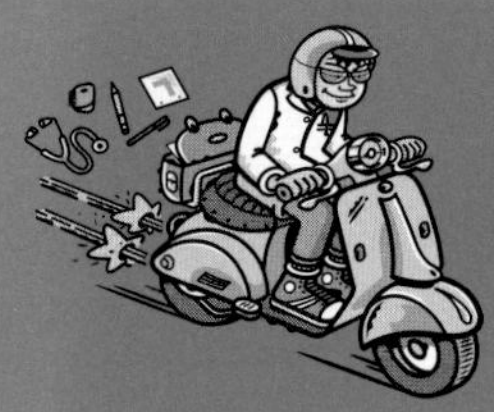

Preface

Welcome to *Crash Course: Nervous System*! Whether you are revising for preclinical exams, coming up for finals or simply looking for an integrated course text, this book should have something for you. It has been designed with tired, stressed out and coffee-deprived students in mind, and contains enough core information to help you sail through your exams. Along with core facts, I have tried to include clinically relevant material to add interest to what can often be a dry and complex topic. There are many unanswered questions in the field of neurology and I hope this book gives you a taste for discovering more about this fascinating topic.

I hope you get as much out of using this book as I have gained from writing it.

Charlie Briar

Crash Course: Nervous System offers an innovative approach to the education of medical students combining, in one text, the basic science required to understand the nervous system with an introduction to its pathology and pharmacology. In addition guidelines on taking a neurological history and performing a neurological examination are also included.

This second edition, updated by a senior medical student, represents the knowledge that a student at the top end of the academic spectrum sees as essential for a good understanding of the nervous system, its clinical problems and clinical neurological assessment. It is sufficiently comprehensive to allow a medical student to become conversant with the essential knowledge needed to understand how the nervous system functions and how it is affected by the various diseases it is vulnerable to. Students will be able to use this book as a revision source and, additionally, as a basis from which to explore the subject further.

Prof Anthony Angel
Faculty Advisor

In the six years since the first editions were published, there have been many changes in medicine, and in the way it is taught. These second editions have been largely rewritten to take these changes into account, and keep *Crash Course* up to date for the twenty-first century. New material has been added to include recent research and all pharmacological and disease management information has been updated in line with current best practice. We've listened to feedback from hundreds of students who have been using *Crash Course* and have improved the structure and layout of the books accordingly: pathology material has been closely integrated with the relevant basic medical science; there are more MCQs and the clarity of text and figures is better than ever.

The principles on which we developed the series remain the same, however. Medicine is a huge subject, and the last thing a student needs when exams are looming is to waste time assembling information from different sources, and wading through pages of irrelevant detail. As before, *Crash Course* brings you all the information you need, in compact, manageable volumes that integrate basic medical science with clinical practice. We still tread the fine line between producing clear, concise text and providing enough detail for those aiming at distinction. The series is still written by medical students with recent exam experience, and checked for accuracy by senior faculty members from across the UK.

I wish you the best of luck in your future careers!

Dr Dan Horton-Szar
Series Editor (Basic Medical Sciences)

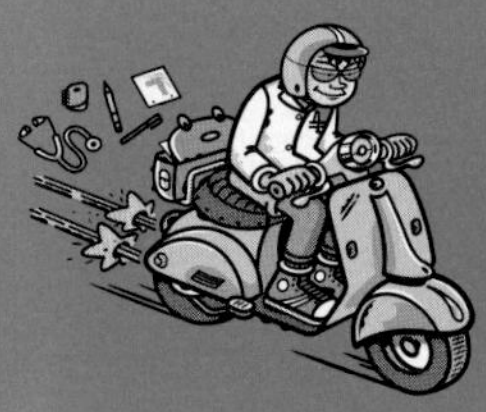

Acknowledgements

Fig 8.1 adapted with permission from C Page, M Curtis, M Sutter, M Walker and B Hoffman. Integrated Pharmacology. Mosby, 1997

Figs 9.1 and 9.2 adapted from A Stevens and J Lowe. Human Histology, 2nd edition. Mosby 1997

Figs 14.5, 14.8, 15.4, 15.8, 15.19, 15.23 and 15.24 adapted with permission from O Epstein, D Perkin, D de Bono and J Cookson. Clinical Examination, 3rd edition. Mosby, 1997

Figs 16.10, 16.11 and 16.18 reproduced with permission from J Weir and PH Abrahams. Imaging Atlas of Human Anatomy, 2nd edition. Mosby, 1997

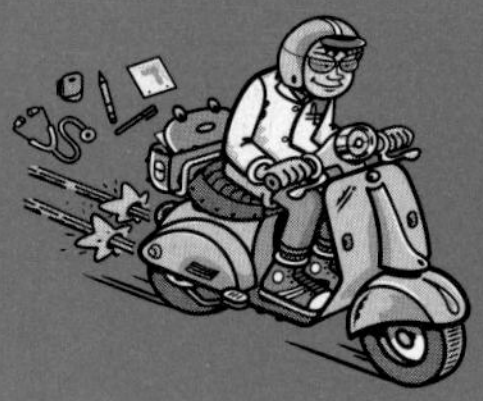

Dedication

To K and D who kept me sane,
and, most of all, to Andrew
who makes it a fulltime job.

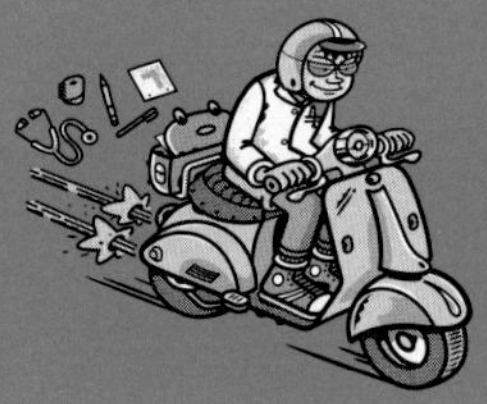

Contents

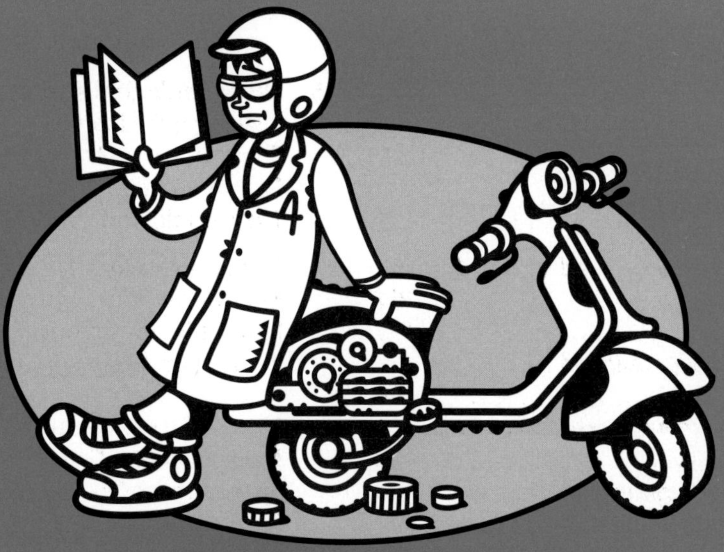

BASIC MEDICAL SCIENCE OF THE NERVOUS SYSTEM

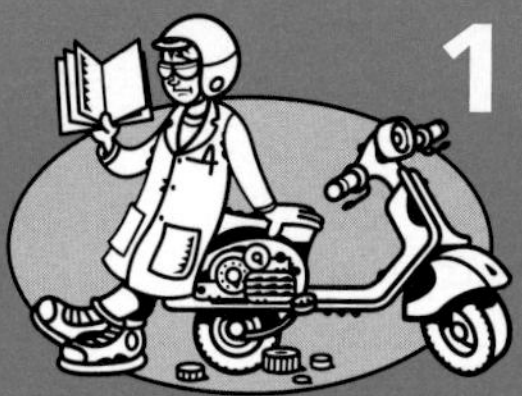

1. Overview of the Nervous System

In this chapter, you will learn about:

- The anatomy of the central nervous system.
- The development of the central nervous system.
- The blood supply, and venous drainage of the central nervous system, cerebrospinal fluid and supporting cells of the central nervous system.

Introduction

The nervous system is divided up into two anatomically different parts. These are:

- Central nervous system, including all the nerves contained within the cranium and spinal column.
- Peripheral nervous system, which contains the nerves and ganglia (groups of nerve cell bodies) outside the brain and spinal cord. The peripheral nervous system is further divided into somatic and autonomic branches:
  - The somatic portion contains the sensory and motor supply to skin, muscles and joints.
  - The autonomic division supplies smooth muscle and glands along with some specialized structures, such as the pacemaker cells of the heart. One of its main function is the control of the internal environment.

The nervous system is designed to detect features of the internal and external environments, to process this information and to use it to direct behaviour and body processes. There are three basic processes that work together to achieve this.

Perception

Specialized receptors in the skin respond to touch, pain and temperature. Those in muscle respond to muscle length and others in joints respond to the position of the joint. These, together with information gathered by the special sense organs (for sight, hearing, smell and taste), provide the brain with information about the immediate and remote external environment and the body's position in space. There are also receptors which monitor the state of the internal environment (e.g. baroreceptors for blood pressure).

Information transfer and processing

Neurons (nerve cells) have specialized projections called axons that can conduct trains of electrical impulses over long distances. The information delivered to neurons can be modified by, or integrated with, other inputs from related areas. In the central nervous system, neurons have many complex connections, allowing the brain to use the information in several different ways at once.

Output to body

Once the information has been collated and processed by the brain, it is then used to drive the outputs of the central nervous system. This includes supply to other excitable cells, such as muscles, internal organs and glands (e.g. the diaphragm, heart and hormone producing centres such as the adrenals). In this way, the brain can control movement of the body and also modify the circulation and respiration.

Anatomy of the central nervous system

The fully developed central nervous system is shown in Fig. 1.1.

The cerebral cortex is divided into four lobes on the basis of the folds (sulci) in the surface, as shown in Fig. 1.2.

- The frontal lobe is separated from the parietal lobe by the central sulcus.
- The temporal lobe is separated from these by the lateral sulcus.
- Demarcation of the occipital lobe is difficult to appreciate from a lateral view but, on the medial (mid-sagittal) view (Fig. 1.3), the parieto-occipital sulcus can be seen. You can also see the leaf-like folia of the cerebellum, sitting behind the midbrain, pons and medulla, can also clearly be seen.

The paired lateral ventricles (Fig. 1.4) are shaped like the jaws of an animal, with anterior, posterior and inferior horns. The lateral ventricles

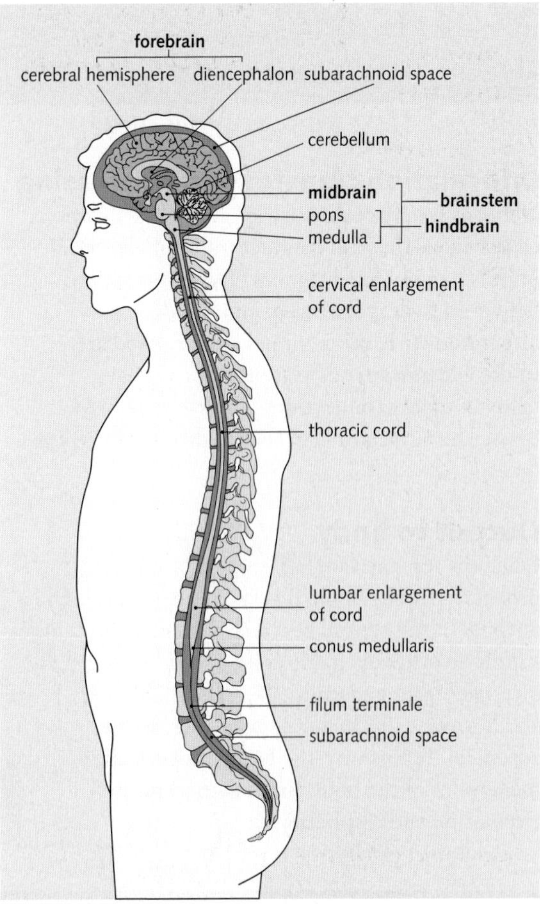

Fig. 1.1 Midsagittal section of the central nervous system showing components of the forebrain, midbrain, hindbrain and spinal cord.

are connected to the third ventricle, which lies posterior and inferior, through the interventricular foramen of Monro. The ventricles of the brain contain cerebrospinal fluid and are joined together to allow the fluid to circulate around the brain.

The ventricles can sometimes be distorted by pressure exerted upon them by, for example, a tumour. Computed tomography or magnetic resonance imaging are good investigations to see this 'mass effect'.

Blood supply to the central nervous system

Fig. 1.5 shows the arteries which provide the blood supply to the brain. These form an anastomosis (different arteries supply blood to the same area), known as the Circle of Willis. Fig. 1.6 shows the territories of the major arteries supplying the cortex. A broad knowledge of these is helpful when assessing a person with a stroke.

Four vessels supply the brain—the right and left internal carotid arteries, and the vertebral arteries.

- The internal carotid arteries send off two branches (anterior and posterior communicating arteries) before becoming the middle

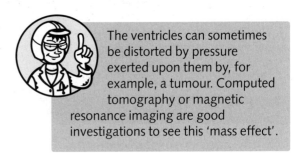

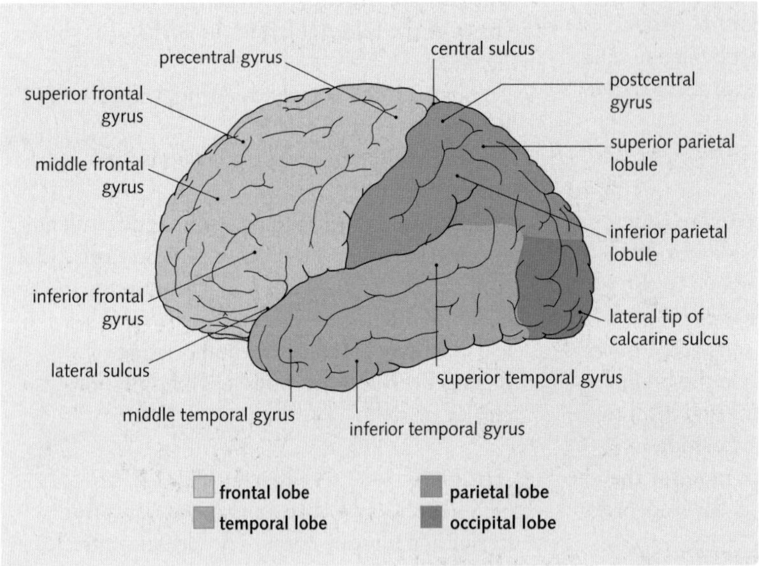

Fig. 1.2 Left cerebral hemisphere, lateral view showing major lobes.

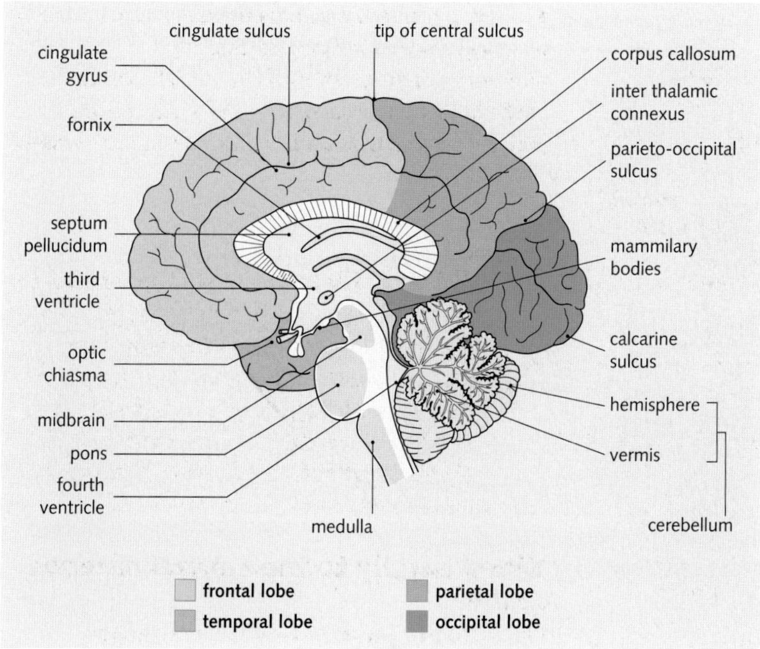

Fig. 1.3 Medial view of the right side of the brain, showing deep structures, midbrain and hindbrain.

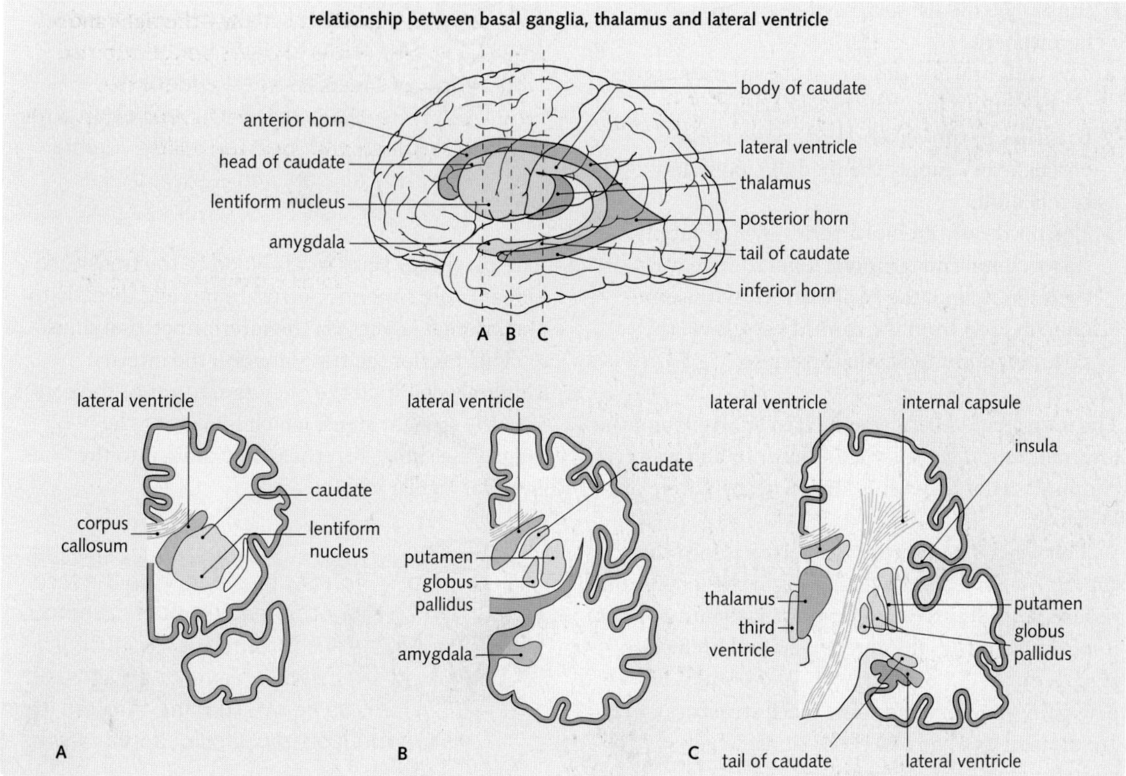

Fig. 1.4 The lateral ventricle, and its relationship to the basal ganglia and thalamus.

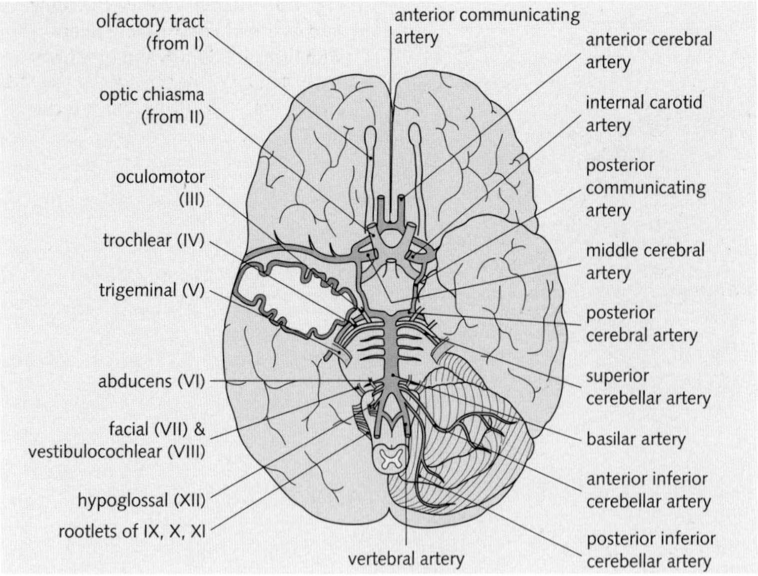

Fig. 1.5 Blood supply to the brain, showing the Circle of Willis and its relationship to the cranial nerves.

cerebral artery. This artery has an extensive territory, covering the majority of the surface of the brain and also some of the basal ganglia.

- The anterior cerebral arteries travel forwards on either side of the longitudinal fissure to supply the medial surface of each cerebral hemisphere.
- The vertebral arteries join at the inferior border of the pons to form the basilar artery. Branches of the vertebral arteries and the basilar artery supply the medulla, pons and cerebellum.
- The posterior cerebral arteries, which supply the occipital and temporal lobes, derive most of their input from the basilar artery, with some contribution from the carotid vessels via the posterior communicating arteries.

The loop formed between the basilar artery and the internal carotid vessels via the anterior and posterior communicating arteries is known as the Circle of Willis.

The venous drainage of the cortex is into the superior sagittal sinus, which runs in the longitudinal fissure. This drains into the transverse sinuses where it joins blood from the cerebellum and brainstem (Fig. 1.7).

Optic, olfactory and some facial structures are drained into the cavernous sinus, which contains many important structures, including:

- Internal carotid artery.
- Cranial nerves III, IV, VI and the ophthalmic and maxillary divisions of V.

Atherosclerosis in the common carotid artery may cause blood clots to travel up the internal carotid artery. Due to its anatomy, it is most likely that the clot will end up in the middle cerebral artery territory and cause a stroke.

The cavernous sinus sends blood to the transverse sinus via the superior petrosal sinus and directly to the internal jugular via the inferior petrosal sinus.

The inferior sagittal sinus and the internal cerebral vein drain the deep structures of the cortex into the straight sinus, which joins with the transverse sinus. Together, they drain into the internal jugular vein.

Infection spread from the face or orbit may result in cavernous sinus thrombosis, producing a red swollen eye, and palsies of the nerves running through it. On fundoscopy, papilloedema may be seen.

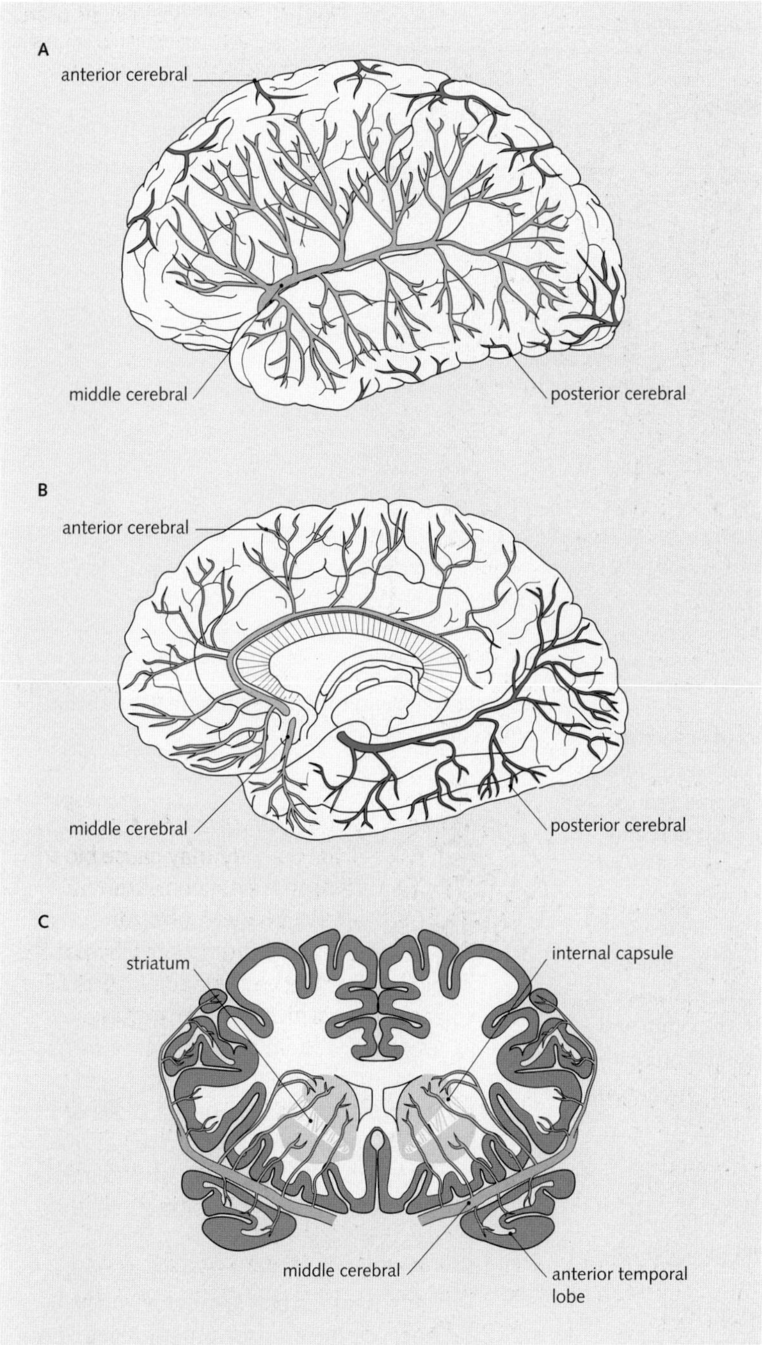

Fig. 1.6 Territories of the cerebral arteries. (A) Lateral and (B) medial views of the left and right cerebral hemispheres respectively. (C) Coronal (transverse) section of the cerebral hemispheres.

Overall development of the nervous system

Development of the nervous system begins early in gestation, at approximately 3 weeks. There are three layers to the embryo at this stage:

- Endoderm (which forms the gastrointestinal tract among other things).
- Mesoderm (which becomes muscles, connective tissues and blood vessels).
- Ectoderm (which forms the whole nervous system and the skin).

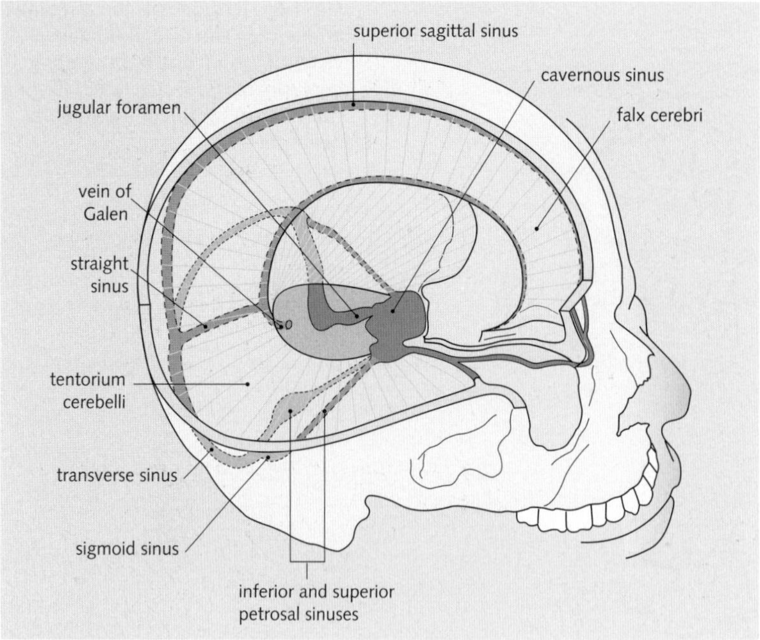

Fig. 1.7 The venous sinuses.

Neurulation

At around day 22 of gestation, an area of ectoderm on the dorsal surface of the embryo, called the neural plate, thickens and folds to form the neural groove. The ridges on either side of the groove expand and begin to fuse in the midline approximately halfway along its length (at the level of the 4th somite). Somites are paired blocks of mesoderm, segmentally arranged alongside the neural groove of the embryo. The very tips of these ridges become the neural crest, and the fused neural tube gives rise to the brain and spinal cord. The tube at the cranial (rostral or head-end) neuropore fuses on day 25, and the caudal (or tail-end) neuropore on day 27. The stages of neurulation are shown in Fig. 1.8 .

Neural crest cells migrate to form most of the cells in the peripheral nervous system, along with autonomic ganglia, cells of the adrenal medulla and melanocytes in the skin.

By the end of development, the segmental arrangement of the nervous system determined by the somites is retained only in the spinal cord.

Embryology of the spinal cord

The neural tube is hollow, with the centre becoming the spinal canal. Neuroblast cells, which surround the canal, divide and move outwards within the neural tube to ultimately form nerve cells and the grey matter of the spinal cord. These cells then send out nerve fibres that grow out peripherally into the marginal zone, and form the white matter of the spinal cord.

If the cranial neuropore fails to close, the fatal condition of anencephaly results—the embryo continues to develop but the brain does not, and the structures which would normally overlie the brain are prevented from forming normally. This normally results in spontaneous abortion. Failure of the caudal neuropore to close results in disruption of the lumbar and sacral segments of the cord. Structures that lie superficial to the cord are also involved (e.g. meninges, vertebral arch, paravertebral muscles and skin) because their development relies upon closure of the neural tube. Malformations involving the vertebral arch and the cord are called spina bifida.

The neuroblasts in the primitive grey matter form two populations—a dorsal alar plate and a ventral basal plate separated by a shallow groove (sulcus limitans).

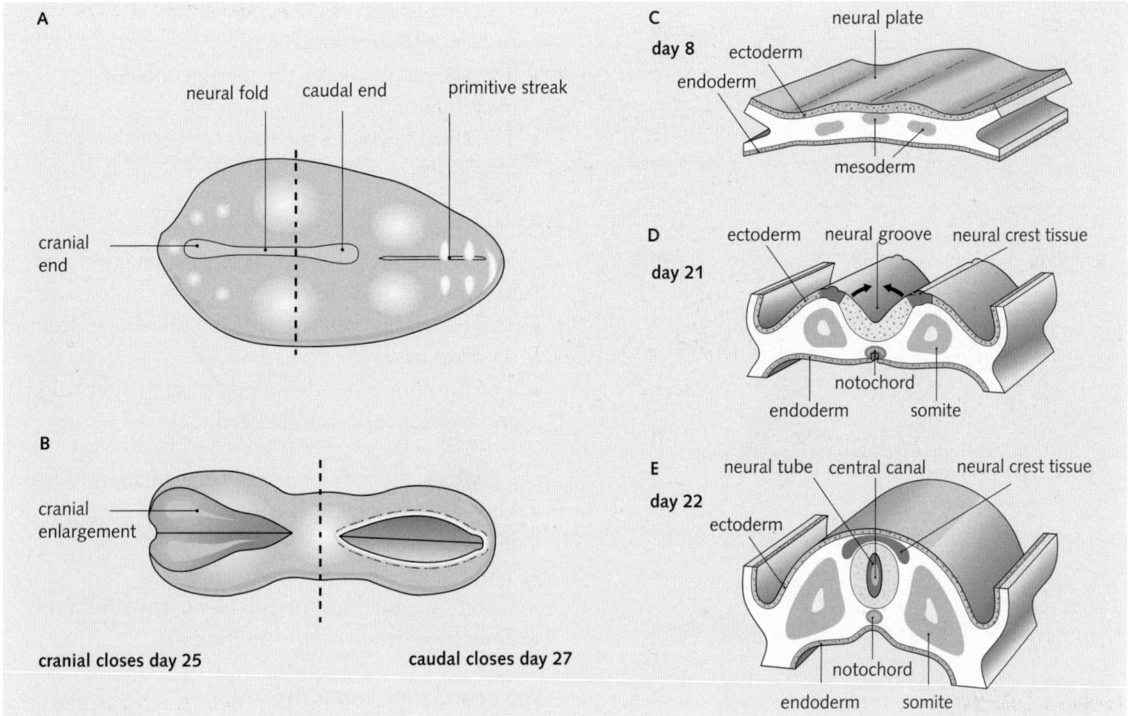

Fig. 1.8 Stages of neurulation. (A) Early embryonic disc. (B) Progression to formation of brain vesicles and spinal canal. (C–E) Transverse sections of neural tube taken at different stages of development.

- The alar plate cells form the sensory cells of the posterior (dorsal) horn.
- The basal plate cells form the motor cells of the anterior (ventral) horn along with sympathetic (in the thoracic region) and parasympathetic (in the lumbar and sacral regions) preganglionic neurons.

Fig. 1.9 shows the formation and development of the alar and basal plates.

The mesenchymal tissue around the neural tube forms the coverings of the brain and spinal cord:

- Pia mater (nearest the neural tube).
- Arachnoid mater.
- Dura mater (outer layer).

In the first 8 weeks of gestation, the spinal cord is the same length as the vertebral column. After this time, the vertebral column grows at a faster rate so that, by 40 weeks of gestation (term), the spinal cord stops at the level of L3 and, in adults, it ends at L1. The spinal nerve roots below this level in the adult descend within the vertebral canal until they reach the appropriate exit foramen. The pia mater remains attached to the coccyx and therefore elongates with respect to the spinal cord. The strand of pia mater between the coccyx and the lower end of the spinal cord is known as the filum terminale, and collectively with the individual nerve roots below L1, as the cauda equina (literally 'horse's tail').

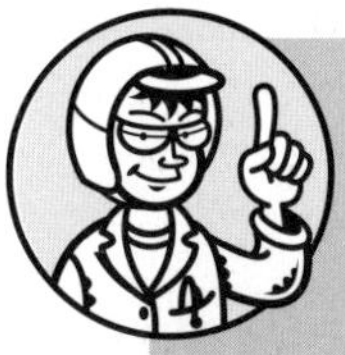

Cauda equina syndrome. A prolapsed intervertebral disc or fracture can cause compression of the cauda equina. The symptoms of this include pain in the nerve distribution of the root affected, saddle anaesthesia (around the anus) and disturbance of bladder/bowel function. It is a neurosurgical emergency and the pressure must be relieved to preserve the function of the nerves.

Embryology of the brain

General arrangement

The neural groove rostral to the 4th pair of somites enlarges before it fuses to form three primary brain vesicles or swellings.

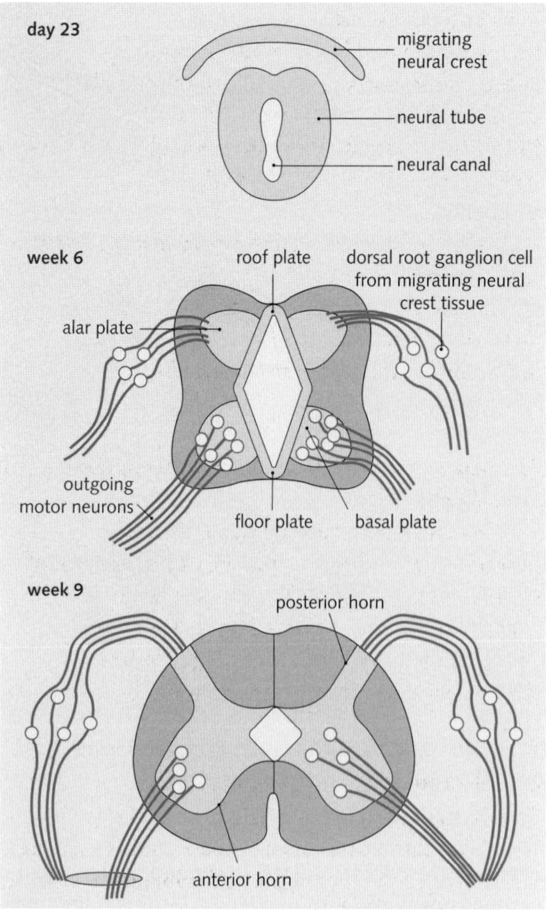

Fig. 1.9 Cross-sections through the developing spinal cord, showing development of alar and basal plates and the primitive beginnings of inflow and outflow tracts.

- The first brain vesicle becomes the prosencephalon or forebrain.
- The second becomes the mesencephalon or midbrain.
- The third becomes the rhombencephalon or hindbrain.

Fig. 1.10 shows the fate of these vesicles.

Before the fifth week of gestation, the first and third vesicles divide in two.

- The forebrain vesicle forms the telencephalon and diencephalon.
- The hindbrain vesicle forms the metencephalon and myelencephalon (or medulla).

The central canal of the neural tube enlarges to form:

- Lateral ventricles in the primitive cerebral hemispheres.
- Third ventricle in the diencephalon.
- Cerebral aqueduct (of Sylvius) in the midbrain.
- Fourth ventricle in the hindbrain.

The neural tube bends to form:

- The cervical flexure (between the primitive spinal cord and the third vesicle). The cephalic flexure (between the first and second vesicles).

Development of the brainstem

The brainstem has the same basic structure as the spinal cord, except that it has to accommodate the large motor and sensory tracts that run between the spinal cord and the brain.

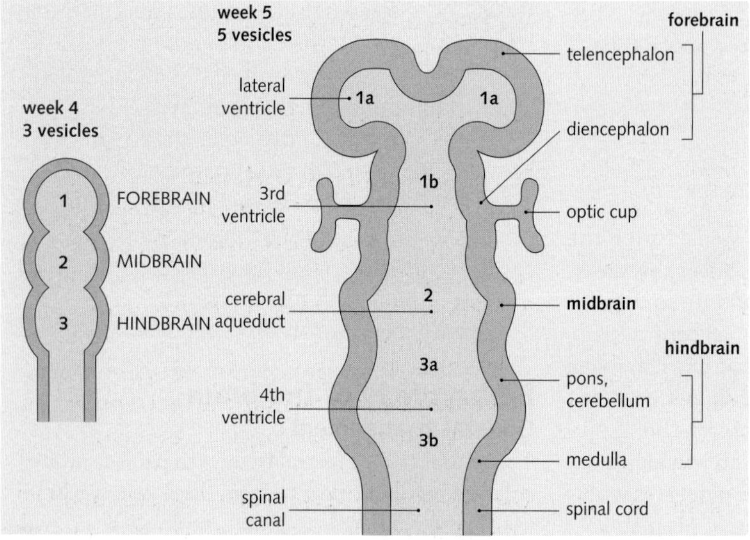

Fig. 1.10 Development of the brain from the three-vesicle stage to adult areas.

Medulla

Initially, the myelencephalon or medulla is organized like the primitive spinal cord with alar and basal plates. As it flattens out further up, forming the floor of the fourth ventricle, the alar plates (sensory cell groups) move outwards until they lie lateral to the basal plates (motor cell groups). Other cells from the alar plate migrate ventrolaterally to form the olivary nuclei. This process is shown in Fig. 1.11.

The cells of the alar and basal plates are arranged in columns according to whether they innervate somatic (body wall) or visceral (internal organ) structures.

- The basal plate forms the motor nuclei for cranial nerves IX, X, XI, XII.
- The alar plate forms sensory nuclei for cranial nerves V, VIII, IX, X along with the gracile and cuneate nuclei (receiving inputs from the spinal cord).

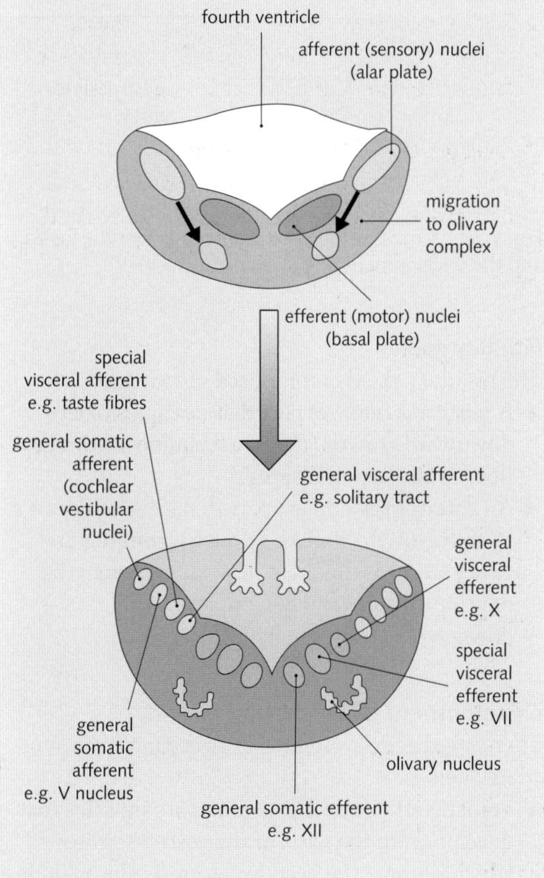

Fig. 1.11 Development of the medulla, with grouping of sensory and motor nuclei.

Pons and cerebellum

The pons is formed by the anterior part of the metencephalon and part of the alar plate of the medulla. It contains a thick band of fibres (important in motor processing) which connect the forebrain with the cerebellum.

The neurons of the ventromedial alar plate at this level form:

- The main sensory nucleus of V.
- A sensory nucleus of VII.
- Vestibular and cochlear nuclei of VIII.
- Pontine nuclei.

The neurons of the basal plate form the motor nuclei of V, VI and VII.

The cerebellum develops from the most posterior parts of the alar plates, above the level of the medulla. The cerebellar growths project over the top of the fourth ventricle and fuse in the midline, with the migrating cells from the alar plates becoming the cerebellar cortex.

Development of the midbrain

The midbrain retains the basic alar/basal plate structure. The neural canal becomes much narrower forming the aqueduct of the midbrain (also known as the aqueduct of Sylvius).

- The cells of the basal plate form the pure motor nuclei of the third and fourth cranial nerves, and possibly the red nucleus, substantia nigra and reticular formation (involved in motor processing).
- The cells of the alar plates become the sensory neurons of the superior and inferior colliculi (involved in visual and auditory reflexes, respectively).

This is shown in Fig. 1.12.

Development of the forebrain

The part of the forebrain rostral to the optic vesicles becomes the telencephalon, containing:

- Cerebral cortex.
- Commisures (made up of cortico-cortical connections).
- Basal ganglia—which develop as swellings that protrude into the cavity of the lateral ventricles, along with the developing hippocampus.

The telencephalon (hemispheres) expands much more than the other parts of the brain, and ultimately

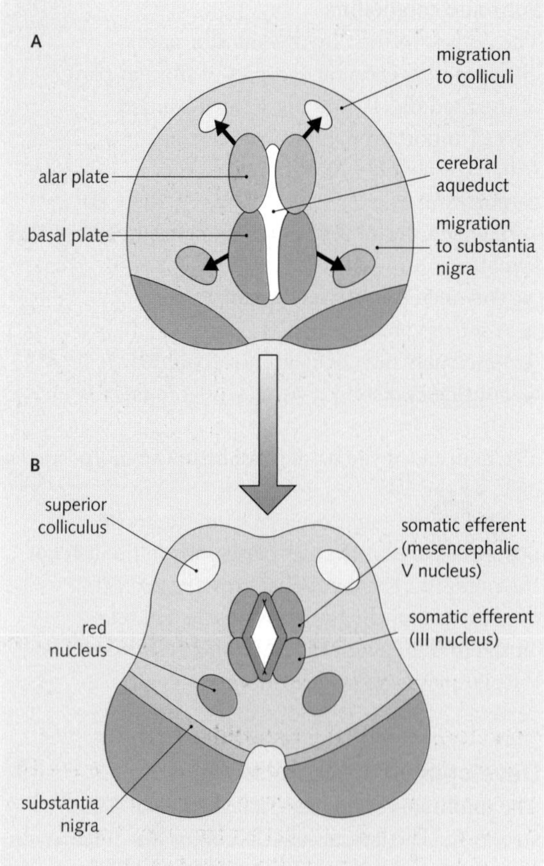

Fig. 1.12 Development of the midbrain, showing proximity to substantia nigra (basal ganglia).

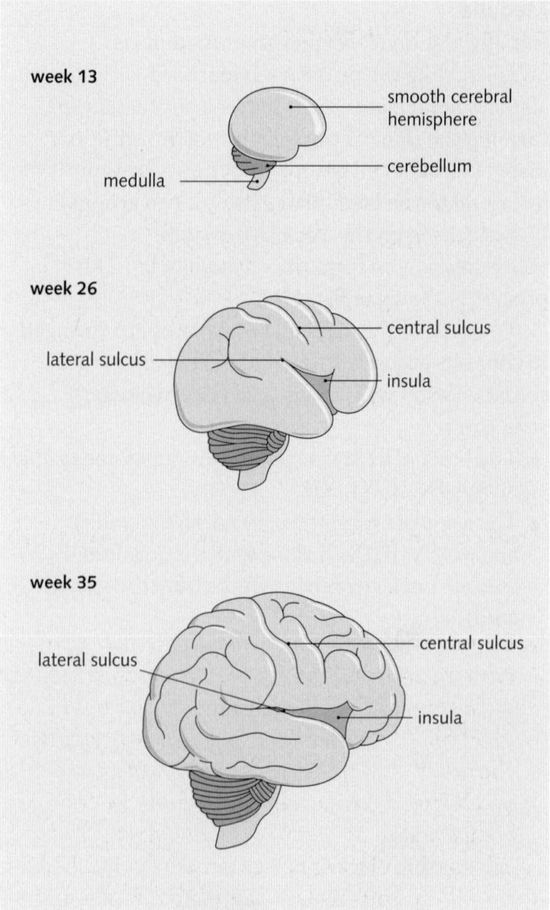

Fig. 1.13 Growth of the cerebral cortex over the insula, and the development of gyri.

covers the diencephalons and midbrain. The two swellings meet in the midline, trapping a small amount of mesenchymal tissue which forms the falx cerebri. The occipital lobes of the hemispheres similarly are separated from the cerebellum by mesenchyme, which becomes the tentorium cerebelli.

Grooves gradually appear on the smooth surface of the hemispheres, which become the sulci. The gyri thus formed allow a much greater volume of cortex (folded up) to be packed into the cranium. The cortex that covers part of the corpus striatum (lentiform nucleus) is called the insula. It remains fixed whilst the temporal, parietal and frontal lobes rapidly grow to bury it within the lateral sulcus. This process is shown in Fig. 1.13.

The rest of the forebrain becomes the diencephalon (Fig. 1.14), which contains:

- Hypothalamus (most rostral/ventral).
- The posterior pituitary gland and its stalk (the infundibulum).
- Thalamus.
- Epithalamus (most caudal/dorsal).

Pituitary gland

The pituitary gland is composed of two parts:

- A posterior (neural) part that develops from a downward growth (the infundibulum) from the floor of the hypothalamus.
- An anterior (glandular) part that develops as an inward growth (Rathke's pouch) from the oral cavity towards the brain. It passes through the developing sphenoid bone to reach the downgrowth from the hypothalamus.

Development of the cranial nerves

There are three developmentally distinct groups of cranial nerves:

- Somatic efferents. These innervate muscles that develop from the parts of the rostral somites which become the head myotomes. This includes cranial nerves III, IV, VI to the ocular muscles, and XII to the tongue muscles.

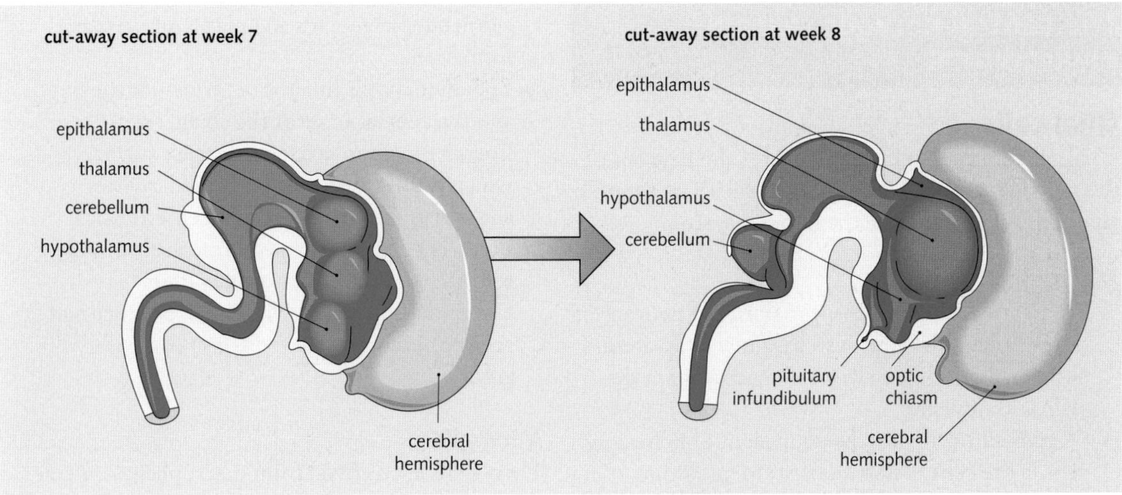

Fig. 1.14 Development of the diencephalons, showing cervical and cranial flexures.

- Pharyngeal arch nerves. These supply motor and sensory innervation to the embryological pharyngeal arches that formed the primitive oral cavity and pharynx. This group includes cranial nerves V (from the first arch), VII (second arch), IX (third arch) and X (fused fourth and sixth arches with the cranial branch of XI, the accessory nerve). The relationship of these nerves is shown in Fig. 1.15.
- Special sensory nerves. These afferent nerves relay information from special-sense receptors to the appropriate central pathway. This group includes cranial nerves I (olfaction), II (vision) and VIII (hearing and balance).

Development of the choroid plexuses

The choroid plexus is formed from two layers—the pia mater and the ependymal lining of the cavities of the ventricles, which together are called the tela choroidea. This surrounds a core of vascular connective tissue that contains the blood supply. The tela choroidea push into the ventricles and develop into the choroid plexuses.

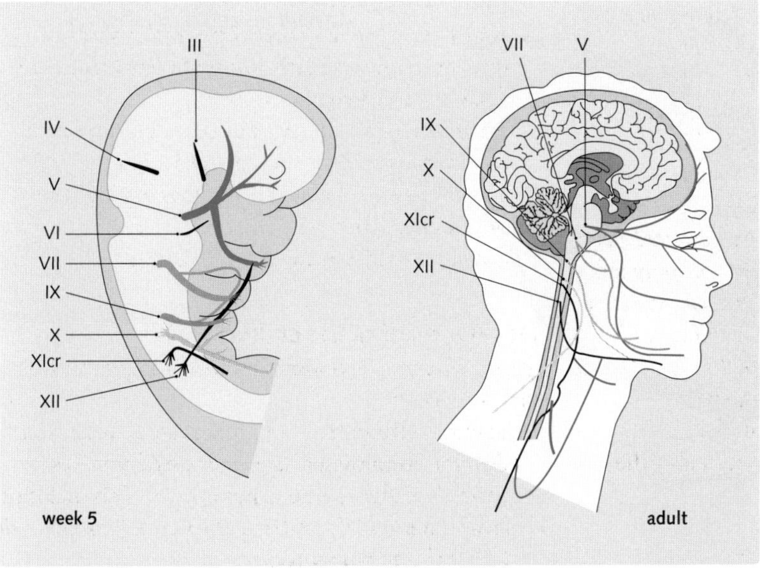

Fig. 1.15 Pharyngeal arch nerves in the embryo and adult.

The central nervous system environment

Glial cells

Glial cells are the supporting cells for the neurons of the nervous system. There are five to 10 times more glial cells than neurons in the nervous system.

Macroglia

- Schwann cells surround the majority of neurons in the peripheral nervous system. They wrap around individual cells like a swiss roll, and insulate the axon with myelin.
- Oligodendrocytes are the equivalent of Schwann cells in the central nervous system, providing myelin insulation. Unlike Schwann cells, each oligodendrocyte can myelinate many axons.
- Astrocytes are small cells with long branching processes that provide the framework for the surrounding neurons (Fig. 1.16). They provide a kind of 'scaffolding' which prevents axons of different nerve cells coming into contact with one another, and their signals suffering interference. Astrocytes also take up neurotransmitters, such as γ-aminobutyric acid (GABA) and glutamate, preventing them from constantly activating postsynaptic neurons. They store glycogen, which can be broken down to glucose in times of high metabolic demand and help to regulate interstitial fluid potassium. They can act as phagocytes and play a role in scar formation.
- Ependymal cells line the ventricles of the brain and the central canal of the spinal cord. Ependymocytes have cilia on their surface which project into the fluid-filled cavities and contribute to the flow of cerebrospinal fluid. They may also have a role in absorbing solutes from the cerebrospinal fluid. Choroidal epithelial cells, which produce and secrete cerebrospinal fluid, also come into this group.

Microglia

These cells are derived from macrophages outside the nervous system. Under normal circumstances, they appear to be inactive, but when there is tissue damage or inflammation they multiply and act as phagocytes. Similar to macrophages, they are antigen-presenting cells and can therefore interact with other elements of the immune system.

Cerebrospinal fluid

Cerebrospinal fluid surrounds the brain and spinal cord in the ventricles, central canal and subarachnoid space. It provides a cushion to prevent the delicate nervous tissue being damaged by the surrounding bones. It also plays an active part in providing nutrition to the central nervous system, and removing waste products.

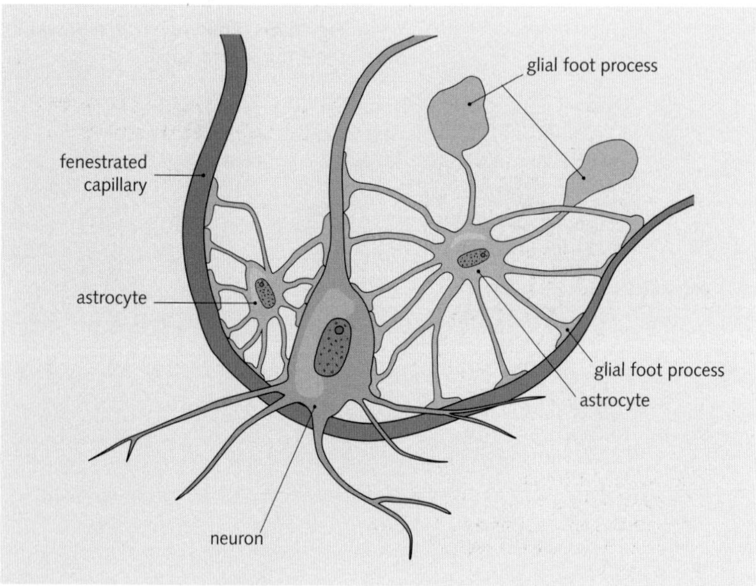

Fig. 1.16 Glia, and their relationship to neurons and capillaries.

The majority of cerebrospinal fluid is formed by the choroid plexuses of the lateral, third and fourth ventricles at the rate of about 500 mL/day. The total cerebrospinal fluid space is approximately 150 mL, and this quantity must be turned over approximately three times a day. Groups of choroid plexus epithelial cells project into the ventricles, giving a folded appearance. These folds contain a leaky fenestrated capillary in the centre, and on their surface have microvilli which project into the ventricles. The flow of cerebrospinal fluid is shown in Fig. 1.17.

Cerebrospinal fluid is produced by a combination of capillary filtration and active transport of solutes. Blood and cerebrospinal fluid are in osmotic equilibrium because water follows the gradients created. The differences between blood and cerebrospinal fluid are shown in Fig. 1.18. These parameters can be measured on lumbar puncture.

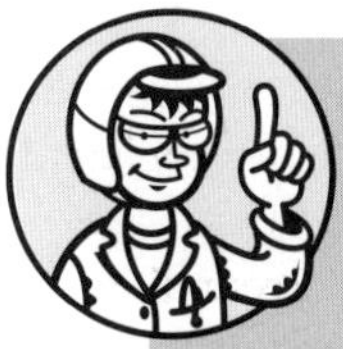

Lumbar puncture should not be performed on any individual who has a raised intracranial pressure because it may cause herniation of the cerebellar tonsils ('coning') and brainstem death—if in any doubt, a computed tomography head scan should be obtained first.

The cerebrospinal fluid flows through the ventricles, through the cerebral aqueduct to the fourth ventricle. From there, it gains access to the subarachnoid space and the central canal of the spinal cord. The cerebrospinal fluid reaches the nervous tissue by travelling along blood vessels in the perivascular (Virchow–Robin) space (Fig. 1.19).

Cerebrospinal fluid is taken back into the circulation by:

- Arachnoid granulations, which are protrusions of the arachnoid space covered by a thin layer of cells that line the venous sinuses.
- Perineural lymph vessels of the cranial and spinal nerves.

Hydrocephalus

This condition results from an increase in pressure within the ventricular system, usually due to a blockage in the flow of cerebrospinal fluid. This is most likely to occur at the outlets from the fourth ventricle (the foramina of Luschka and Magendie), which are very narrow. It may also occur at the level of the cerebral aqueduct (of Sylvius). This is known as non-communicating hydrocephalus. Causes include:

- Tumours (either blocking the ventricular drainage or producing excess cerebrospinal fluid).
- Congenital malformations.
- Infection (e.g. tuberculous meningitis).

Communicating hydrocephalus is caused by a blockage outside the ventricular system in the arachnoid space. This can be caused by:

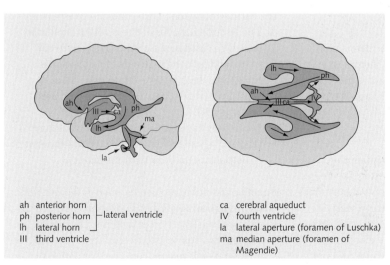

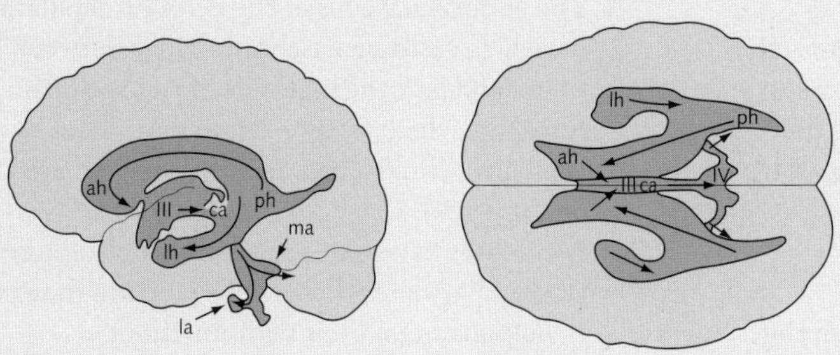

Fig. 1.17 The ventricular system and the flow of cerebrospinal fluid.

Differences between blood plasma and cerebrospinal fluid (CSF)		
	Plasma	CSF
Protein (mg/dl)	7000	35
Glucose (mg/dl)	90	60
Na (mmol/l)	138	138
K (mmol/l)	4.5	2.8
Osmolarity (mOsm/l)	295	295
PH	7.41	7.33

Fig. 1.18 The differences between blood and cerebrospinal fluid.

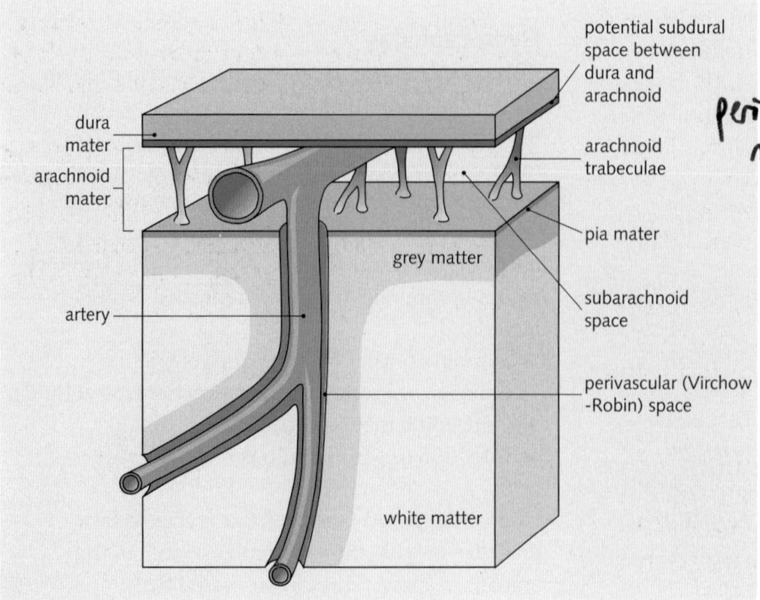

Fig. 1.19 Spaces filled with cerebrospinal fluid—subarachnoid and perivascular.

periosteal/endosteal meningeal .

- Meningitis.
- Subarachnoid haemorrhage.

The ventricles rostral to the blockage dilate and put pressure on the brain tissue. This increases intracranial pressure and, in the newborn, can distort the skull bones (as the sutures have not fused at this stage).

The blood–brain barrier

The blood–brain barrier exists to maintain the environment of the brain in a steady state, protected from extracellular ion changes, peripheral hormones (such as adrenaline) and drugs. It also prevents neurotransmitters from the central nervous system entering the peripheral circulation (except at the pituitary where the blood–brain barrier is absent).

There are two factors that combine to maintain the balance between plasma and cerebrospinal fluid:

- The endothelial cells of the cerebral capillaries have high resistance tight junctions between them, and lack the methods of transcellular transport which are present in peripheral capillaries (fluid-phase and carrier-mediated endocytosis).
- Astrocytes have foot processes which adhere to the capillary endothelial cells (and are thought to help maintain their tight junctions).

Small lipid-soluble molecules, such as diamorphine, cross this barrier easily, but hydrophilic molecules rely on specific transporter systems. D-glucose, for example, has a stereospecific membrane transporter that facilitates diffusion from the circulation to the cerebrospinal fluid at high rates because the brain relies heavily on glucose for energy. However, in situations where there is a dramatic fall in plasma glucose levels (e.g. in diabetic hypoglycaemic states), glucose may diffuse back out of the cerebrospinal fluid into the plasma. This is a medical emergency as the brain needs glucose to survive.

Other transport systems include those for amino acids—one each for basic (e.g. arginine), neutral (e.g. phenylalanine) and acidic (e.g. glutamate) amino acids. Clinically, the neutral transporter is important, as it will transport L-dopa (used as a treatment for Parkinson's disease, to replace dopamine lost from the substantia nigra). However, dopamine cannot be given as a treatment because it does not have a transporter.

Abrupt changes in the ionic concentration can be damaging to neurons. The blood–brain barrier not only helps to protect the brain from such changes in plasma levels, but also helps to remove excess ions from the cerebrospinal fluid. For example, intense neuronal activity can increase the cerebrospinal fluid potassium concentration, and there is a high concentration of K^+ channels on endothelial cells which clear the excess.

Brain ischaemia, brain tumours, haemorrhage, systemic acidosis or infections such as bacterial meningitis may break down the blood–brain barrier.

> In diabetic ketoacidosis (where plasma glucose becomes excessively high), pH of the plasma may fall below 7, at which point the blood–brain barrier is compromised and neuronal death occurs.

Metabolic requirements of the central nervous system

The mechanisms within the blood–brain barrier provide the substrates for cellular metabolism in the brain via the cerebrospinal fluid.

The brain is vulnerable to interruptions in its blood supply because it can store neither oxygen nor glucose, and cannot normally undergo anaerobic metabolism. It has a high metabolic rate due to the energy demand of Na^+/K^+ ATPase pumps in the neuronal membranes. The brain consumes 20% of the body's oxygen and 60% of its glucose.

Under conditions of starvation for several days, the central nervous system can adapt to use ketones (fat derivatives acetoacetate and hydroxybutyrate) as its main energy source. These compounds normally make up approximately 30% of the fuel for the brain in adults but, after fasting for 40 days, this can rise to 70%.

- In infants, blood–brain barrier transport of glucose is 30% of the adult level, whereas ketone transport is approximately seven times as high. Amino acid transport in children is also higher than in adults, reflecting a higher rate of protein synthesis in the developing brain.

- What structures make up the brainstem?
- Describe the ventricular system within the brain.
- How is the neural tube formed? How might failure of fusion present?
- How does the diencephalon develop from the primitive forebrain?
- What are the functions of glial cells? How do macroglia and microglia differ?
- Explain the production and circulation of cerebrospinal fluid with reference to hydrocephalus.
- Compare the composition of plasma with that of cerebrospinal fluid.
- What is the blood–brain barrier? Why is it important?

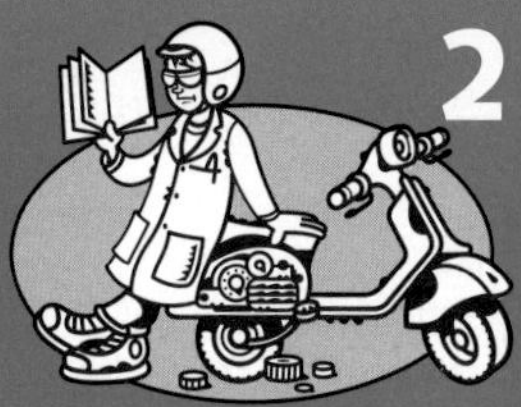

2. Cellular Physiology of the Nervous System

In this chapter, you will learn about:

- The structure of neurons and their networks.
- The action potential and transmission of impulses.
- Synaptic transmission.
- The effect of damage to the nervous system at the cellular level.

Neuronal structure and function

Introduction

The nervous system is highly complex, but the basic principles which underlie its function are fairly simple. Understanding these concepts is the first stage in appreciating the way in which the whole system works.

Neurons

Neurons are excitable cells that can conduct electrical impulses and communicate with other excitable cells via specialized junctions called synapses. Although they vary considerably in their structure according to their location and function, a typical neuron is shown in Fig. 2.1.

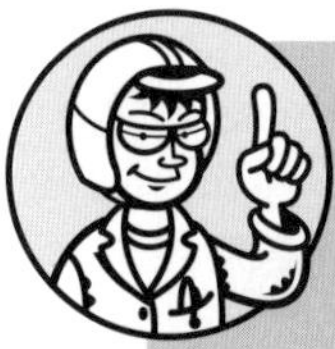

Certain viruses can exploit the retrograde transport of transmitter fragments from the axon to the cell body to gain access to the nervous system. These include the herpes simplex viruses, herpes zoster, rabies and the polio virus.

The cell body has a series of branching processes called dendrites which collect information from surrounding excitable cells and conduct it to the cell body. The number of dendrites it has reflects the way information is processed in that pathway. For example, a cell with many inputs may condense information from several pathways, whereas a cell with few inputs may be part of a highly conserved parallel pathway.

The output of the nerve cell is a binary signal (meaning that it is an all-or-none impulse or train of impulses). The output is generated at the axon hillock when the cell's electrical threshold potential is reached. The output travels down another process extending from the cell body—the axon. In contrast to the dendrites, there is only one axon per neuron (although the axon may divide into numerous branches).

The axon transmits the output of the neuron (the action potential), to the terminal boutons, which are presynaptic swellings containing vesicles of neurotransmitter. Different arrangements of the cell body and its processes are shown in Fig. 2.2 .

Arrangement of neurons

According to the function of the area, neurons can be arranged as:

- Layers (e.g. in the cerebral and cerebellar cortices) (Fig. 2.3).
- Rods (e.g. motor neurons in the spinal cord).
- Clumps (nuclei) (e.g. cranial nerve nuclei in the brainstem).

There are two classes of neuron:

- Projection neurons (called Golgi type-1 neurons) influence cells located in a different part of the nervous system and so have long axons (e.g. cortical motor neurons). The long axons often give off small collateral branches that further help to spread information in the central nervous system. These are distinct from projection neurons which have connections outside the nervous system. Such neurons may be either afferent (or sensory) axons (e.g. from skin receptors) or efferent (motor) axons (e.g. to muscles or glands).
- Local interneurons (termed Golgi type-II neurons) have shorter axons that do not leave their cell group, and so provide more opportunities for cells in a group or circuit to communicate with each other. Often, the axons give off many collateral branches. This will increase the ability of the cells in the circuit to process information. Humans have a much larger number of these types of neuron compared with their closest evolutionary relatives.

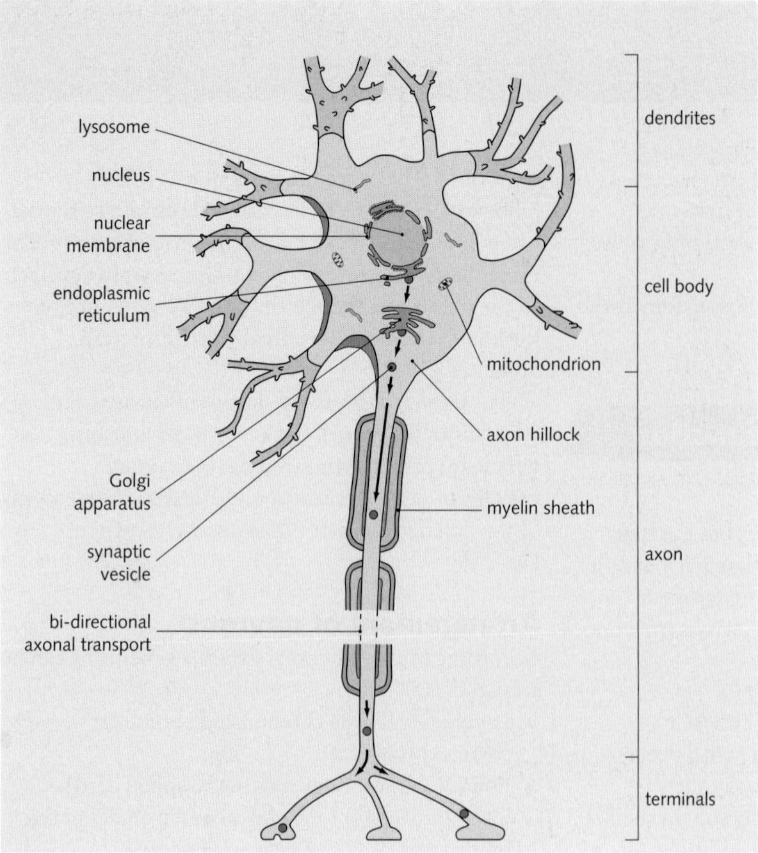

Fig. 2.1 Cellular features of a typical neuron. Note that although only anterograde transmitter transport is shown, retrograde movement of molecules also occurs.

Neuronal excitation and inhibition

All nerve cells are electrically polarized (there is an electrical potential gradient across their membranes). The value of this potential determines whether a cell will or will not generate an action potential. It depends on the relative membrane permeabilities to the ions in the extracellular fluid (mainly Na^+ and Cl^-) and intracellular fluid (mainly K^+). The signal to alter permeability comes from neurotransmitter interaction with receptors at the synapse or direct electrical excitation of the neuron.

Similarly, the neuron may be inhibited from firing when the membrane potential is moved further away from the threshold value, usually by increasing permeability to Cl^-.

Ionic basis of resting potentials

In the resting neuron, there is a great deal more potassium within the cell than outside, and much less sodium. The cell membrane is relatively impermeable to ions (although there is some leak of K^+). If there were no active channels at work, and no other ions crossed the membrane, then potassium ions would have a tendency to move out of the cell down their concentration gradient, leaving a relatively negative charge behind. This would continue until the electrical force attracting the positive K^+ ions into the cell is equal (and opposite) to the chemical force of the concentration gradient. The electrical potential at which this equilibrium is reached for an ion is calculated by using the Nernst equation:

$$E_x \cong \frac{RT}{zF} \ln \frac{[Xo]}{[Xi]}$$

Where E_x is the equilibrium potential for ion X, R is the international gas constant, T is the temperature in °Kelvin, z is the valency of X, F is Faraday's constant, X_o is the concentration of X

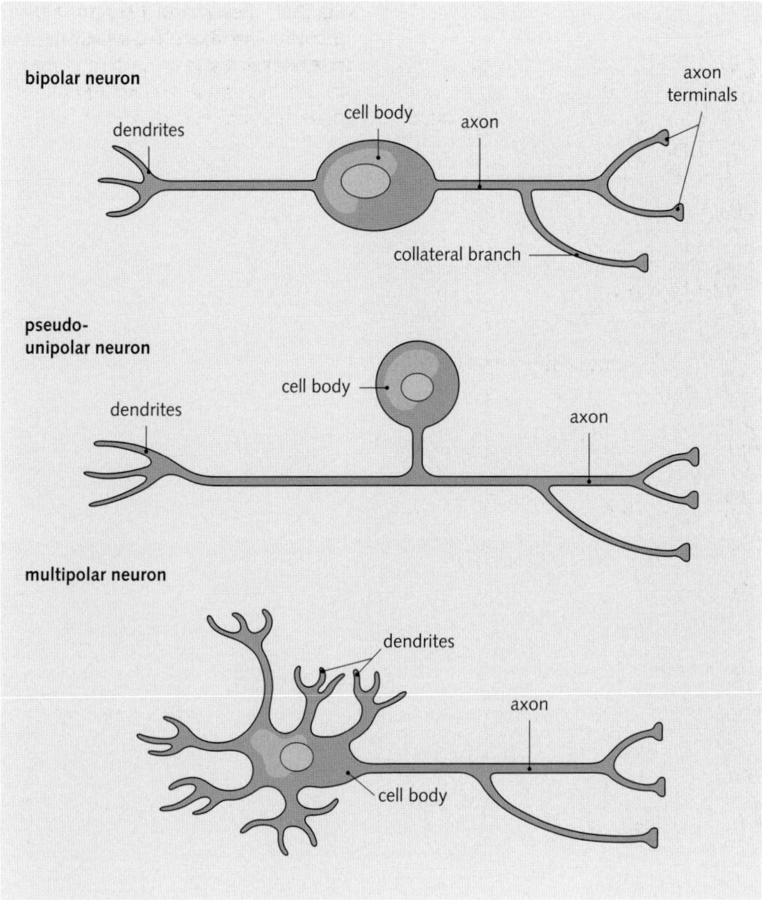

Fig. 2.2 Different neuronal shapes (morphologies).

outside the cell, X_i is the concentration of X within the cell.

The equilibrium for potassium is –74.8 mV. The overall potential difference across a resting cell membrane when taking into account all the ions involved is more positive (around –65 mV) as there is a small sodium leak in the membrane too (the equilibrium potential for sodium is around +55 mV). The Goldman equation is a modified version of the Nernst equation, which takes into account the relative permeabilities of all the ions involved in generating the membrane potential. Fig. 2.4 shows how the Goldman equation predicts the actual membrane potential more accurately than the Nernst equation.

Because there is a small inward leak of sodium ions then the potential would eventually reach a level halfway between –74.8 mV and +55 mV. This does not occur because the membrane contains a Na^+/K^+ ATPase exchange pump that moves Na^+ ions out of the cell against both their electrical and chemical gradient. It pumps 3 Na^+ ions out in exchange for 2 K^+ ions in, which is an energy-requiring process. There are many of these pumps in the membranes of all excitable cells, and they are largely responsible for the high metabolic requirements of neurons.

Generation and propagation of the action potential

In the 1950s, Hodgkin and Huxley discovered the ionic mechanism for the action potential by studying the squid giant axon. Since then, it has proven to hold good for many other excitable cells.

In nerve cells an action potential may be produced as a result of inputs from other nerve cells or inputs from sensory neurons. Whenever there is an excitatory input, this causes an influx of Na^+ ions, which pass down their electrical

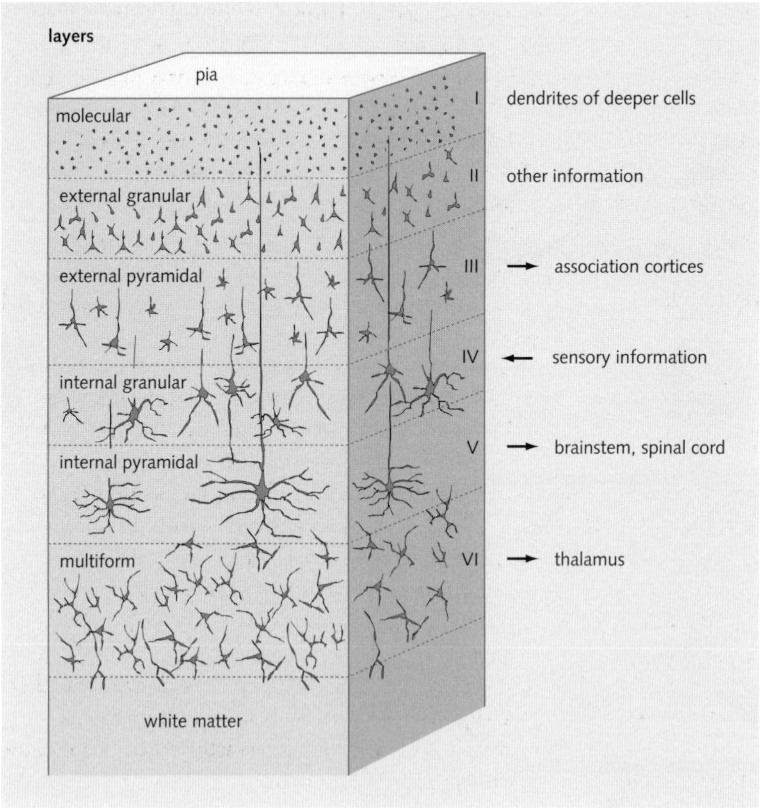

Fig. 2.3 Schematic diagram showing the layers in a typical area of cerebral cortex.

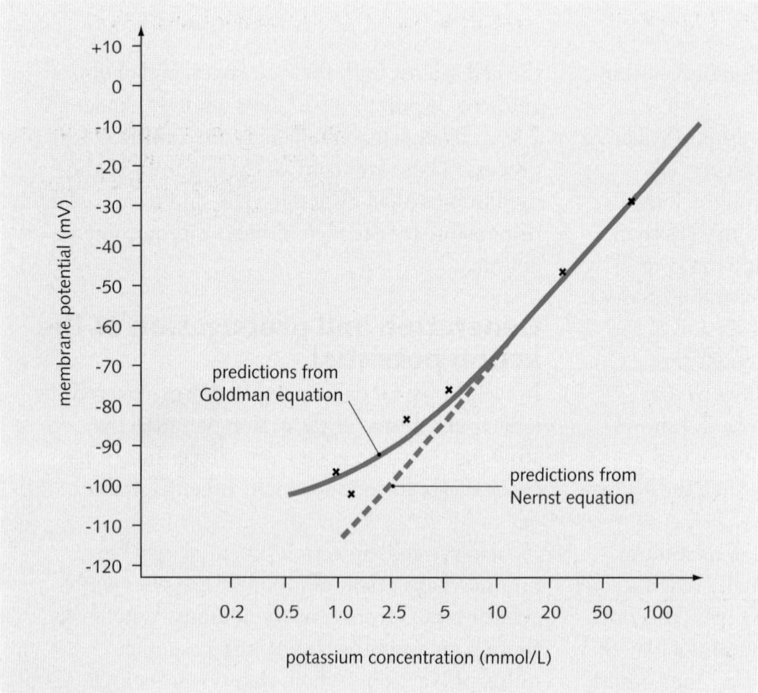

Fig. 2.4 Effect of changing external potassium concentration on the resting potential of a neuron (as determined by experimental electrophysiology). The predictions made by the Goldman equation are more accurate because it takes into account more of the ions involved than the Nernst equation does.

and chemical gradients through voltage-gated Na^+ channels bringing the membrane potential closer to zero. This is known as depolarization.

If the influx of Na^+ is sufficient to reach the threshold potential for the membrane (generally around –55 mV) there is a sudden and massive increase in the number of open voltage-gated Na^+ channels. This causes the membrane potential to shift towards the value of the Nernst equation for sodium (+55 mV).

- An action potential is an all-or-nothing reaction of the cell to an influx of positively charged ions.
- Because the size of the action potential is constant, intensity of the stimulus is coded by the frequency of firing of a neuron.

The sodium channels are only open briefly, and will not reopen until the membrane potential is restored to its resting level. This causes an absolute refractory period in which the cell cannot fire again.

Potassium channels also open at the time of depolarization, but are much slower. Once they are open they begin to return the membrane potential to the Nernst equation value for potassium (as the Na^+ channels have now shut). These channels are also slow to close, and therefore the resting potential of –65 mV is 'overshot', and there is a brief period of hyperpolarization. The slow closing of the K^+ channels cause a relative refractory period, which means that the neuron will only fire to greater than normal stimulation, as the efflux of K^+ offsets the influx of Na^+. Fig. 2.5 shows the contributions of the Na^+ and K^+ channels to the action potential.

The action potential is generated at the axon hillock as it has a high concentration of sodium channels and a reduced threshold for action potential generation.

- Current passes along the axon from the active region to the neighbouring resting region, which has a more negative membrane potential. At this site the current flows outwards across the membrane causing the axon to depolarize.This causes the opening of voltage-gated sodium channels in that region, and consequent depolarization. In this way, the action potential is propagated down the length of the axon.
- Current does not pass backwards to cause further action potential in the axon hillock as the membrane there is in a refractory state. Current is therefore unidirectional.

Myelin is an electrical insulator which surrounds the axons of many neurons, meaning that most of the axon is not in contact with extracellular fluid. In these cells, depolarization occurs only at nodes of Ranvier, where the majority of the sodium channels are

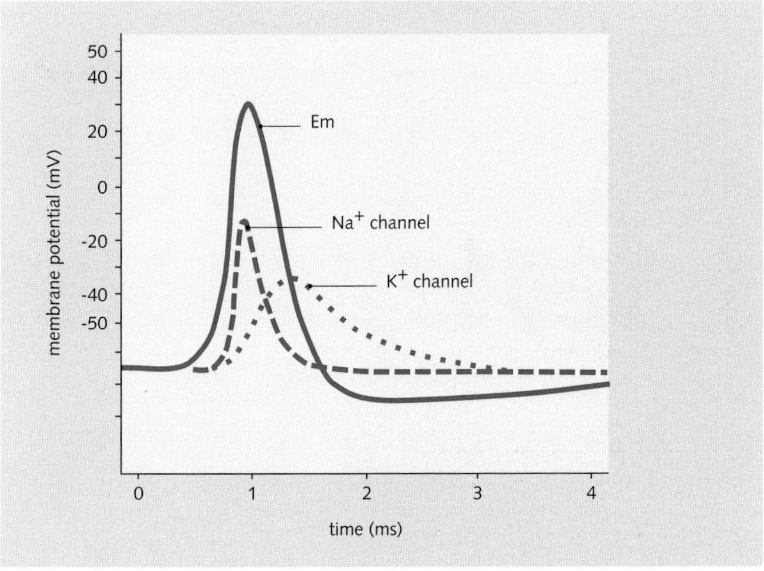

Fig. 2.5 Relationship between the opening of ion channels and the timing of the action potential (Em, membrane potential).

located. The current therefore travels along between nodes, and this is known as 'saltatory' (literally jumping or leaping) conduction. This is a much faster means of conduction—six times quicker than in non-myelinated neurons. This is shown in Fig. 2.6.

Nerves can be tested by stimulating them at their distal end, and recording the action potential from a more proximal part of the axon. For example, nerves in the fingers can be electrically stimulated and the action potential in the median nerve at the wrist examined to assess its function. This is useful in median nerve compression which occurs in carpal tunnel syndrome.

Velocity of action potentials

The factors limiting the movement of the action potential along the axon are:

- Axonal diameter—the larger the diameter, the lower the internal resistance.
- Membrane conductance—if poorly insulated, the axon leaks charge.
- Membrane capacitance—current is used up charging the membrane.

Myelin reduces both membrane conductance and membrane capacitance. Less charge is lost through the membrane if the axon is myelinated.

As an approximate guide, the velocity of an action potential in a myelinated axon (in metres per second) is six times the diameter (in microns).

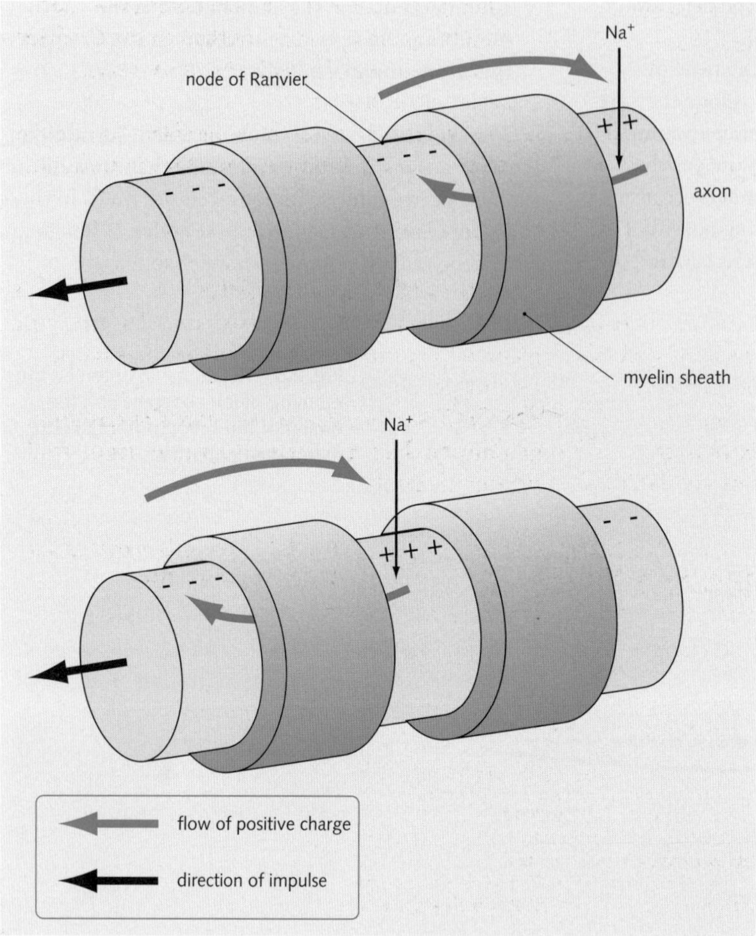

Fig. 2.6 Saltatory conduction in a myelinated axon .

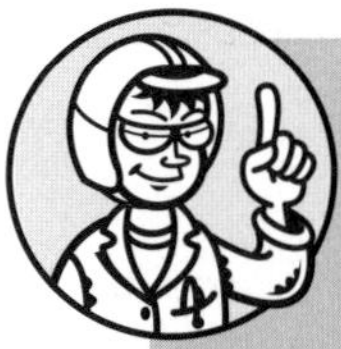

Neurons can be demyelinated by diseases such as Guillain–Barré syndrome and multiple sclerosis. This causes slowing of conduction, and may even prevent neurons from conducting impulses at all. Both conditions may result in paralysis or even death, although these changes are reversible in Guillain–Barré syndrome.

Synaptic transmission

Introduction

Synapses are junctions between the terminal boutons of neurons and target cells (which may be another nerve, muscle or gland cell). The junction comprises the membranes of both cells, a tiny gap between them, and the basement membrane in between. Synapses alter the membrane potential of the postsynaptic cell and may be:

- Chemical (where a neurotransmitter is required).
- Electrical (where there is a cytoplasmic connection between the cells).

The differences between these types are shown in Fig. 2.7.

For chemically operated synapses (which make up the vast majority of junctions in the nervous system), the postsynaptic site contains specific receptor proteins that bind the released chemical. This is essential for amplifying the signal from the neuron, as the extracellular current generated in the presynaptic neuron is not sufficient to cause a significant depolarization of the postsynaptic cell.

Types and location of synapses

Synapses (Fig 2.8) may be:

- Excitatory (depolarizing—increasing the membrane permeability to Na^+ (E_x = +55 mV) and hence dragging the membrane potential towards threshold level).
- Inhibitory (hyperpolarizing—increasing the membrane permeability to Cl^- (E_x = –65 mV) or K^+ (E_x = –75 mV) thereby taking the membrane potential further from the threshold).

Their location can enhance their action—the closer a synapse to the axon hillock, the greater its effect.

The most common sites for synapses are:

- Axodendritic. These comprise the 'standard' form of synapse between neurons).
- Axosomatic. These are usually inhibitory, and when placed close to the axon hillock will more effectively inhibit cell firing than an axodendritic synapse as the cell body is the site of action potential generation.
- Axoaxonic synapses, which can affect (modulate) the release of transmitter from the presynaptic cell.

Process of transmission

Fig. 2.9 shows the steps between arrival of the action potential, transmitter release and termination of transmitter effect.

Step 1: Action potential arrives at the terminal bouton and the depolarization opens voltage-gated calcium channels.

Comparison of electrical and chemical synapses		
Feature	**Electrical**	**Chemical**
cytoplasmic continuity	yes	no
delay	none	0.8–1.5 ms
agent	ion	neurotransmitter
space between cells	2 nm	30–50 nm
direction of signal	one way or both ways	one way
variation in function	either on or off	modifiable activity levels

Fig. 2.7 Comparison of electrical and chemical synapses.

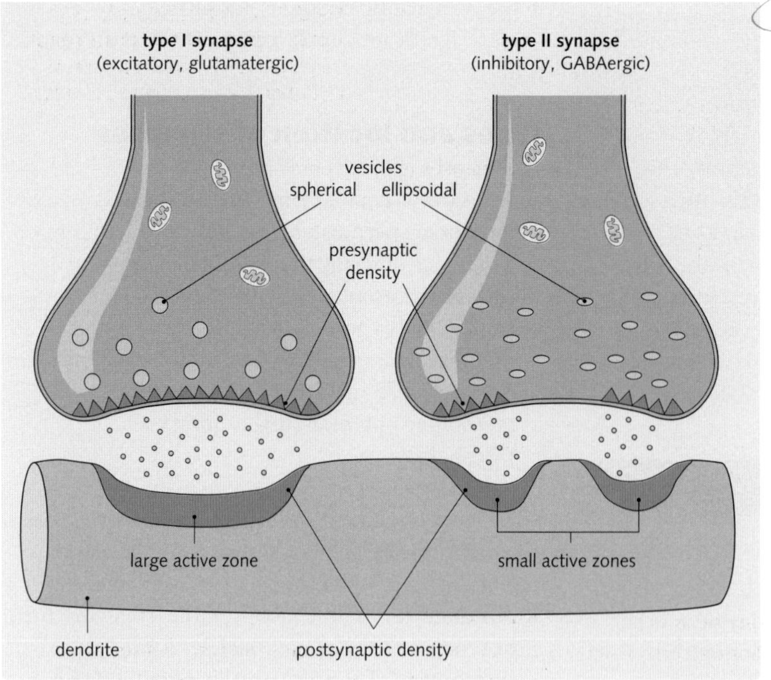

Fig. 2.8 Excitatory (depolarizing) synapse and inhibitory (hyperpolarizing) synapse.

Step 2: Calcium ions enter the terminal bouton and allow the vesicles to attach to presynaptic releasing sites via an intracellular framework of actin filaments.

Step 3: The vesicle membrane then fuses with the presynaptic membrane and the contents are released into the synaptic cleft. The vesicle membrane is then invaginated back into the presynaptic terminal and recycled to form more vesicles which are filled with transmitter for re-use. This is a dangerous process because it allows extracellular contents to gain access to the interior of the nerve cell (e.g. poliovirus or herpes virus).

Step 4: The transmitter diffuses across the cleft to postsynaptic receptors and, in some systems, to presynaptic receptors to regulate transmitter release.

Once the transmitter has bound to the postsynaptic receptors it causes a change in the postsynaptic membrane potential (either an excitatory or inhibitory postsynaptic potential, EPSP or IPSP). The size of this change is very small if only one vesicle has been released containing a fixed amount of transmitter. However, if many vesicles are released, these EPSPs are summed, and may cause a change in membrane potential which is sufficient to reach the postsynaptic cell's threshold. This theory of small, identical EPSPs corresponding to individual vesicle release is known as the quantum hypothesis (the amount of transmitter in each vesicle being the quantum). The effects of EPSPs and IPSPs on the membrane potential are shown in Fig. 2.10.

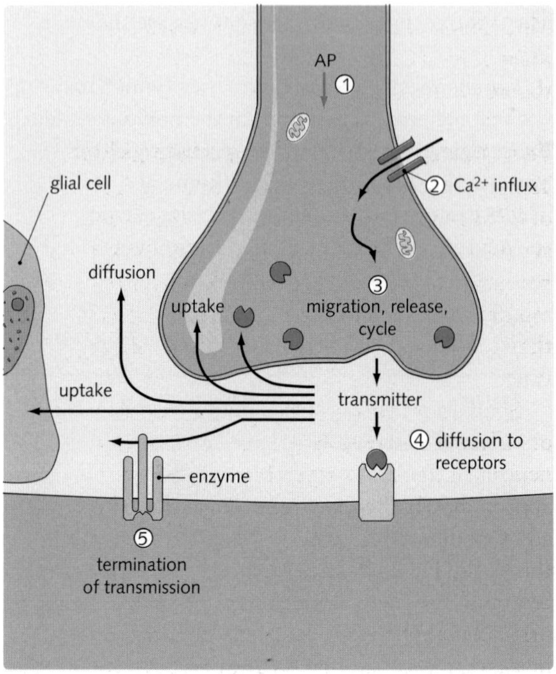

Fig. 2.9 Synaptic transmission.

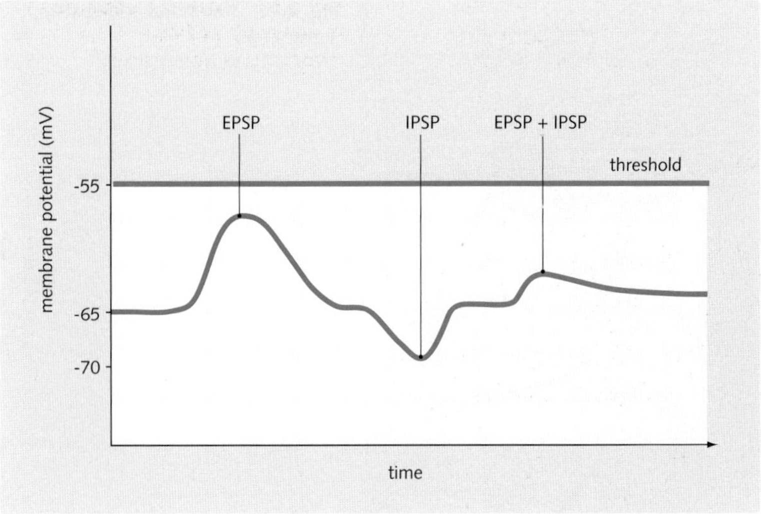

Fig. 2.10 Effects of excitatory postsynaptic potential (EPSP) and inhibitory postsynaptic potential (IPSP) on the membrane potential.

The effect of the chemical transmitter is terminated (Step 5) by one or more of the following mechanisms:

- Enzymatic destruction of the transmitter in the cleft (e.g. acetylcholinesterase in cholinergic neurons).
- Re-uptake of the transmitter into the terminal bouton.
- Uptake of transmitter into glial cells.
- Diffusion out of the cleft.

Modulation of these mechanisms forms the main basis of central nervous system therapeutics.

Temporal and spatial summation

Temporal summation occurs when a number of EPSPs caused by transmission at the same synapse add together to bring the membrane potential to threshold. These EPSPs have to occur rapidly one after another as the fluctuations they cause individually die away after a short time.

Spatial summation occurs when a number of different synapses located on the same neuron all transmit a signal for an EPSP at approximately the same time. All the EPSPs can add together to bring the membrane potential to threshold. Fig. 2.11 shows the difference between temporal and spatial summation. The same principles apply to IPSPs, except that the membrane potential moves away from its threshold level.

Facilitation

If a number of action potentials reach a terminal bouton in a short space of time, then gradually the effect of the transmitter on the postsynaptic cell is enhanced (i.e. either more excitation or more inhibition occurs). This may be because of a build-up of Ca^{2+} within the presynaptic bouton causing increased exocytosis, as a result of increased Ca^{2+} entry outstripping the removal mechanism. Facilitation can only be sustained as long as there is transmitter in the vesicles. The enzymes that generate transmitter molecules and peptide transmitters are synthesized in the cell body and must be transported along the axon, which takes time. The facilitatory effect is therefore not sustained indefinitely.

Neurotransmitters and their receptors

There are five major types of neurotransmitter. An example of the synthesis of each is given in Fig. 2.12:

- Acetylcholine. This is the transmitter at the neuromuscular junction (NMJ) and also at many points in the autonomic nervous system. The cholinergic pathways in the brain may be important for memory formation, as anticholinesterase drugs seem to help people with Alzheimer's disease and anticholinergics make their symptoms worse.
- Amines (dopamine, noradrenaline, 5-hydroxytryptamine). The central pathways of the neurons containing these transmitters come mainly from the brainstem, and they have

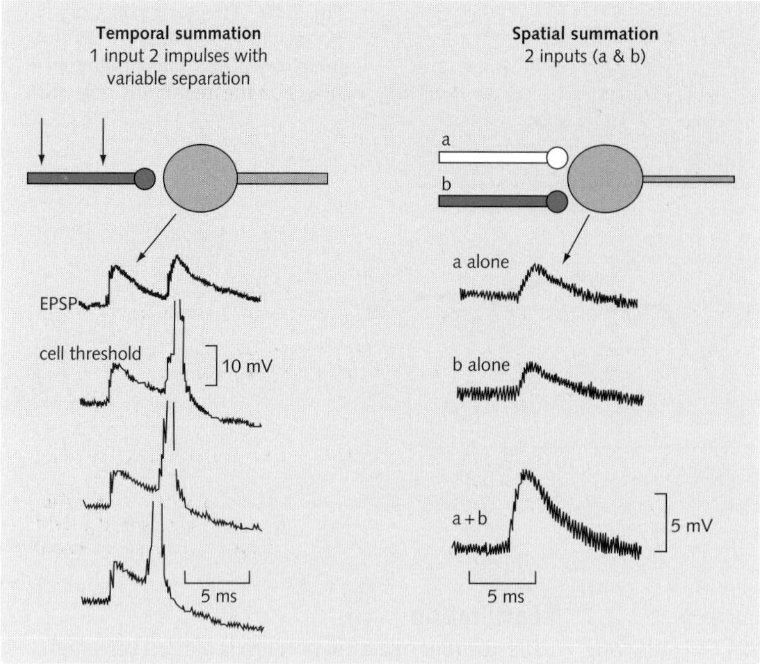

Fig. 2.11 Temporal and spatial summation.

important actions on all parts of the brain. The monoamine pathways are often modified when treating people with depression, but it is not known exactly why the drugs work.

- Excitatory amino acids (glutamate, aspartate). Glutamate is the most important excitatory amino acid, and is extremely widespread throughout the central nervous system. There are two main classes of glutamate receptor: the AMPA receptors and the NMDA receptor. The latter is thought to be an important component in long-term potentiation and the formation of memory. Glutamate is highly toxic to the brain in large quantities, possibly mediated by Ca^{2+} influx through the NMDA receptors, which are widespread throughout the cortex. This may be the cause of neuronal cell death in status epilepticus.
- Inhibitory amino acids (GABA, glycine). GABA is a derivative of glutamate and is widespread throughout the central nervous system, whereas most of the glycine-containing cells are interneurons in the spinal cord. Both are thought to cause hyperpolarization via the influx of Cl^- ions thereby taking the neuron further from its threshold potential.
- Peptides (opioids, neuropeptide-Y, substance-P, somatostatin). This is an extremely diverse group, with equally wide-ranging functions. Some have hormone activity (somatostatin, insulin), others modulate nociceptive pathways in the spinal cord and brainstem (opioids). They are commonly released along with small molecules which themselves have neurotransmitter-like actions (e.g. ATP).

Myasthenia gravis is a condition caused by antibodies to the postsynaptic acetylcholine receptor. It is characterized by weakness which becomes progressively worse with exercise. This is known as fatiguability. Diagnosis is made by the improval of symptoms when given a short acting anticholinesterase (the tensilon test).

The effect of a neurotransmitter depends upon the type of receptor that is present at the synapse. Thus, one neurotransmitter can have different effects throughout the central nervous system, depending on the receptors it acts upon.

Receptors can be classified according to the second messenger system that they use to alter the

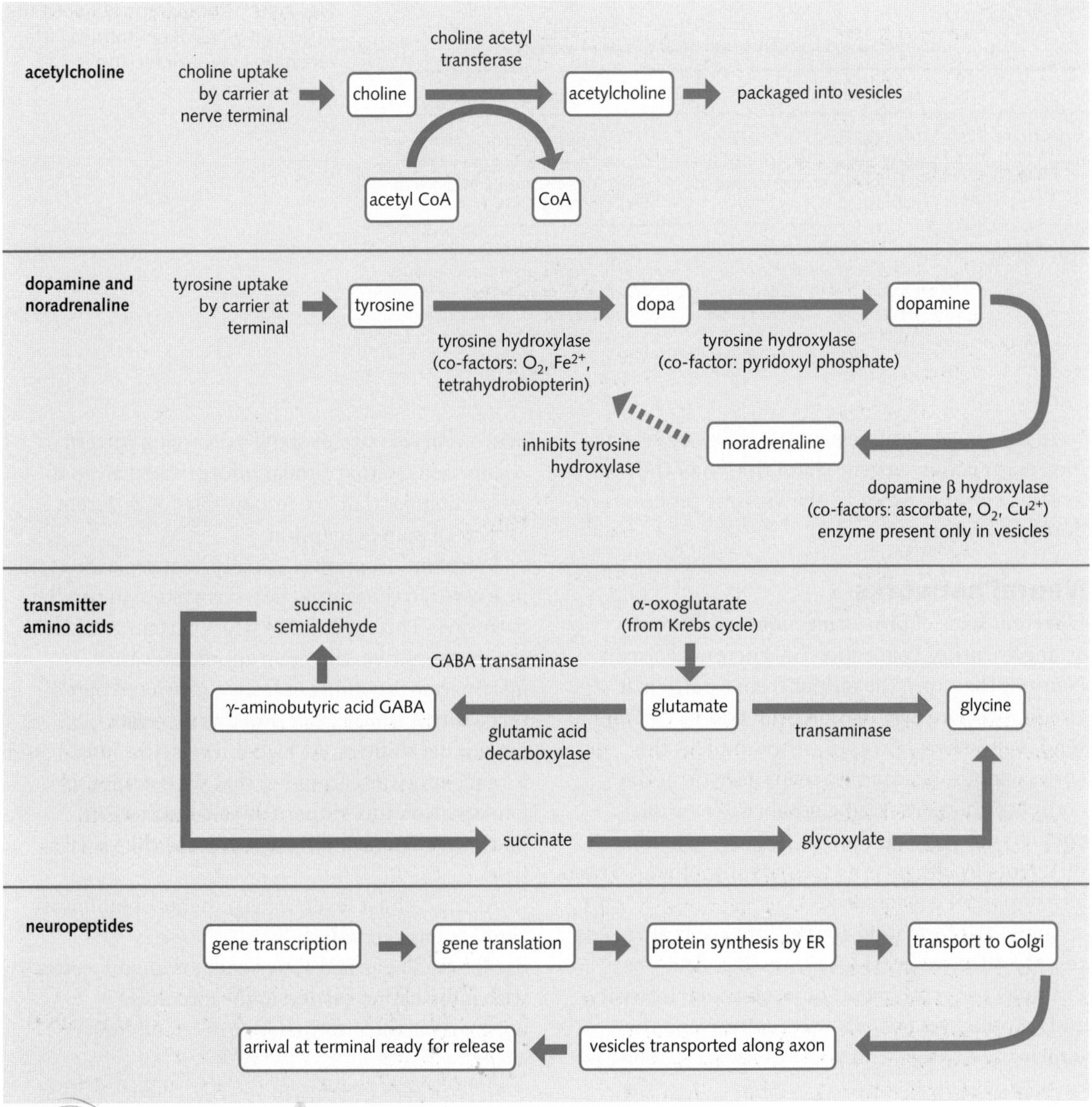

Fig. 2.12 Neurotransmitter synthetic pathways.

membrane potential. Two main classes of receptor are outlined in Fig. 2.13:

- The ionotrophic receptor that is coupled with an ion channel for cations or anions. When these receptors are simulated, they have a direct effect on membrane potential.
- The metabotrophic receptor that is coupled to a G-protein and uses cAMP (cyclic adenosine monophosphate) or IP_3 (inositol 1,4,5-triphosphate) as second messengers that can then have intracellular effects to bring about changes in ion channels to alter the membrane potential.

Receptor diversity for the major neurotransmitters is shown in Fig. 2.14.

Regulation of transmitter synthesis

Transmitter synthesis can be regulated in the short term at the terminal bouton by the intracellular calcium level. If the neuron fires many action potentials, Ca^{2+} will build up at the bouton and increase the activity of Ca^{2+}-dependent protein kinases that can influence the enzymes in the transmitter pathway.

Structure and function of two main classes of receptor		
	Ionotrophic	**Metabotrophic**
structure	transmembrane ion channel composed of five subunits; binding sites for ligand and modulators outside cell	single transmembrane protein with sites for interaction with ligand outside cell and interaction with G-protein inside cell
functional units	each subunit has four transmembrane domains, and subunits create a charge field to attract either cations or anions; e.g. AChα subunit attracts Na^+, $GABA_B$ subunit attracts Cl^-	seven transmembrane domains with specific amino-acid residues within domains important for ligand binding; e.g. D_1 receptor has aspartate in domain 3 for dopamine binding

Fig. 2.13 Comparison between the two main types of neurotransmitter receptor—ionotrophic and metabotrophic.

In the longer term, regulation occurs by second messenger action on gene transcription of the rate-limiting enzyme. Fig. 2.15 shows these processes for dopamine regulation.

Neural networks

Different sorts of processing require different arrangements of connections in a neuronal circuit. Neurons that form the output from a particular circuit integrate information from that circuit and send it elsewhere. An extreme example is the cortical motor neuron that sends its axon in the corticospinal tract. A large number of neuronal contacts converge on the cell; because a number of different circuits govern voluntary movement. This is an example of convergence.

Sensory information coming into the brain needs to go to different areas for processing. Pain, for example, has components of localization, intensity and emotion, yet only a few receptors send this information to the central nervous system. The neurons in this circuit show a diverging pattern of connections so that similar information can go to different areas that are responsible for different aspects of pain perception.

Visual information is initially kept separate as it is processed in the central nervous system in parallel pathways. This means that when certain neuronal groups are active, the brain appreciates that information is coming in from a restricted part of three-dimensional space and this increases our perceptual abilities. At higher levels, this information is much more integrated so that we consciously perceive a picture rather than a collection of lines and colours in different areas of the visual field.

At the cellular level, arrangements of inhibitory connections can reduce ‘noise’. Noise is background neuronal activity that is unconnected with information carried in the circuit (i.e. noise makes the information in a circuit less clear).

Receptor diversity for the major neurotransmitters					
Transmitter	**Cation channel**	**Anion channel**	**Increased cAMP by G-protein**	**Decreased cAMP by G-protein**	**Increased IP_3 by G-protein**
ACh	nicotinic			M_2, M_4	M_1, M_3
dopamine			D_1	D_2	
glutamate (channels classified according to experimental agonists)	NMDA (Na^+, K^+, Ca^{2+}), kainate and AMPA (Na^+, K^+)			mGluR2	mGluR1
GABA		$GABA_A$ (Cl^-)		$GABA_B$	
opioids				μ, δ	

Fig. 2.14 Receptor diversity for the major neurotransmitters.

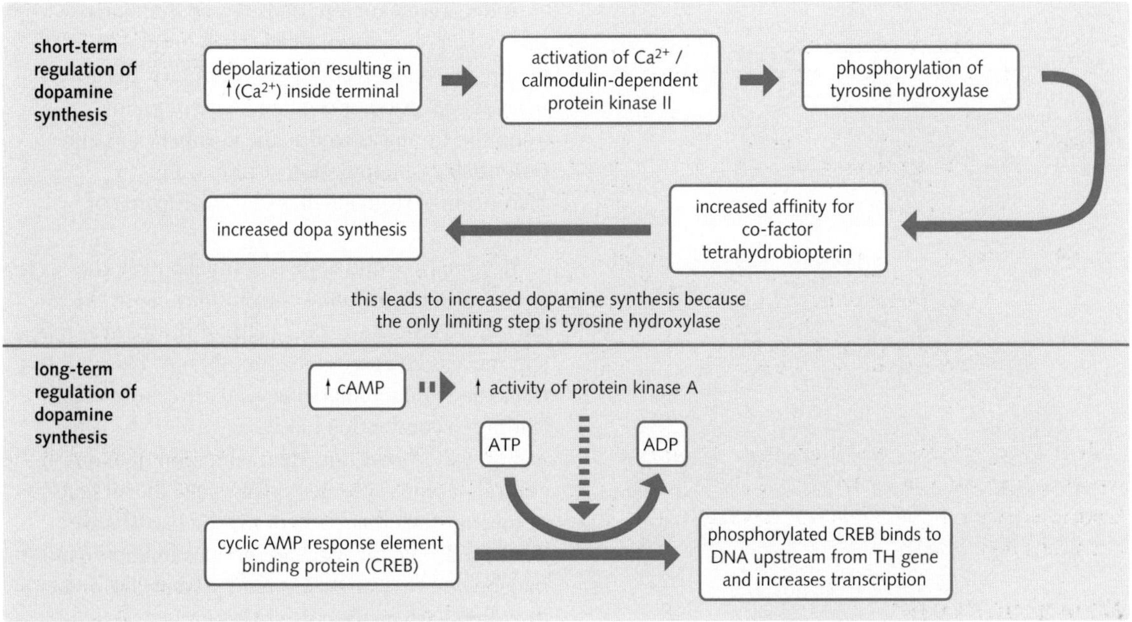

Fig. 2.15 Short- and long-term regulation of dopamine synthesis (TH, tyrosine hydroxylase).

There are many patterns of inhibition with different functions:

- Recurrent inhibition is shown in Fig. 2.16. It permits a stable discharge without sudden surges in activity which could be damaging. An example is seen in the spinal cord where spinal motor neurons are prevented from firing too often by connections with Renshaw cells. The most active cells activate the Renshaw cells maximally, thereby causing a global inhibitory feedback onto the group of cells they belong to. In this way, only the most stimulated cells continue to fire, and the output of the group of cells becomes more focussed.
- Lateral inhibition is shown in Fig. 2.17. Inhibitory interneurons can be used to 'sharpen' a response, to give a distinct border between the 'on' and 'off' part of a receptive field.
- Presynaptic inhibition is shown in Fig. 2.18. An inhibitory synapse placed on a terminal bouton can reduce the membrane depolarization caused by an incoming action potential, probably by increasing the permeability to Cl^- so that when the inside of the cell becomes more positive with Na^+ current, Cl^- starts to move into the bouton. This will reduce the inward flow of Ca^{2+} and therefore also reduce exocytosis.
- Signalling by disinhibition also occurs. A neuron at the end of a chain can be excited by inhibiting an inhibitory neuron earlier in the chain.

Inhibition is used in the creation of receptive fields, as shown in Fig. 2.17. A receptive field is the area which, when stimulated, causes a particular neuron to fire. It can be altered by inhibitory connections with neighbouring sensory units. This can produce a receptive field where the receptor responds to stimulation in one area but is inhibited by stimulation immediately around that area, a so-called 'on' centre and an 'off' surround (e.g. in retinal ganglion cells).

Looking at a higher level, there are connections between large groups of cells. Feedback loops between circuits encourage stable patterns of firing within individual circuits. Parallel pathways occur where there is more than one route that leads between two groups of cells. This arrangement may allow different processing to occur along the pathways (e.g. in relay nuclei), or may simply be an example of redundancy (useful if one pathway is damaged).

Connections

Commissural fibres connect neurons in different hemispheres. Association fibres connect neurons in the same hemisphere. There are vast numbers of connections in the central nervous system and there are many inputs modulating the effects of all

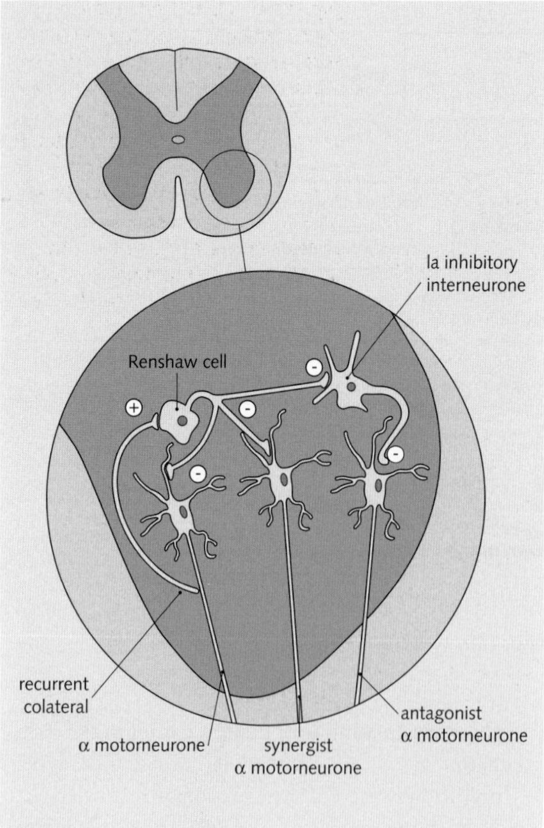

Fig. 2.16 Recurrent inhibition. When the alpha motor neuron is activated, it also activates the Renshaw cell, which in turn inhibits the motor neuron and synergistic motor neurons. It also relieves antagonistic motor neurons of their inhibition.

connections. This means that even the simple reflex is under many other influences and is not that 'simple'.

Damage and repair in the nervous system

A damaged nerve will not conduct action potentials to its terminal boutons. This block of conduction usually occurs either after section of the axon or demyelination of the axon.

The effect of demyelination

In myelinated axons, sodium channels are only present at the nodal regions, with the rest of the axon being electrically insulated.

Fig. 2.19 shows that if myelin is removed, the current density at the nodal regions will be reduced because current will escape across the bare membrane.

A decreased current density will depolarize the nodal region more slowly than normal, leading to reduced conduction velocity. Because normal activation of the target site depends upon the timing as well as the number of action potentials in a population of fibres, any disruption in timing will lead to disruption of function.

If more than one node is demyelinated, the severe decrease in longitudinal current may cause the current to fade along the length of the axon as more and more is lost across the membrane. This will stop the axon from depolarizing to its threshold level, leading to conduction block.

Fig. 2.20 shows how demyelination of axons in the central nervous system explains the clinical features of multiple sclerosis, where myelin sheaths are destroyed. The mechanism remains unknown but it may be due to an immune-mediated attack or an infection with an obscure pathogen.

Responses of peripheral axons to different types of trauma

Fig. 2.20 shows the relationship between a peripheral axon, its associated Schwann cells and thin connective-tissue covering—the basal lamina—which forms a continuous tube containing the axon–Schwann cells complex.

Fig. 2.21 shows that, after trauma, the main factors influencing restoration of function are the integrity of the axon itself, the integrity of the basal lamina and the length of time needed for regrowth to the site of innervation (i.e. distal muscles may atrophy completely before a nerve sectioned far away grows and reaches them).

Responses of the central nervous system to damage

The central nervous system is hostile to axonal regrowth. Neurons will not grow through glial scars, and inhibitory molecules, associated with oligodendrocytes, cause a collapse of the growing tip of the axon.

It is possible that cells secreting antibodies to the inhibitory molecules could be inserted locally in the tissue protecting the growth cone from inhibitory signals. Alternatively, in the case of spinal-cord injury, a piece of peripheral nerve could be inserted above and below the transection to provide a growth-friendly bridge across the gap. However, these therapies are a long way from entering current practice.

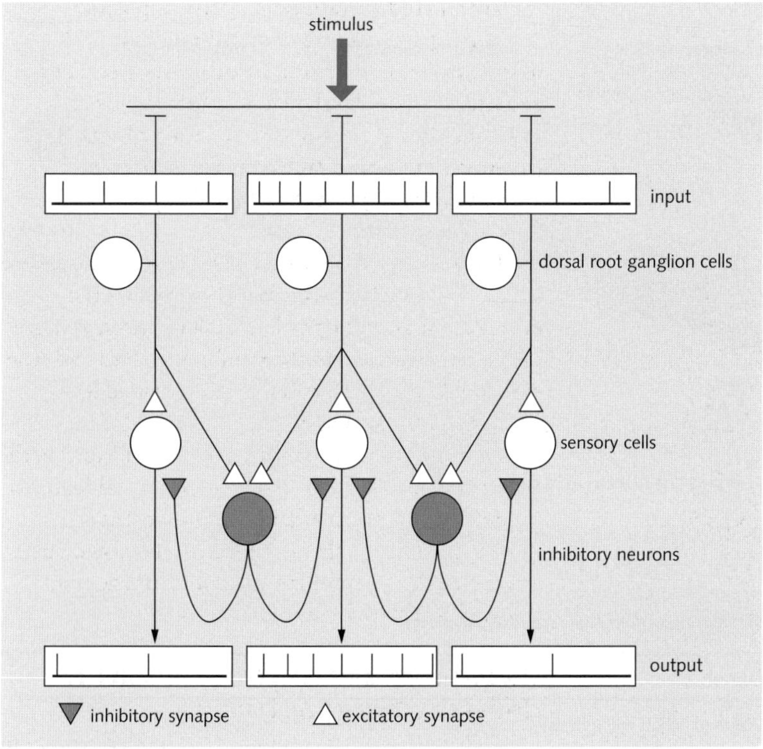

Fig. 2.17 Lateral inhibition. A stimulus causes a response in one receptor maximally and, to a lesser extent, in neighbouring receptors. If solely excitatory neurons link the inputs (level one), the signal becomes blurred. However, if inhibitory interneurons are introduced, then the cells which are not maximally stimulated will cease to fire. This sharpens the border between 'off' and 'on' (level 2) in a receptive field.

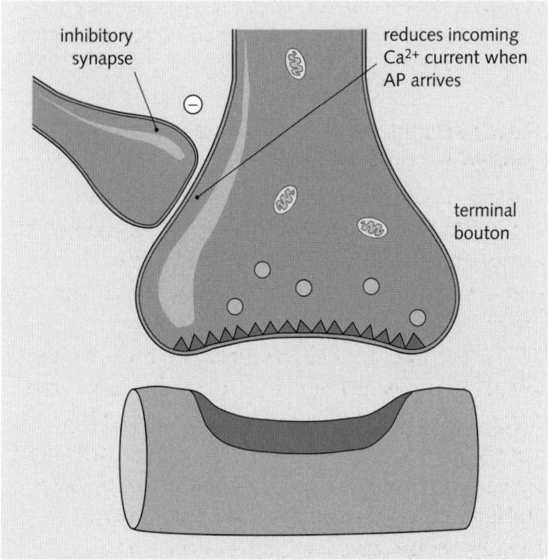

Fig. 2.18 Presynaptic inhibition preventing vesicle mobilization and release by decreasing calcium influx.

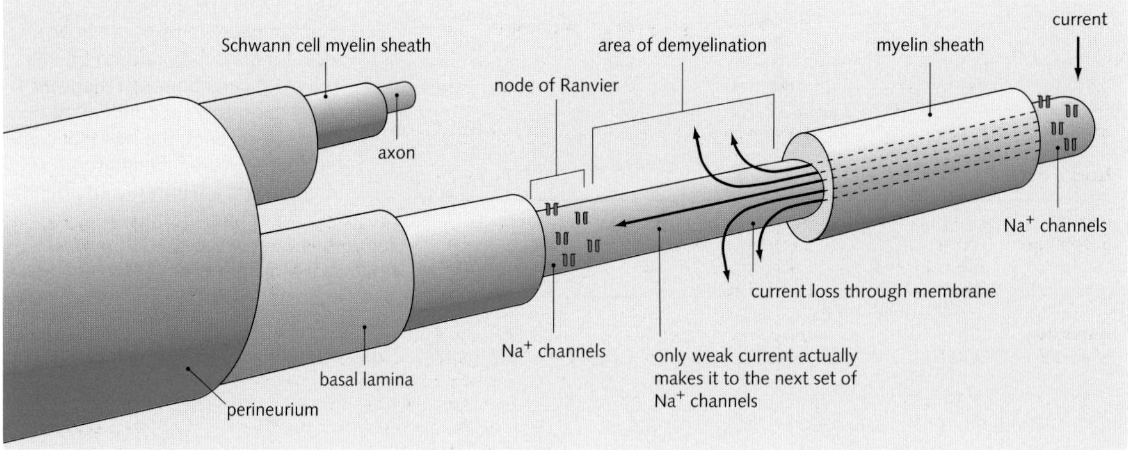

Fig. 2.19 The effect of demyelination on current flow in an axon.

Pathophysiology of multiple sclerosis symptoms	
Symptoms	**Cellular explanation**
blindness, numbness, weakness, paralysis	Block in conduction of action potential caused by dissipation of current after demyelination
paraesthesia (tingling)	Extracellular potassium builds up at sites of demyelination as channels exposed that leak potassium. This raises membrane potential to threshold and action potential generated spontaneously (Nernst equation)
remission of symptoms	Caused by: (A) remyelination by oligodendrocytes (B) use of alternative neural pathways (C) new sodium channels produced
relapse	(A) extension of existing lesion with exposure of membrane with few sodium channels (B) new lesion site
Lhermitte's sign (feeling of electric shock in limbs upon stretching)	Lesions often form in areas of CNS that are constantly being moved, such as the part of the spinal cord in the region of the cervical vertebrae. When lesioned axons are stretched they generate impulses. (A similar problem occurs in the optic nerve and flashes are seen at night when there is much less light to mask the effect of these spontaneous impulses.)

Fig. 2.20 Pathophysiology of multiple sclerosis symptoms.

Effects of peripheral nerve injury				
	Compression	**Crush**	**Severed nerve**	**Severed limb**
axon	intact	discontinuous	discontinuous	discontinuous
basal lamina	intact	intact	discontinuous	discontinuous
regrowth possibilities	no regrowth needed, full remyelination within a few weeks	trophic factors released by distal part of axon, and proximal axon (still attached to cell body) regrows at 1 mm/day	trophic factors released by distal part of axon, but can grow into wrong basal lamina, previously occupied by nerve with different function	no distal part of axon present; nerve forms a neuroma
restoration of function	complete	dependent on lengthof axonal growth needed for reinnervation	four possibilities: 1. grows into original basal lamina 2. grows into basal lamina of same modality—altered function 3. grows into basal lamina of different modality—no function 4. forms neuroma—no function	no function; disturbed sensation and chronic/ transient pain

Fig. 2.21 Effects of peripheral nerve injury.

- Describe the basic structure of a neuron and comment on the function of the individual elements.
- What is the difference, anatomically and functionally, between projection neurons and interneurons?
- What is meant by the 'resting potential' of a cell, and how is it maintained?
- Describe the sequence of events involved in an action potential.
- How is an action potential propagated along an axon?
- How do electrical and chemical synapses differ?
- What is the series of steps involved in chemical synaptic transmission from the action potential arriving at the terminal bouton?
- Explain the difference between temporal and spatial summation.
- What patterns of inhibition do you know? Describe them.
- What is the effect of demyelination on the conduction of action potentials?
- Name the common types of peripheral nerve function and the cellular processes of repair which allow restoration of function.

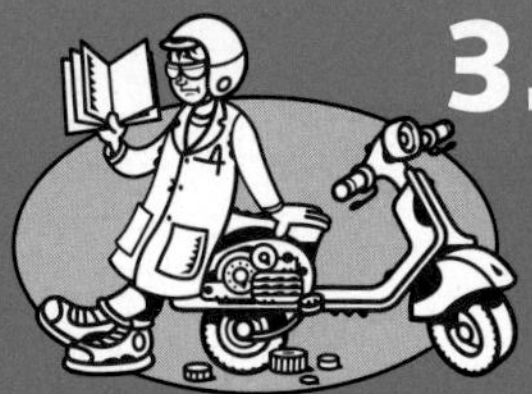

3. The Spinal Cord

In this chapter, you will learn about:

- The anatomy of the spinal cord.
- The tracts within the cord, and the modalities they subserve.
- The effect of damage to the spinal cord.

The spinal cord

The spinal cord is a segmentally organized tube with a central cellular area surrounded by nerve-fibre tracts. The tracts carry information between different levels of the spinal cord, and also to and from the supra-spinal structures.

Fig. 3.1 shows the relationship between the spinal cord, its coverings and its bony housing in the vertebral column. In adults, the cord ends at vertebral body level L1/L2 and so a lumbar puncture needle can be inserted into the subarachnoid space below this level (e.g. L3/L4) without damaging the cord.

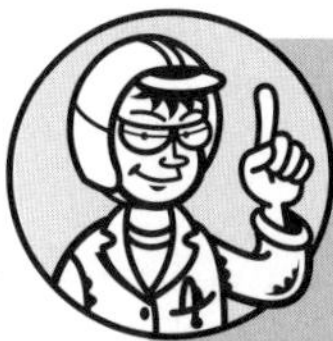

The presence of oligoclonal bands of protein in the cerebrospinal fluid on electrophoresis suggests the presence of large quantities of immunoglobulins. This is a feature of multiple sclerosis.

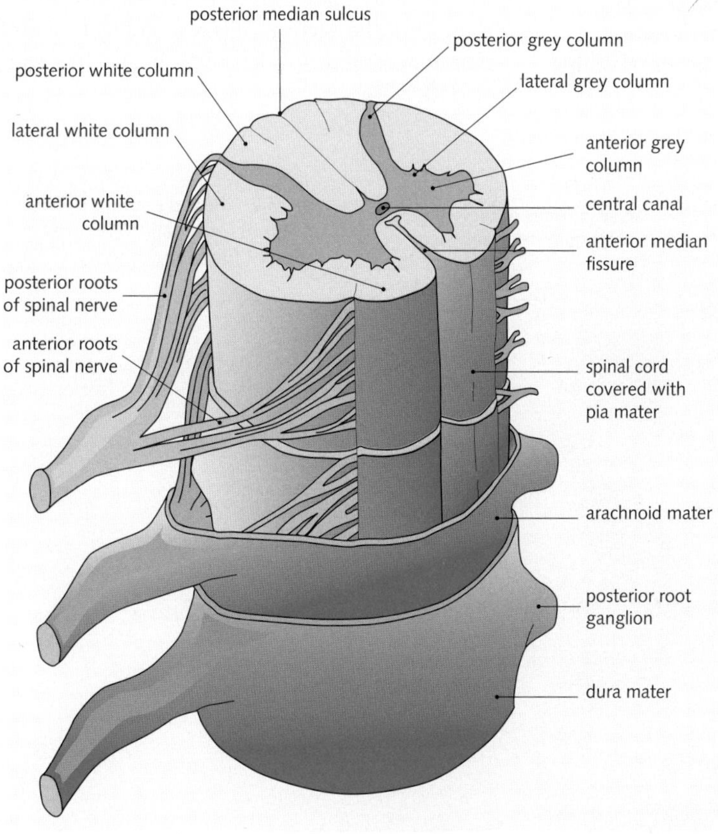

Fig. 3.1 Spinal cord above the level of L1, showing the meningeal coverings (dura mater, arachnoid mater and pia mater).

Cells

Fig. 3.2 shows that the cells in the central grey matter can be divided up as a series of layers in the dorsal horn and as a series of columns in the ventral horn. These layers and columns are known as Rexed's laminae (numbered I–X) and are based on groupings of similarly shaped cell bodies.

- The dorsal horn layers are involved in sensory pathways and are the target sites for some sensory afferent nerves, particularly for pain, temperature and crude touch.
- The ventral columns are made up of pools of motor neurons innervating skeletal muscle. Medial motor columns supply proximal muscles and lateral motor columns supply distal muscles.
- In between the dorsal and ventral horns lies the interomedio-lateral column where the cell bodies of preganglionic sympathetic neurons are found.

The spinal tracts

As a general rule, in the white matter, the ascending sensory tracts run in the periphery and descending motor tracts occupy a more central position, as shown in Fig. 3.3. Sensory inputs from the skin terminate in laminae I–IV, with some fibres travelling to the segments above and below in Lissauer's tract.

Ascending

The major difference between the main sensory tracts is that fine touch information (dorsal column tract) is conveyed up the cord on the same side as it enters, whereas pain, temperature and crude touch (spinothalamic tract) are conveyed upwards on the opposite side of the cord. The point at which the tract crosses to the contralateral side is known as the decussation.

The sensory tracts are both arranged segmentally (i.e. fibres from the same level run upwards together in the tract). At the top of the dorsal columns, the segments are arranged in a coherent pattern from medial (sacral) to lateral (cervical), maintaining the body pattern. The pattern is distorted by divergence and convergence in the dorsal column nuclei so that distal structures (such as the hands) have a greater representation.

The dorsal column pathway

One of the functions of this pathway is to re-arrange the input from the dermatomal input of the primary sensory fibres into the grossly distorted map of the body surface seen in the primary sensory cortex (the sensory homunculus). Here, the body surface is seen as grossly distorted with most of the cortical cells responding to sensory exploratory structures such as the hands, feet and lips.

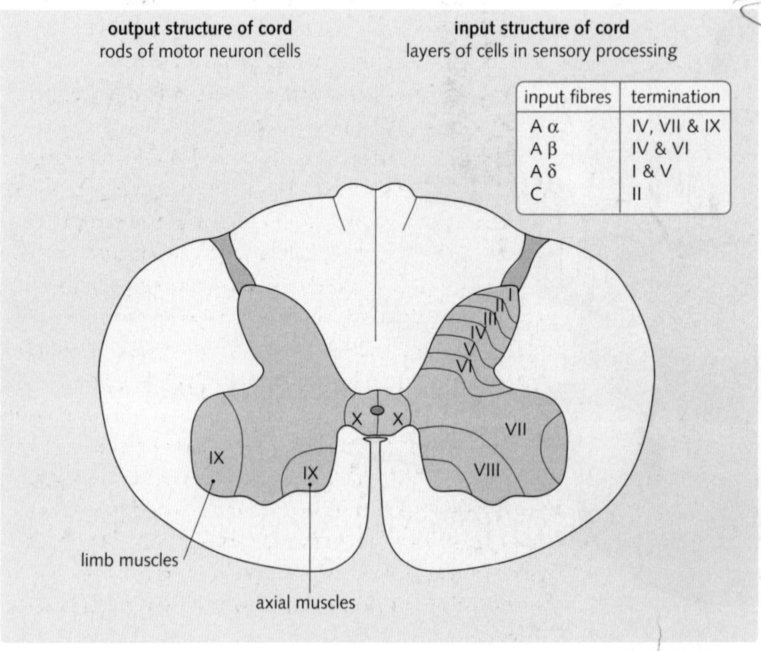

input fibres	termination
A α	IV, VII & IX
A β	IV & VI
A δ	I & V
C	II

Fig. 3.2 Rexed's laminae. The different termination patterns of afferent fibres are shown.

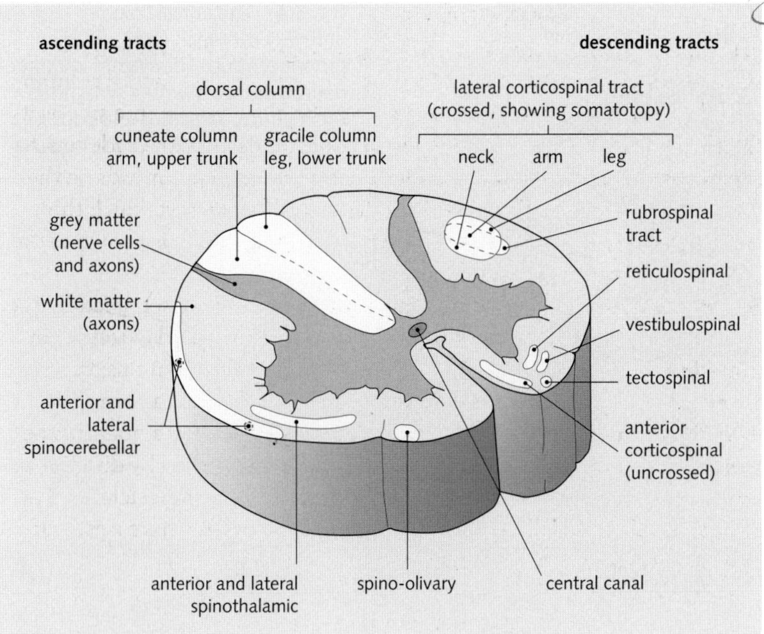

Fig. 3.3 Ascending and descending spinal tracts.

This pathway:

- Segregates information into modality-specific pathways for touch, hair movement, pressure and joint rotation.
- Contains feedback mechanisms to gate the amount of incoming information to the cortex.

These functions are carried out in the areas where the pathway is interrupted by synapses, to allow for re-organization, segregation and suppression. Fig. 3.4 shows the dorsal column system as a three-neuron pathway. The first neurons in the pathway synapse in the dorsal column nuclei (gracile and cuneate).

- Sensory input from the leg and lower trunk travels to the gracile nucleus.
- Sensory input from the arm, upper trunk and neck to the cuneate nucleus.
- Sensory input from the face goes via the trigeminal nerve (cranial nerve V) to the trigeminal nucleus.

The next synapse is in the contralateral ventropoterolateral nucleus of the thalamus (or VPL) or the contralateral ventroposteromedial nucleus (VPM) for trigeminal inputs. The inputs reach here via the medial lemniscus.

The homuncular organization which began in the dorsal columns and trigeminal nuclei is amplified here and reaches its climax in the cortex.

The neurons from the VPL and VPM nuclei project to the cortex via the thalamocortical radiations.

Spinothalamic tract and pain signals

In addition to pain, the spinothalamic tract also carries crude touch and thermal information. Pain information is also carried in the spinoreticular and spinomesencephalic tracts.

Noxious and thermal information is carried into the dorsal horn by fast myelinated Aδ fibres (conveying sharp, stabbing pain) and slower unmyelinated C fibres (conveying dull, nagging pain as well as thermal information).

Aδ fibres terminate in laminae I and V. The axons from these cells cross over to the opposite side of the cord (decussate) and ascend in the anterolateral white matter, forming the spinothalamic tract.

C fibres influence the firing of the spinothalamic dorsal horn cells via interneurons, because they terminate in a different layer of the cord—lamina II. This provides further synaptic steps in the pain pathway, which may comprise targets for modulation of pain signal transmission by higher centres.

Fig. 3.5 shows that the spinothalamic fibres join the medial lemniscus in the medulla and project to the thalamus. The thalamic termination of the tract is in the ventroposterior nuclei and also in the intralaminar nuclei, from which there is a relay to the cortex.

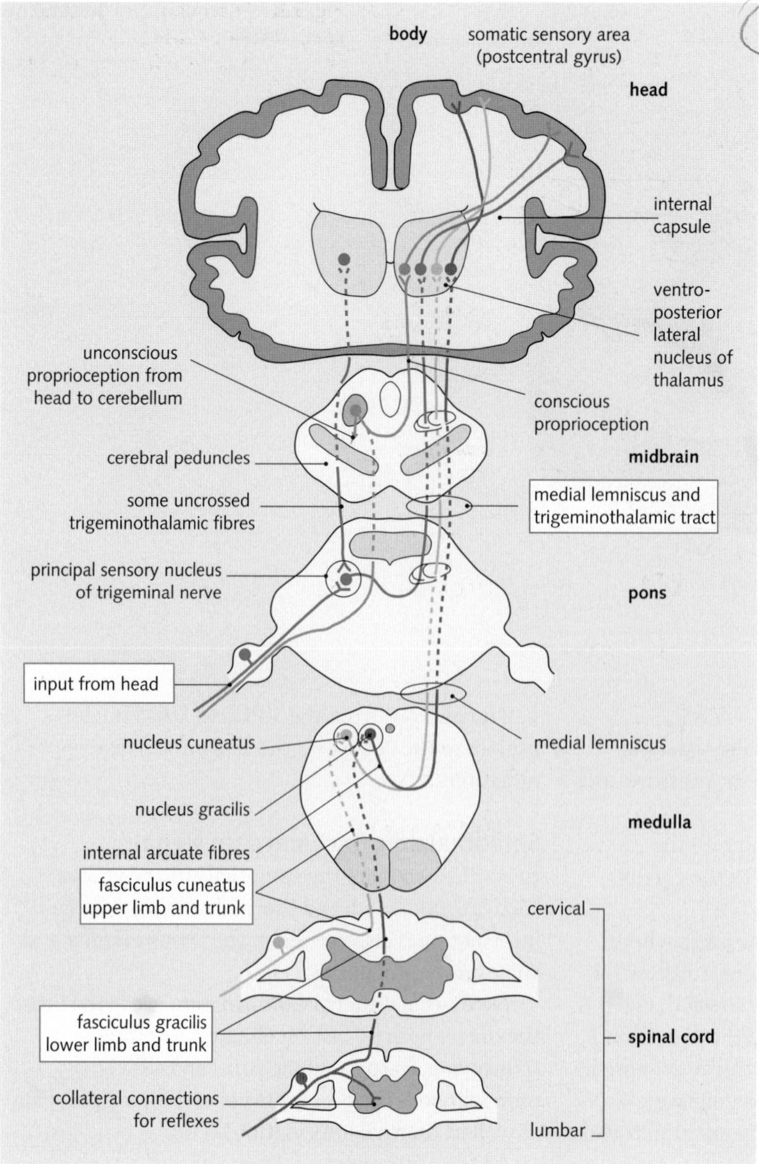

Fig. 3.4 The dorsal column pathway for touch and proprioception. The system is a three-neuron pathway with a synapse in the medulla, thalamus and cortex. Note the decussation in the medulla.

As with fine touch, nociceptive afferent nerves from the face are carried in the trigeminal (V) nerve to the spinal trigeminal nucleus (which takes over the function of dorsal horn laminae I and II). The ascending fibres from the spinal nucleus of V cross over to the other side of the medulla and pass up to the thalamus to join the nociceptive spinothalamic inputs from the rest of the body.

Noxious input also projects to a variety of brainstem structures; some of which are implicated in generating sensations of agonizing pain (spinomesencephalic) and others being involved in arousal mechanisms (spinoreticular).

Spinocerebellar tract

The spinocerebellar tract (Fig. 3.6) deals with proprioceptive information and can be divided into two parts:

- The dorsal spinocerebellar tract is formed by the axons of cell bodies that lie in a column at the base of the dorsal horn (Clarke's column) running from T1 to L2. These cells receive information from muscle spindles and tendon organs. Below L2, the fibres ascend in the dorsal

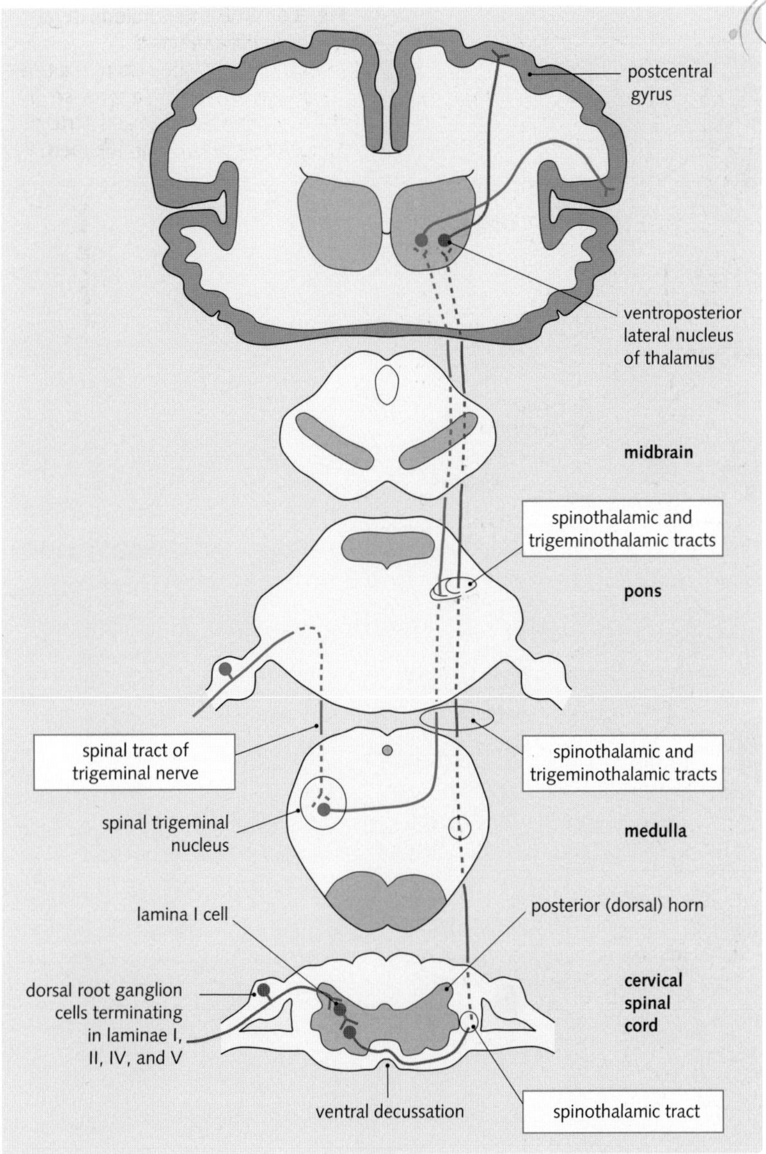

Fig. 3.5 The spinothalamic tract. Note the decussation at the same spinal level as the afferent fibres enter the cord.

columns before they synapse with the cells in Clarke's column. This tract conveys information about body movement, from the trunk and lower limb, to the cerebellum via the inferior cerebellar penduncle. The same kind of information from the upper limb is transferred via the external cuneate nucleus located laterally in the medulla.

- The ventral spinocerebellar tract receives its input from cell bodies in lamina VII (the spinal interneuron layer). Most of the axons cross to the other side of their segment then up to the cerebellum via the superior cerebellar peduncle where most of the axons cross over again. This tract sends information primarily about inhibitory interneuron activity.

Descending

The corticospinal tract

The corticospinal (sometimes called the pyramidal) tract is the major controller of skeletal muscle activity. It has two branches:

- The decussating lateral tract controls the precision movements of the limbs (innervating lateral motor neuron pools).

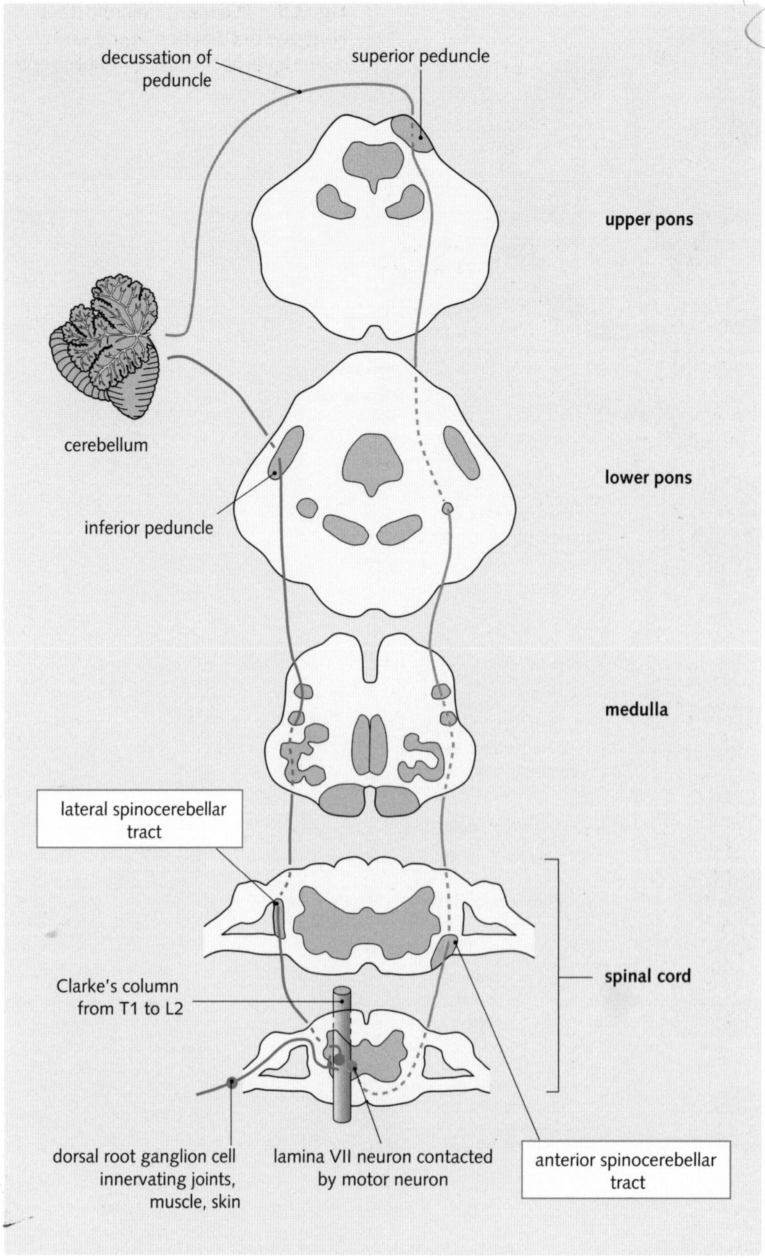

Fig. 3.6 The anterior and lateral spinocerebellar tracts.

- The uncrossed anterior tract controls the less precise movements of the trunk (innervating medial motor neuron pools).

The fibres that influence motor neurons innervating muscles in the head (e.g. extraocular muscles, tongue muscles and facial muscles) run in the corticobulbar tracts to the appropriate cranial nerve nuclei. The somatotopic arrangement of the descending motor fibres from the cortex includes the head in the cerebral peduncles, but not at the level of decussation in the medulla (Fig. 3.7).

The motor fibres carry signals for highly skilled voluntary movements. To achieve this:

- The tract needs to be highly somatotopic.
- The fibres must have few collaterals so that excitation from one fibre is communicated to the minimum number of spinal motor neurons (this allows a great deal of control over the execution of movement).

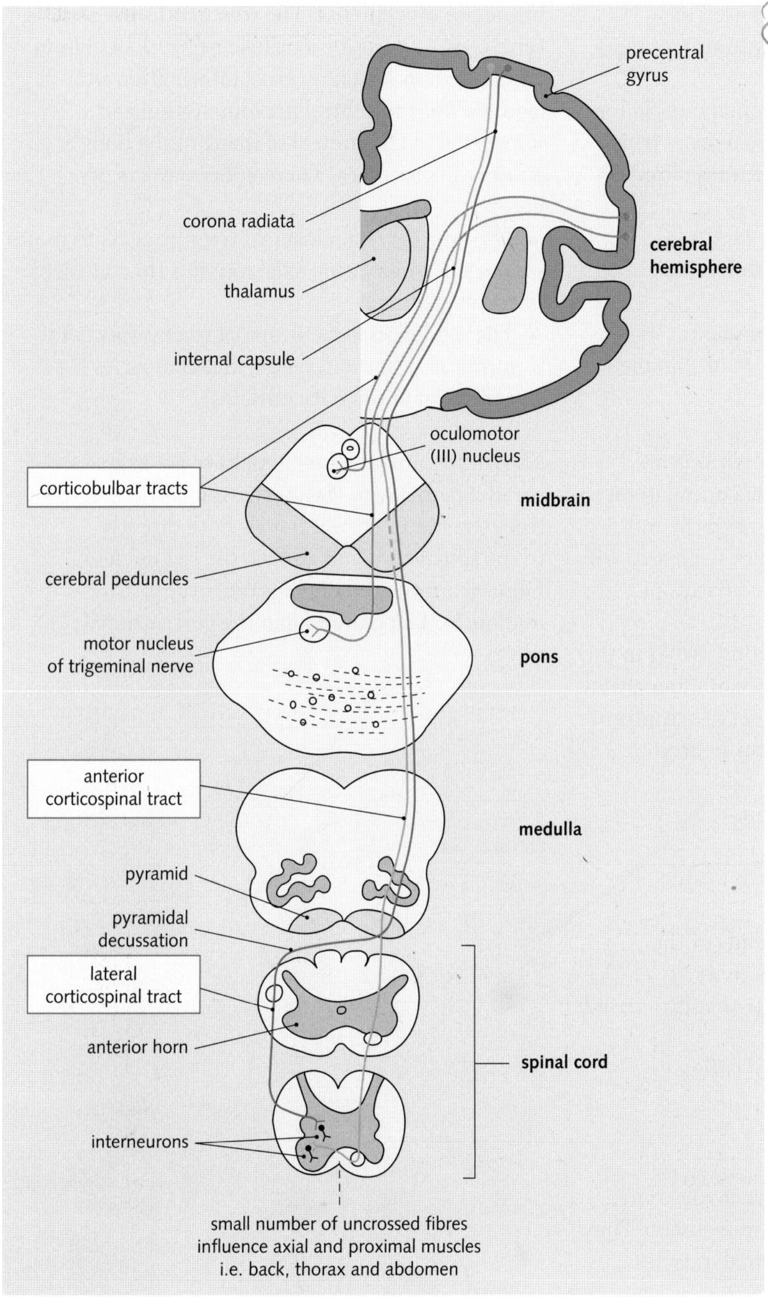

Fig. 3.7 The corticospinal and corticobulbar tracts. Note the decussation in the spinal cord.

As well as motor axons, there are fibres that regulate spinal reflexes in the tract and feedback to the dorsal horn sensory circuits from the sensory cortex.

Upper and lower motor neuron lesions

Damage to the motor cortex leads to an absence of volitional movement but experimental evidence from cutting just the pyramidal tract in the medulla of monkeys results in very little motor deficit.

In humans, damage to the motor cortex and premotor areas after a cerebrovascular accident (or stroke) in the middle cerebral artery territory leads to a set of symptoms and signs affecting some of the contralateral muscles in the limbs and face. Because upper (i.e. cortical) motor neurons are involved, the effect is termed an 'upper motor neuron lesion', although other cells are involved too.

Voluntary paresis (weakness) is caused by loss of corticospinal input. The symptoms and signs are:

- Spasticity or abnormal distribution in muscle tone which affects flexors more than extensors (this may be caused by disruption of extrapyramidal systems).
- Stronger deep reflexes (e.g. knee jerk).
- Loss of superficial reflexes (e.g. abdominal, cremasteric).
- Positive Babinski's sign—extensor plantar response to stroking the lateral part of the sole from heel to toe.

The effects of an upper motor neuron lesion are typically seen on the side of the body contralateral to the lesion. If there is localized damage to the motor cortex or pyramidal tract, all the input to an area will be affected due to homuncular and somatotopic organization.

Damage to the spinal motor neurons, either in the cord or along their pathway to the site of innervation of the muscle, produces a different set of symptoms and signs, referred to as a lower motor neuron lesion:

- Weakness caused by loss of nervous innervation.
- Atrophy as a result of disuse (this is a late sign).
- Fasciculation (squirming movements of the muscle) caused by increased sensitivity at receptor level to any acetylcholine that is released from intact terminals.
- Absent reflexes caused by loss of reflex output.

Other descending tracts

The other descending tracts are more involved in automatic or involuntary control of movement. They largely deal with the axial and proximal muscles which control posture.

The tectospinal tract controls head and neck posture. The tract begins with cells in the superior colliculus and their axons cross the midline in the midbrain, but only go as far as motor neurons in the cervical cord.

The vestibulospinal tract acts with the tectospinal to keep the head balanced on the shoulders as the body moves through space and to turn the head in response to sensory stimuli.

The reticulospinal tract (Fig. 3.8) controls posture and helps in the control of crude imprecise movements. The reticular formation is a term used to describe a diffuse network of cells in the brainstem which receives information from a large part of the central nervous system and is involved in the control of many of the body's automatic processes. There are two tracts of note:

- The pontine reticulospinal tract projects to motor neurons innervating axial muscles (in control of trunk posture).
- The medullary reticulospinal tract projects to motor neurons innervating distal muscles (in control of antigravity muscles).

The rubrospinal tract is thought to act as a parallel pathway to the corticospinal tract. Output from the motor cortex travels both directly to the spinal cord and also via the red nucleus. Fibres from the red nucleus cross the midline in the pons and join the corticospinal tract.

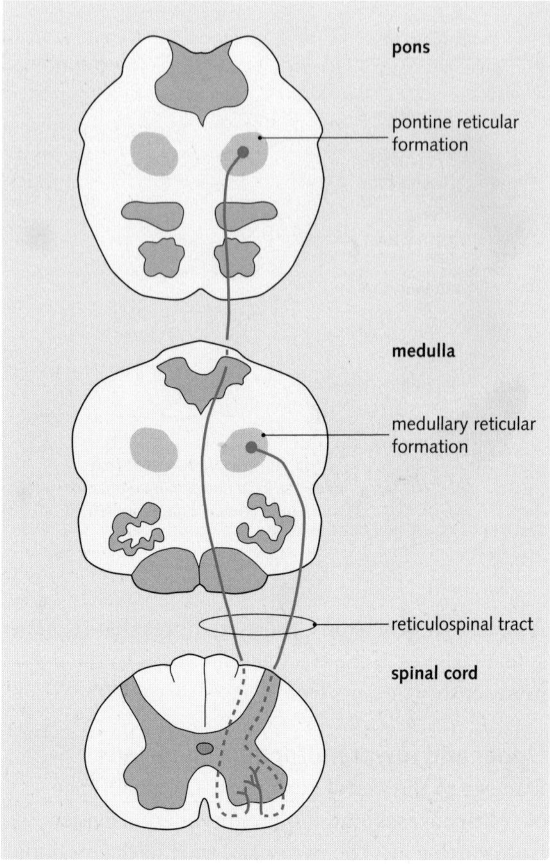

Fig. 3.8 The reticulospinal tract.

Damage

Fig. 3.9 shows that damage to the cord at different levels will produce different degrees of deficit in both motor and sensory function. Lesions to the VPL nucleus in the thalamus and somatosensory cortex show similar deficits to dorsal column lesions, but on the contralateral side of the body.

> After transection of the spinal cord, there may be an initial period where no reflexes can be elicited below the level of the lesion (when you would expect exaggerated reflexes). This coincides with a period of 'spinal shock', which may persist for several weeks.

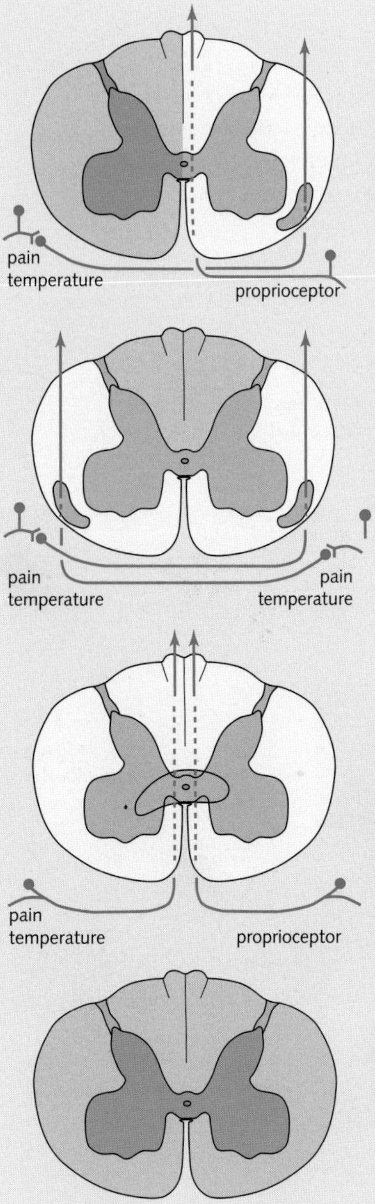

Lesion – hemi-section through cord (Brown-Séquard syndrome)
Tracts affected – ipsilateral spinothalamic, dorsal column and corticospinal
Symptoms and signs – no pain and temperature sensation below lesion contralateral to side of lesion. No fine touch or position sense below lesion ipsilateral to side of lesion. Weakness of ipsilateral body below lesion with the same distribution of upper motor neuron signs

Lesion – tabes dorsalis (3° syphilis)
Tracts affected – dorsal columns bilaterally
Symptoms and signs – no perception of fine touch bilaterally. No proprioceptive feedback about movement bilaterally below level of lesion–stamping gait results producing mechanical damage to joints

Lesion – syringomyelia (cavitation from central canal into grey and white matter)
Tracts affected – initially spinothalamic bilaterally. May extend to include motor neurons in the anterior horn and the corticospinal tract
Symptoms and signs – bilateral loss of pain and temperature sensation below lesion. Variable degree of lower motor neuron (anterior horn) and upper motor neuron (corticospinal tract) signs

Lesion – complete section through whole cord (trauma, transverse myelitis)
Tracts affected – all tracts below level of lesion
Symptoms and signs – paralysis with upper motor below level of lesion. No sensation in any modality below level of lesion

Fig. 3.9 Effects of spinal cord lesions in different areas. The area of lesion is shaded.

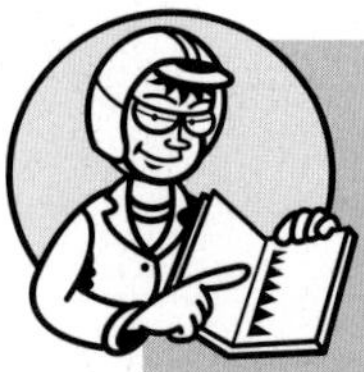

- Where can a lumbar puncture needle be inserted in the adult with the smallest risk of damage to the spinal cord?
- What are the differences between the dorsal and ventral columns?
- What are Rexed's laminae?
- Explain the three-neuron relay in the dorsal column pathway.
- What information is transferred in the spinocerebellar tracts?
- Describe the corticospinal tract and its two branches.
- How would you distinguish an upper motor neuron lesion from a lower motor neuron lesion?

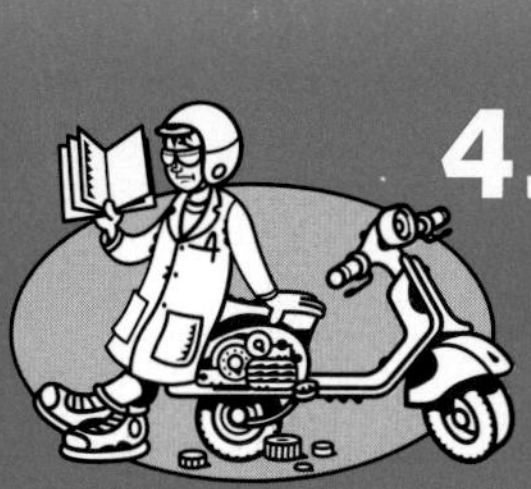

4. Somatosensation and the Perception of Pain

In this chapter, you will learn about:
- Somatosensation and the primary sensory cortex.
- Nociception and the perception of pain.
- Common analgesics and local anaesthetics.

Somatosensation and the sensory cortex

Sensation

Sensation is a remarkably important part of life. Patients who have lost sensation in some way end up unable to perform simple tasks such as undoing buttons and manipulating coins. In severe forms of sensory disturbance (such as the neuropathy that occurs with diabetes), patients may sustain severe injuries—particularly to the feet in diabetics—partly because they cannot feel the pain.

There are four sensory modalities—touch, thermal sensation, pain and proprioception. In this chapter, we will not look at proprioception, which is covered in Chapter 5.

There are individual receptors for submodalities within these groups. For example, the body can differentiate between light touch and pressure, between hot and cold and between mechanical and thermal pains.

In humans, no matter how a receptor is activated (electrically or electromagnetically), the subjective sensation reported is always that of its modality. This has proved particularly useful for physiologists studying the processes!

They have shown that there are modality-specific channels that convey information of one modality from the skin to the sensory receiving area.

Receptors

Receptors are formed by the peripheral terminations of the axons of dorsal root ganglion cells.

Receptors in the skin may be free nerve endings, or associated with different connective-tissue structures (e.g. Pacinian corpuscles).

Receptors can be divided into slowly adapting and rapidly adapting types. These two categories work in harmony to send different information about the same stimulus. The different signalling depends either on the linkage of the receptor to its incident energy or on a property called adaptation (i.e. a decline in receptor responsiveness even though the stimulus is still present). As a general rule, slowly adapting receptors signal the magnitude or location of a stimulus, whereas rapidly adapting receptors signal its rate of change and duration.

The receptor membrane depolarizes in response to its modality stimulus, causing a generator potential. If sufficient, this causes the axon to depolarize to its threshold level and produce an action potential. Because the axon recovers after its refractory period, a long-lasting generator potential will cause the axon to fire a train of impulses whose frequency will be proportional to the magnitude of the generator potential. To accommodate the wide range of sensory experience, different unimodal receptors have different thresholds, and the generator potential has a logarithmic relationship between stimulus intensity, frequency of firing and ultimately perceived sensation.

Fig. 4.1 shows different fibre types for different modalities and their conduction speeds and axonal diameters.

The axons of these receptors enter the spinal cord via the dorsal root ganglion, with the fibres signalling modalities of touch travelling in the dorsal column pathway, and the fibres signalling thermal and pain information travelling in the spinothalamic tract (along with some information about crude touch). The dorsal column pathway and spinothalamic tract are discussed in detail in Chapter 3.

The site of the sensory cortex and its organization are shown in Fig. 4.2. The homunculus is distorted because more of the cortex is used to process information from body areas used for exploration. Areas of greatest organized receptor density (i.e. other than free nerve endings) have the biggest representation in the sensory cortex.

The sensory cortex has an homunculus for each modality (i.e. there is a map for touch, another for pressure, etc., all lying next to each other). Within each homunculus, there is a columnar organization from the cortical surface to the corpus callosum. Within each column, the cells have similar receptive fields and modality. The layers in the column send

Sensory afferent fibres				
Class	**Modality**	**Axonal diameter (μm)**	**Conduction speed (m/s)**	**Pattern of termination in Rexed's laminae**
myelinated				
Aα	proprioceptors from muscles, tendons	20	120	III, IV, V
Aβ	mechanoreceptors from skin	10	60	III, IV, V
Aδ	nociceptor, cold thermoreceptor	2.5	15	I, II, V
unmyelinated				
C	nociceptor, heat thermoreceptor	<1	<1	I, II

Fig. 4.1 Sensory afferent fibres.

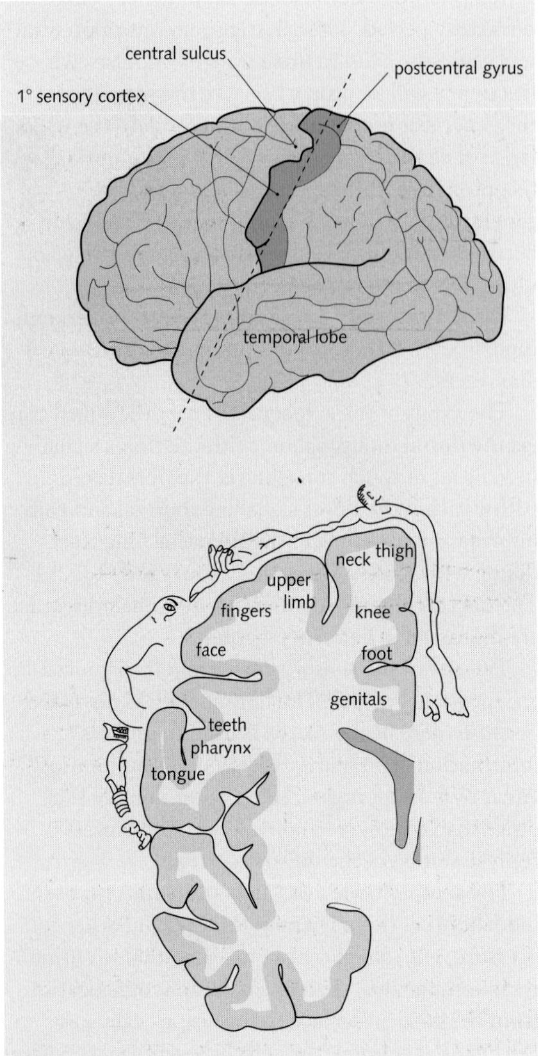

Fig. 4.2 Homuncular organization and location of primary sensory cortex (S1).

and receive fibres from different areas of the cortex and thalamus. This is shown in Fig. 4.3.

Nociception

Nociception is the sensory process detecting overt or impending tissue damage. Pain is the perception of irritating, sore, stinging, throbbing or painful

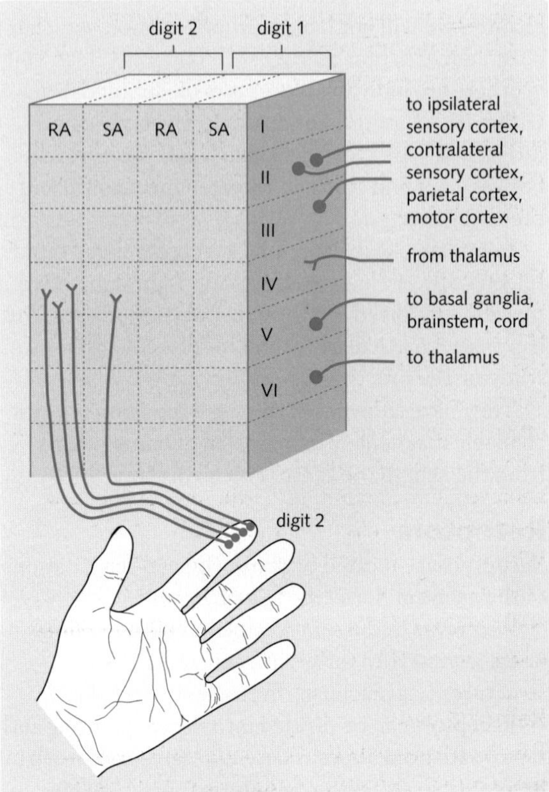

Fig. 4.3 Columnar organization of primary sensory cortex (RA, rapidly adapting; SA, slowly adapting).

sensations arising from the body. The way the body perceives pain not only depends on nociceptor input, but also on other pathways giving information about, for example, emotional components. Thus, pain is an 'experience' rather than a simple sensation.

Although nociceptors do not show adaptation (i.e. they fire continuously to tissue damage), pain sensation may come and go and pain may be felt in the absence of nociceptor discharge. They rely on chemical mediators around the nerve ending which indicate tissue damage. Pain is somehow related to itch. Itch is also mediated by Aδ and C fibres; people born without a sense of pain show no sense of itch, but itch is unaltered by opiate drugs.

Hyperalgesia is the phenomenon of increased sensitivity of damaged areas to painful stimuli:

- Primary hyperalgesia occurs within the damaged area.
- Secondary hyperalgesia occurs in undamaged tissues surrounding this area.

After damage, blood vessels become leaky and the damaged tissue cells release a variety of chemicals that give a local response—inflammation (e.g. histamine, which directly excites nociceptors, and prostaglandin, which sensitizes nociceptors).

Nociceptor afferent nerves release not only the excitatory transmitter glutamate (as do all sensory afferent nerves), but also the cotransmitter substance-P. This causes a very long-lasting excitatory postsynaptic potential and helps sustain the effect of noxious stimuli.

Processing of nociceptive afferent nerves begins in the circuits in the dorsal horn and a certain amount of descending control is exercised over the firing of spinothalamic cells in lamina I. Pain information is then transmitted to the cortex in the spinothalamic tract (see Chapter 3). Whether the cortex is the ultimate site of pain sensation is a matter for debate. Certainly, subjects who are awake during neurosurgery do not report pain sensations when electrodes are passed through areas of the cortex. When those areas are stimulated, subjects may report tingling or thermal sensation, but not pain. It is likely then that the conscious sensation of pain has a large subcortical component.

Referred pain

Pain from internal organs (viscera) is felt as pain in a more superficial region of the body. Nociceptor fibres from viscera and from cutaneous structures converge on the same pain pathway (i.e. spinothalamic cells). The central nervous system can make no distinction between superficial pain and deep pain and consequently interprets all pain as superficial. For example:

- Pain of myocardial infarction is classically felt centrally just behind the sternum, radiating down the left arm and up the root of the neck into the jaw.
- Inflammation affecting the diaphragm is felt in the tip of the shoulder (phrenic nerve root values C3–C5).

Regulation of pain

Peripheral regulation

Pain can be regulated by sensory input—it can be reduced by activity in low-threshold mechanoreceptors as their afferent nerves inhibit spinothalamic cell discharge, the phenomenon of 'mummy rubbing it better'.

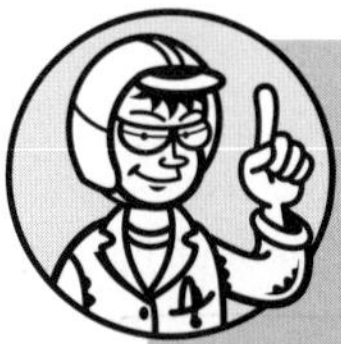

Transcutaneous electrical nerve stimulation (TENS) can be used to activate large-diameter fibres to decrease the sensation of pain. This is particularly useful in chronic pain states (e.g. lower back pain) and increasingly is being used as non-invasive pain relief for women in labour.

Central regulation

Pain can sometimes be suppressed by 'willing it to go away'. A possible reason for this is that there are regions in the central nervous system that have been implicated in pain suppression (Fig. 4.4).

Electrical stimulation of the periaqueductal grey matter in the midbrain causes profound analgesia. This area receives information from higher structures processing emotional states and projects to the midline reticular and raphe nuclei, which in turn project to the dorsal horns.

Two other parts of the reticular formation—the nucleus reticularis paragigantocellularis and the locus coeruleus—are also implicated in modulating nociceptive neuronal activity in the dorsal horns.

Opiates are thought to produce their antinociceptive action by activating these central regulating structures.

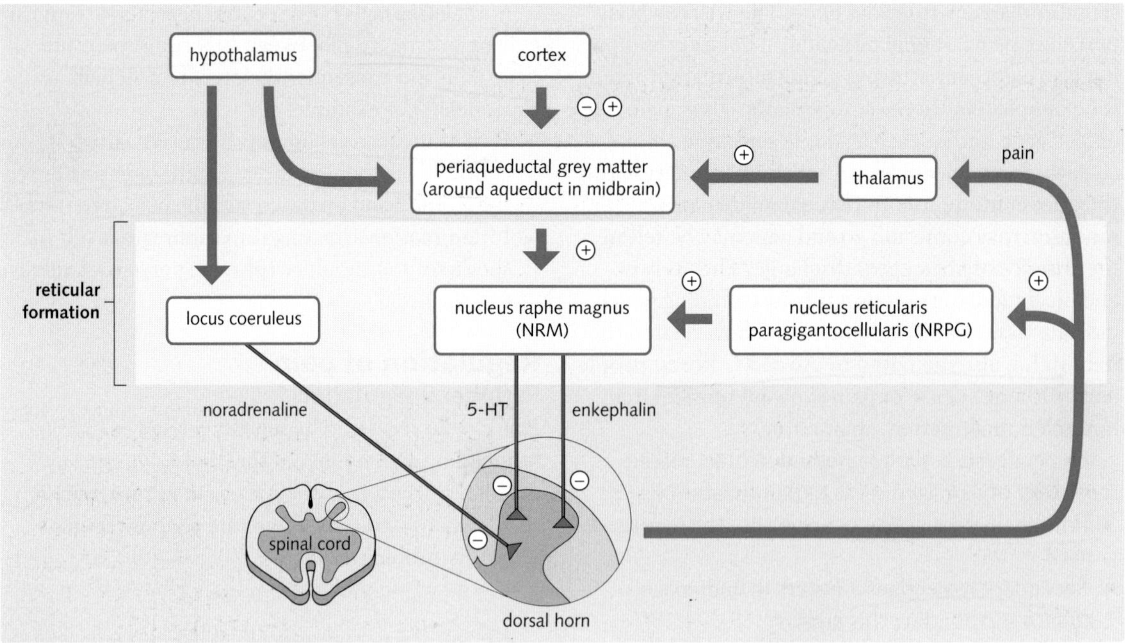

Fig. 4.4 Central regulation of pain.

Some of these regions contain endogenous opioid peptides, although pain modulation also involves 5-hydroxytryptamine (5-HT) from the raphe nuclei and noradrenaline from the locus coeruleus.

There are three classes of endogenous peptides (shown in Fig. 4.5).

There are three major classes of opioid receptor:

- μ (mu)
- δ (delta)
- κ (kappa)

Morphine is a potent μ agonist and naloxone an antagonist. Endogenous enkephalins are active at both μ and δ receptors. Both receptor types are found in the periaqueductal grey matter and in laminae I and II of the dorsal horn.

Note that each of these receptors is found throughout the central nervous system, suggesting that they are involved in processes other than pain perception. This explains the other effects of opiates, such as euphoria and hallucinations.

Analgesia

Analgesia is relief from the psychological state of pain, whereas antinociception is simply the blockage of nociceptive inputs. The main analgesics in clinical use are:

- Opioid analgesics acting on the endogenous system of pain control.
- Non-steroidal anti-inflammatory drugs, which reduce the production of inflammatory mediators that sensitize nociceptors to bradykinin and 5-HT.
- Simple analgesics (e.g. paracetamol).
- Local anaesthetics, which block action potential conduction along axons.
- Miscellaneous drugs (e.g. sumatriptan, a 5-HT_{1D} agonist) in migraine; carbamazepine (antiepileptic) in trigeminal neuralgia; tricyclic antidepressants (amitryptyline) in some types of chronic pain.

Opioids

Opioid drugs bind to the receptors of the endogenous opioid transmitters. There are two classes of opioids:

- Opiates, which include morphine and analogues that are structurally similar to morphine and usually synthesized from it (e.g. diamorphine, codeine).
- Synthetic derivatives structurally unrelated to morphine (e.g. pethidine, fentanyl).

Opioids block pain information from being transmitted up the spinothalamic tract (antinociceptive action) but they also act in the brain to reduce the unpleasantness of the pain state (analgesic action).

Opioid peptides			
Parent peptide	**Opioid peptide**	**Amino acid sequence**	**Location**
proenkephalin	enkephalins	Leu^5, Met^5, and longer sequences	spinal cord, brainstem
prodynorphin	dynorphins	all contain Leu^5 within longer sequences	spinal cord, brainstem
pro-opiomelanocortin	β-endorphin	Met^5 in 31 amino acid sequence	hypothalamus

Fig. 4.5 Opioid peptides.

- The weaker opioids (such as codeine) are widely used in over-the-counter pain preparations, and often in conjunction with a simple analgesic in presciption medications (e.g. co-codamol is codeine and paracetamol).
- Stronger opioids (such as morphine and pethidine) are used in post-operative pain and sometimes in severe chronic pain (such as cancer pain).
- Either fentanyl or morphine are commonly used as part of general anaesthesia.

The main effect of opioids is on the μ receptor, causing:

- Analgesia and antinociception.
- Euphoria and drowsiness—depending on the circumstances of administration.
- Respiratory depression—reducing the sensitivity of the brainstem to $PaCO_2$.
- Miosis—pupillary constriction caused by stimulation of parasympathetic component of cranial nerve III.
- Nausea—stimulation of the chemoreceptor trigger zone in the brainstem which sends signals to the vomiting centre.
- Constipation—increased tone and reduced motility of gastrointestinal tract.

There are problems with repeated administration of opioids:

- Tolerance—a gradual reduction in effect over repeated administration of the same amount of drug. Doses of morphine therefore need to be increased over time to produce the same degree of pain relief, but this causes a greater degree of constipation.
- Dependence—this can be physical (where a withdrawal syndrome of physical symptoms and signs like influenza occurs when the drug is not administered) or psychological (where compulsive drug-seeking behaviour develops). Often, it is a combination of both.

> The opiate class of opioids (morphine, diamorphine, codeine) also inhibit histamine release from mast cells and are cough suppressants, but these effects are not mediated by opioid receptors. This is exploited by codeine-based cough linctuses.

The most common drug of abuse in this class is diamorphine (otherwise known as heroin), but it should be remembered that many patients will be taking opioids which are legitimately prescribed and will develop these side effects and may be at risk from overdose.

The main danger of opioid abuse is from overdose, which presents with:

- Coma.
- Respiratory depression.
- Pin-point pupils (there is no tolerance to pupillary constriction even in the hardened addict).

Treatment is with intravenous μ-antagonists, such as naloxone (rapidly acting and short duration of action) or naltrexone (longer to act but longer duration of action). Note that antagonists may stimulate an acute withdrawal state and supportive therapy alone (e.g. ventilation) may be appropriate in some cases of opioid overdose.

The main opioids are shown in Fig. 4.6 with their different pharmacological properties and clinical uses.

Opioid drugs					
μ Agonist	Bioavailability and administraion	Metabolism	Potency and length of action	Clinical use	Notes
morphine	Poor availability when given orally due to high rate of first-pass metabolism. Intravenous administration gives reliable dosing	active metabolite morphine-6-glucuronide	$t_{1/2}$ 3 h	acute and chronic pain	cannot be given in labour as fetal liver cannot conjugate
diamorphine (heroin)	More lipid soluble. Given orally or by intramuscular, intravenous or subcutaneous injection	partly to morphine	very potent, rapid onset, $t_{1/2}$ 2 hrs	acute and chronic pain	
codeine	High oral bioavailability	to other opioids including morphine	one-sixth potency of morphine	mild pain, headache, dental pain	potent antitussive, low side effect profile
pethidine	High lipid solubility. Given orally and by intramuscular injection	metabolite norpethidine interacts with MAOIs	one-tenth potency of morphine	acute pain, labour	does not cause miosis
fentanyl	High lipid solubility. Given intravenously, epidurally, transdermally		very potent, short acting	intra-operative pain	intra-operative analgesia
buprenorphine	Increased first-pass metabolism. Given sublingually, intra-thecally		$t_{1/2}$ 12 h, slow onset	acute and chronic pain	partial agonist and difficult to reverse effects in overdose
methadone	Given orally or by injection		$t_{1/2}$ >24 h, very slow onset	maintenance of drug addicts	does not produce euphoria

Fig. 4.6 Opioid drugs and their pharmacology (MAOI, monoamine oxidase inhibitors—a type of antidepressant).

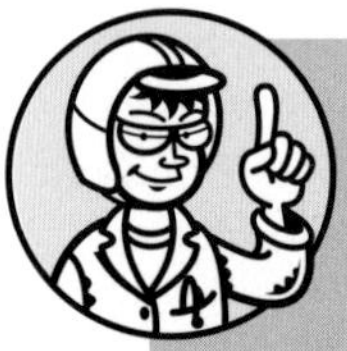

Naloxone is widely used in an emergency setting to treat acute overdose, but its duration of action is much shorter than most opioids which are abused. Therefore, it is important to carry on monitoring the patient to look for signs of relapse.

Non-steroidal anti-inflammatory drugs

Non-steroidal anti-inflammatory drugs relieve pain by reducing the sensitization of nociceptors that occurs in inflammation. NSAIDs are also anti-inflammatory and antipyretic (decrease fever). They inhibit:

- Cyclooxygenase (which metabolizes arachidonic acid to prostaglandins).
- Leukotrienes (which have roles in continuing the process of inflammation).

The prostaglandins, PGE_1 and PGE_2, lower the threshold of polymodal nociceptors to stimulation by the inflammatory mediators bradykinin and 5-HT.

The production of prostaglandins in these normal circumstances is by a subtype of cyclooxygenase, cyclooxygenase-1. The other type, cyclooxygenase-2 (COX-2), is inducible and metabolizes arachidonic acid in inflammatory cells. Side effects of these drugs can result from interference with the physiological role of prostaglandins in the regulation of blood flow. For example, interfering with blood flow in the gastric mucosa reduces HCO_3^- production. Gastric acid can then attack the mucosal surface causing ulceration and potentially fatal bleeding.

This has lead to the introduction of selective COX-2 inhibitors which are marketed as being less damaging to the gastric mucosa (recent BMJ articles may not be protective!).

Fig. 4.7 shows the main NSAIDs in clinical use with their effects and side effects. Fig. 4.8 shows the site of action of NSAIDs.

Generally, NSAIDs are considered to be very safe drugs and are widely available. However, aspirin use has been linked to Reye's syndrome in children (causing liver damage and encephalopathy after a

Non-steroidal anti-inflammatory drugs	
Drug	**Uses and side effects of NSAIDs**
aspirin	for mild pain; causes gastrointestinal upset, haemorrhage, salicylism (tinnitus, dizziness, nausea), Reye's syndrome in children (postviral encephalopathy and liver disorder)
paracetamol	no great analgesic effect in inflammatory conditions but efficacious for headache; liver failure in overdose. Most effective if taken regularly
ibuprofen	inflammatory joint disease, dental pain; much milder side effect profile
mefenamic acid	moderately effective-especially for menstrual cramps; may cause gastrointestinal tract upset and diarrhoea

Fig. 4.7 Uses and side-effects of non-steroidal anti-inflammatory drugs (NSAIDs).

viral illness). Chronic NSAID use may also cause an interstitial nephritis, with lasting kidney damage in some patients.

Local anaesthetic agents

Local anaesthetic agents block the ability of axons to conduct action potentials by blocking Na^+ channels in the axonal membrane. The blocking site on the Na^+ channel is on its intracellular portion. Local anaesthetics are weak bases that can exist, depending on their pK_a (the dissociation constant, calculated by the Henderson–Hasselbach equation), in either a hydrophilic state, when bound to H^+, or in hydrophobic state without H^+.

- In the hydrophobic state, they can pass straight through the lipid membrane to gain access to the blocking site, whether the channel is closed or open.
- In the hydrophilic state, they can enter only through the open mouth of the Na^+ channel, and therefore need to wait until the channel opens to gain access to the blocking site. The hydrophilic route of the drug leads to 'use-dependent' block—the block of channels increases as more channels open.

Fig. 4.9 shows both hydrophilic (XH^+) and hydrophobic (X) blocking of a Na^+ channel.

At low concentrations of local anaesthetic agents, only small-diameter myelinated and unmyelinated fibres are affected. This means that administration of local anaesthetic agents can be used to produce a differential nerve block affecting only Aδ and C fibres. This reduces pain and temperature transmission, leaving proprioception, fine touch and motor functions intact.

The common local anaesthetic agents in use are shown in Fig. 4.10.

Chronic pain

Chronic pain is pain that continues when the causative stimulus is no longer present. Characteristic features are:

- Hyperalgesia—more pain is felt for a given amount of noxious stimulation.

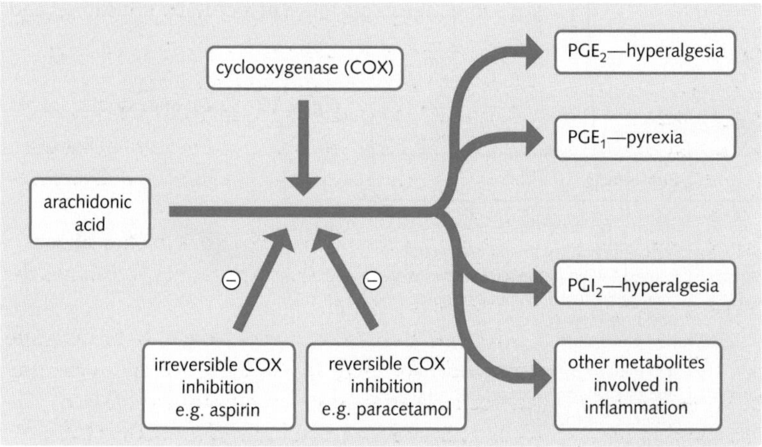

Fig. 4.8 Site of action of non-steroidal anti-inflammatory drugs (COX, cyclooxygenase).

To increase the effect of a given amount of local anaesthetic agent, a vasoconstrictor (e.g. adrenaline) can be given with the local anaesthetic to reduce the rate at which the local anaesthetic is washed out of the tissue being anaesthetized. This is not advisable when the tissue being anaesthetized relies on end arteries for supply (e.g. digital arteries in fingers and toes in a ring block) because ischaemic necrosis will result.

- Allodynia—pain caused by innocuous stimuli such as light touch.
- Spontaneous pain spasms—pain felt in the absence of any stimulation.

The chronic pain state is caused by a hyperactive acute pain pathway.

Increased responsiveness of nociceptors is caused by sensitization by inflammatory mediators such as bradykinin, prostaglandins and nerve growth factor.

Increased excitability of neurons in the dorsal horn and thalamus is due to increases in synaptic transmission that occur after prolonged stimulation. This means that high nociceptor firing frequencies will set up a state of hyperexcitability in dorsal horn neurons. The process that facilitates this increase in synaptic effect is thought to involve the NMDA (*N*-methyl-D-aspartate) receptor, as NMDA antagonists can block the initiation of hyperexcitability.

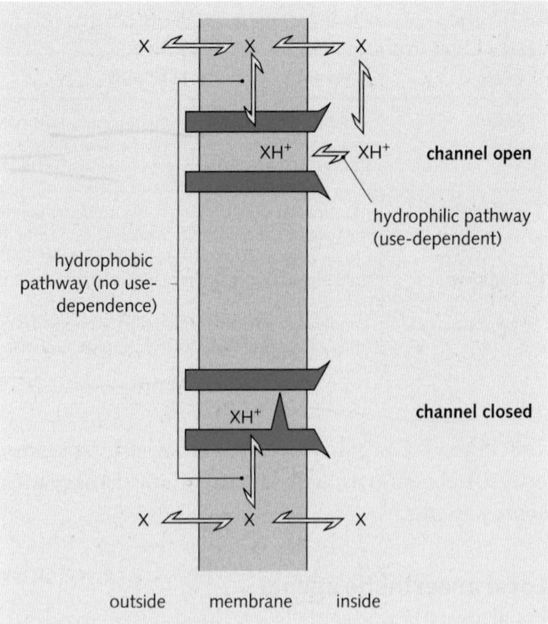

Fig. 4.9 Mechanism of action of local anaesthetics. Local anaesthetic agents (X) interact with ion channels. They can do this in an ionized (hydrophilic form—XH+), which passes through the open channel. This leads to use-dependent block. Alternatively, the uncharged species (X) can gain direct access to the membrane from the outside.

Neurological disease can affect the pain pathway and produce neuropathic pain, a form of chronic pain caused by damaged sensory neurons. Often, α-adrenergic receptors are expressed on the neurons and, as a result, sympathetic activity can cause severe pain.

Psychological aspects of pain

There are many social and psychological influences on pain perception and pain behaviour because pain is a subjective experience affected by emotional and

Local anaesthetic agents

Drug	Use	Side effects
lignocaine	nerve-block anaesthesia, e.g. dentistry; spinal anaesthesia—injection into subarachnoid space for surgery to lower trunk and legs	spinal procedure affects many nerve roots—hypotension and bradycardia caused by sympathetic block, urinary retention caused by block of pelvic autonomic fibres
bupivacaine	epidural anaesthesia to block spinal roots for pain of labour	less than for spinal, as injection into epidural space minimizes diffusion to other nerve roots

Fig. 4.10 Local anaesthetic agents.

social cues. Chronic pain that is resistant to any drug therapy may be responsive to psychological treatments such as cognitive behavioural therapy. If these do not help to relieve the pain, the patient may be provided with coping mechanisms to deal with it on a day-to-day basis.

- What receptors in the skin exist for the perception of touch? Comment on the different modalities they serve, and their location.
- Explain the term 'rapidly adapting receptor'. Give an example.
- List the different classes of somatosensory axon; what information do they convey, and what is their relative speed of transmission?
- Explain the phenomenon of referred pain.
- How might nociceptive inputs be modified non-pharmacologically?
- Discuss the different classes of analgesics, and give an example of when each one might be used.
- List the side effects of opioid analgesics. How would you recognize an overdose?
- Describe the features of chronic pain. What strategies may be employed to treat it?

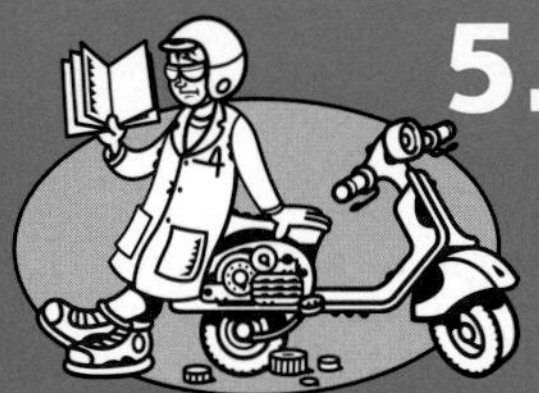

5. Motor Control

In this chapter, you will learn about:

- The control of movement.
- Proprioception.
- Motor units and the control of muscle.
- The motor cortex.
- The basal ganglia.
- The cerebellum.

Movement control

Types of movement

There are three basic types of movement.

- Reflex responses (e.g. the gag reflex)—stereotyped, involuntary responses graded to the eliciting stimulus.
- Rhythmic motor patterns (e.g. walking)—sequences of stereotyped repetitive responses which are largely automatic, but that require voluntary control to start and stop.
- Voluntary movements—these are goal directed, usually learnt, and improve with practice.

Movements may also be categorized according to their speed: slow, or ramp movements are controlled by sensory feedback, very fast or ballistic movements are not.

Muscle contraction is used to produce stabilization of the body (to provide the correct posture against gravity), as well as to produce movement.

- If the external force is smaller than that produced by the muscle, then movement occurs and an isotonic contraction is produced.
- When the external force is greater than that produced by the muscles an isometric contraction is produced.
- If the external force is greater than the muscle contraction, then muscle lengthening occurs as is the case in walking down a flight of stairs.

The importance of sensation

Sensory information can be used in a feedback or feedforward control system.

- In feedback control, the nervous system generates a movement and sensory information is used to obtain an error signal, which is the difference between the desired position and the current position. It is our sense of proprioception, which gives us information about the position of our bodies (joints and muscles) and the movements of muscle groups. These sensations are transferred to the brain in both the dorsal column tract and the spinocerebellar tract. Patients who have lost their sense of proprioception due to a large-fibre sensory neuropathy do not know where their limbs are in space unless they can see them.
- In feedforward control, sensory information is used to derive advance information and direct the movement towards a predicted position (e.g. picking up a drink).

Motor programmes and voluntary movement

Definitions

A 'motor programme' is a sequence of nerve impulses that, when sent to a group of muscles, will execute a movement. The same motor programme can be scaled and timed differently and sent to different muscle groups—for example, it is possible to hold a pen and write with either hand (with different levels of success!). Motor programmes are abstract concepts that help us understand how the motor system executes movement.

A 'motor strategy' is a set of motor programmes that have been selected and sequenced to achieve a recognized goal. An example of this may be playing a tennis shot. A motor programme is needed for the arm holding the racket, the legs to give the correct footwork and to the truncal muscles to give the correct swing.

Development of motor programmes

Motor programmes are time-saving for the motor system because they enable fast accurate movement.

The following stages in the process of learning motor programmes show how proprioceptive feedback is used to adjust the motor output until the precise motor commands are developed. As a motor task is learned, the pattern of muscle activity changes.

- Initially, discontinuous movement occurs where the muscles working to achieve the task (agonists) move the limb nearer and nearer towards a target, judging the end-point with feedback. This gives a slow movement, which is not terribly smooth.
- Faster, continuous movement then develops, with a single agonist burst stopped by an antagonist, then smaller adjustments guided by feedback made with agonist muscles. This is a smoother movement, which gets closer to the target in a shorter time.
- Eventually, the movement becomes ballistic, with a single agonist burst to move the limb towards the target and a single antagonist burst to stop the limb moving so that it comes to rest at the target.

Hierarchy of movement control

There are three levels of motor control arranged hierarchically and in parallel. The lowest level is at the spinal cord. The interneurons in the cord play a major role in sequential operations of muscles that can produce complex movements under sensory control.

The intermediate level is at the brainstem containing medial, lateral and aminergic systems. These project to and regulate segmental networks of the spinal cord and are responsible for the integration of visual, vestibular and somatosensory inputs in the control of posture. In addition, some brainstem nuclei control eye and head movements.

The highest level is in the cortical control of voluntary movement.

- Processes that generate the desire to move in response to recognized demands can be localized to the frontal lobes and limbic system.
- Processes generating strategies to achieve motor aims, by selecting motor programmes, can be localized to the complex of the premotor and supplementary motor areas. Each area projects onto the primary motor cortex and thence to the spinal motor neurons via the corticospinal tract. There is also an indirect pathway via the brainstem, which is also arranged somatotopically both for input and output. The basal ganglia also have a role in motor planning in the scaling and initiation of motor programmes.
- Processes that guide movement are carried out by the primary motor cortex and descending motor tracts. The pyramidal tract governs highly skilled movement involving few muscles. The cerebellum improves the accuracy of movements by comparing descending motor commands with information about resulting motor activity, and also helps to maintain body position through postural muscles.
- The process of execution of movement is carried out by spinal cells that innervate skeletal muscle.

Motor units and the recruitment of muscle fibres

Motor units

A motor unit consists of a motor neuron and all the muscle fibres that it innervates. One motor neuron may innervate many fibres but a single fibre receives input from only one motor neuron (Fig. 5.1).

The innervation ratio of a motor unit is the number of muscle fibres that a single motor neuron innervates.

- A high innervation ratio means that one motor neuron controls many fibres—such a motor unit produces coarse strong movements (e.g. the motor units in gastrocnemius have a ratio of 1 : 2000).
- A low innervation ratio means that only a few fibres are controlled by a motor neuron—such a motor unit produces fine well-controlled movement (e.g. the motor units in the extraocular muscles have a ratio of 1 : 10).

Motor units differ in their properties owing to variation in types of motor neuron and variation in types of fibre innervated.

There are two types of motor neuron—large diameter α-motor neurons that innervate the muscle itself, and small diameter γ-motor neurons that innervate the intrafusal fibres of the muscle spindle (see section on reflexes below).

Recruitment

Two functional types of motor unit can be distinguished by their histochemical features:

- Fast twitch (pale) muscle, involved in quick, phasic movements such as running and walking. This class can be further divided into fast fatiguable and fast fatigue-resistant categories.
- Slow tonic (dark red) muscle, involved in slow sustained contractions, such as those involved in the maintenance of posture.

Any muscle has a variable number of each different type of motor unit, as seen by staining techniques that pick up enzyme quantities (e.g. myosin ATPase). For example, postural muscles have many slow, dark

Properties of motor neurons and function, histology, and biochemistry of muscle fibres			
Motor unit	**Properties of motor neuron**	**Functional properties of muscle fibres**	**Histology and biochemistry of muscle fibres**
slow fatigue-resistant	constant low-frequency firing rate with steady-state depolarization; smaller cell body, smaller diameter axon with slower conduction velocity	longer contraction and relaxation times, lower force (10% of fast fatiguable), very resistant to fatigue	many mitochondria, high levels of oxidative enzymes (succinic dehydrogenase), high levels of myoglobin
fast fatigue-resistant	intermediate firing rate response to steady-state depolarization; intermediate cell body size, axon diameter and conduction speed	slightly slower than fast fatiguable contraction and relaxation times, twice force of slow units, very resistant to fatigue	many mitochondria, high levels of glycolytic and oxidative enzymes, high levels of myosin ATPase
fast fatiguable	progressive drop in firing rate with steady-state depolarization; large cell body, large-diameter axon with high conduction velocity	fast contraction and relaxation times, high force during tetanus, fatigue after repeated stimulation	few mitochondria, high levels of glycolytic enzymes (phosphorylase), high levels of myosin ATPase

Fig. 5.1 Properties of motor units—the firing characteristics of their motor neurons and properties of the muscle fibres.

red fibres, whereas extraocular muscles have mainly fast, pale fibres.

Recruitment describes the order in which types of motor units are activated when making any movement, whether it is reflex or voluntary. Slow units are activated first, then fast fatigue-resistant units and finally fast-fatiguable units.

This allows the motor system to grade simply the amount of force used in a movement. A small amount of excitatory input to a pool of different types of motor neurons in the anterior horn will only produce firing of the slow-unit motor neurons. Greater amounts of stimulation are required to activate the faster and more powerful units.

Tetanic contraction

Tetanic contraction occurs when successive muscle contractions are so rapid that they fuse together resulting in a sustained maximally forceful contraction. This phenomenon has only been seen *in vitro*.

Responses of motor units in damage and disease

Diseases affecting the different parts of the motor unit disrupt their normal function, as shown by changes in the pattern of motor unit arrangement, the size of muscle fibres and electrical recordings from muscle when active and at rest (electromyogram) (Fig. 5.2).

Repeated activation of muscle fibres causes depletion of intracellular ATP stores, meaning that the muscle produces less force. However, the fibres remain in a state of some contraction for some time because relaxation is also an active process requiring ATP. This slow relaxation time has the effect of decreasing the force available to sustained contraction, but not that of single twitches (in early fatigue).

In myasthenia gravis, muscles (particularly those of the eyelid, neck and shoulders) are particularly fatiguable. This is caused by a defect in the neuromuscular junction where there are autoantibodies to the acetylcholine receptor. This fatigue can be overcome temporarily by the use of acetylcholinesterase inhibitors, which is the basis of the diagnostic 'Tensilon' test.

Tetany occurs where hypocalcaemia or alkalosis reduce the threshold for action potential generation and neurons fire spontaneously, characteristically producing a spasm of the hands with the fingers and thumbs adducted and hand flexed at the metacarpophalangeal joints. It should not be confused with tetanus, which is a disease caused by a toxin from a soil-dwelling bacterium. The symptoms of this disease include muscle contractions and 'lock-jaw'—it may be fatal if not swiftly treated.

Reflex action and muscle tone

Clinical relevance

Neurological examination of patients' limbs includes testing stretch reflexes. Tapping the patella tendon and observing the results indicates whether the spinal cord segments L2 and L3 are intact, excluding

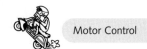

Clinical features and effects on motor units of diseases of the motor neuron cell body, peripheral axon, and muscle fibre				
Part of motor unit affected	**Typical clinical features**	**Example**	**Effect on muscle fibres**	**EMG changes**
motor neuron cell body	weakness, atrophy affecting distal muscles more than proximal, fasciculation [lower motor neuron lesion signs although hyperreflexia is seen in amyotrophic lateral sclerosis (ALS)]	amyotrophic lateral sclerosis (motor neuron disease)	atrophy and disappearance of groups of muscle fibres, with other fibres innervated by new collaterals from remaining motor neurons; this produces 'fibre clumping' where areas of muscle contain fibres of only one type (fibre type is determined by motor neuron type—response to disease results in collaterals of one motor neuron innervating many nearby fibres)	spontaneous activity at rest (fibrillation), discrete pattern of potentials during voluntary contraction as fewer motor units active, potentials are larger as motor units innervate more fibres than usual; no change in axon conduction velocity
motor neuron axon	chronically—weakness, atrophy distally, loss of tendon reflexes, sensory symptoms (loss, paraesthesia) as all types of peripheral nerve are affected	Guillain–Barré syndrome		fibrillation, discrete large potentials; demyelinating neuropathies (Guillain–Barré syndrome) result in reduced axon conduction velocity
muscle fibre	weakness initially affecting walking and lifting, proximal larger muscles involved more than distal ones	Duchenne's muscular dystrophy	no change in spread of type of motor unit; dead fibres and regenerating fibres are present; inflammatory cells and fat sometimes present	no spontaneous activity at rest, shorter smaller potentials as there are fewer remaining fibres in each motor unit; the overall pattern is still smooth as there is no reduction in the number of motor units firing

Fig. 5.2 Diseases affecting the motor neuron cell body, peripheral axon and muscle fibres—clinical features.

peripheral nerve damage, and can also indicate if the spinal motor neurons are receiving an abnormal drive from higher centres. In upper motor neuron lesions, there is a loss of descending inhibition, causing an increase in drive, and therefore brisk reflexes.

Passive movement of a limb provides the examiner with information about the tone of the muscles in the limb; the greater the tone, the more resistance to movement.

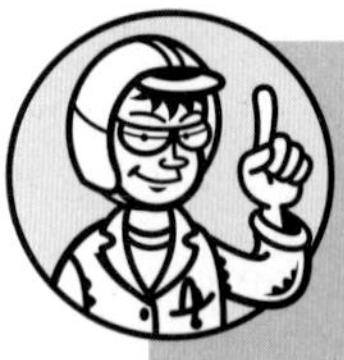

A stretch reflex can be 'reinforced' by performing a valsalva manoeuvre or pulling the hands outwards against each other. This is useful in patients whose reflexes are hard to elicit.

Definitions

'Reflex action' is an automatic motor response (simple or highly coordinated) that is elicited by a stimulus. The stretch reflex (such as that ellicited on tapping the patellar tendon) is simple because the stretch detector (the muscle spindle) makes a monosynaptic connection with the output spinal motor neuron. Other reflexes have neurons between the sensory input and the motor output (interneurons) and can produce more complex responses. The magnitude of the reflex can be influenced by higher centres.

'Muscle tone' is the resting tension in muscle. It is produced by tonic firing of spinal motor neurons and their firing frequency is set by various inputs from stretch receptors and from higher centres through corticospinal, vestibulospinal, cerebellospinal and rubrospinal tracts.

In parkinsonism, there is 'rigidity' where all muscles have increased tone but there is no change in the strength of the reflexes. Thus, there is no alteration in the reflex circuit but there is an alteration in the direct corticospinal input.

A stroke may cause cell death in the motor cortex due to haemorrhage or ischaemia. This leads to 'spasticity' on the contralateral side, where tone is increased more in limb flexors than extensors, and this is known as a pyramidal distribution of weakness. Stretch reflexes elicit stronger responses, and this may produce stretch-induced rhythmic involuntary muscle contractions known as clonus. Reduced cortical input to the reflex circuit frees it from inhibition and its activity is increased, both at rest and when appropriately stimulated.

Proprioceptors and reflexes

Muscle spindles

Spindles consist of muscle fibres enclosed in a connective tissue capsule (the fibres are called 'intrafusal' muscle fibres; all the normal fibres outside the spindles are 'extrafusal'). Only the ends of these fibres can contract.

Sensory endings from dorsal root ganglion cells enter the capsule and innervate the non-contractile middle part of these fibres. Different types of fibres are named according to their cellular appearance:

- Nuclear chain fibres have their nuclei spread in a line. The sensory endings which supply these fibres are sensitive to the absolute length of the muscle.
- Nuclear bag fibres have a clump of nuclei at the centre. The afferents which supply these fibres may be dynamic (signalling the rate of change in the length of the muscle) or static (performing a similar function to the nuclear chain fibres) (Figs 5.3 and 5.4).

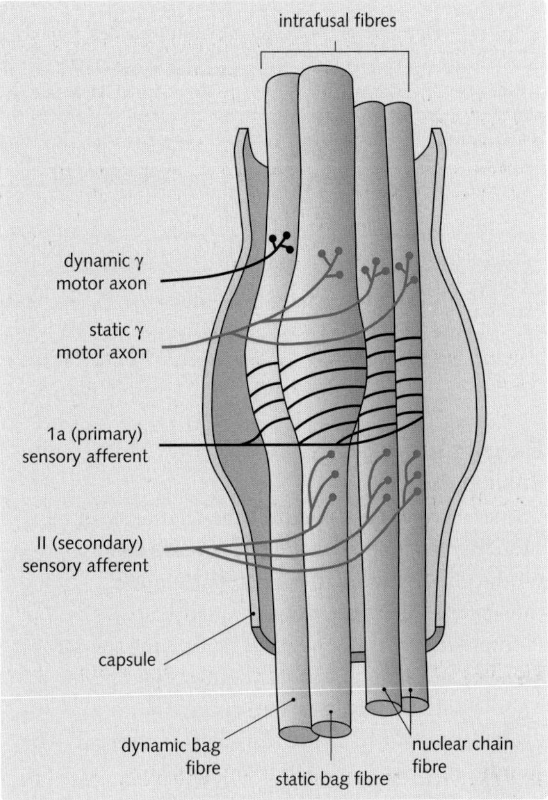

Fig. 5.3 Innervation and contents of a muscle spindle. Ia afferents are large, myelinated, fast fibres which are rapidly adapting. II afferents are small, myelinated, slower fibres which are slowly adapting.

The afferents which innervate muscle spindles have either large myelinated axons (group I) or small myelinated axons (group II). Group Ia afferents have a slightly larger diameter than the Ib afferents which innervate the Golgi tendon organs.

The contractile parts of the intrafusal fibres are innervated by γ-motor neurons which serve to alter the sensitivity of the fibres to stretch and to velocity. Dynamic γ-motor neurons innervate dynamic bag fibres and static γ-motor neurons innervate static bag and chain fibres. The γ-motor neuron is generally activated at the same time as the α-motor neuron to ensure that both intra- and extrafusal fibres contract simultaneously. In some cases, the γ-motor neuron may fire independently in situations of motor learning.

Spindles and α-motor neuron firing

Increasing the activity of γ-motor neurons contracts the ends of the intrafusal fibres, thereby stretching the middle of the fibres. The middle is innervated by stretch-receptor afferent nerves which are connected via the spinal cord to α-motor neurons. Therefore, α-motor neurons can be made to discharge by activation of γ-motor neurons through the reflex loop.

Also, α-motor neurons and γ-motor neurons are often activated together, resulting in the muscle spindle being very sensitive when the muscle is in use, and this provides very accurate feedback for error detection in voluntary movement.

Golgi tendon organs

Golgi tendon organs are found at the junction between muscle and tendon. They are composed of a network of collagen fibres inside a connective tissue capsule with a sensory axon winding around the collagen.

The firing rate of the Ib afferent fibre increases when the tendon organ is stretched, with greater outputs for active contraction rather than passive stretch of the muscle. These organs provide information mainly about active changes in tension in the muscle. This information may also be used to prevent injury to the muscle from excess tension.

Other receptors

There are various joint receptors present in capsules and ligaments that respond to length and changes in joint angle.

Properties of the two types of sensory ending from the muscle spindle			
Type	**Contact**	**Response to linear stretch**	**Encoding**
Ia (primary) ending	dynamic bag, static bag, nuclear chain	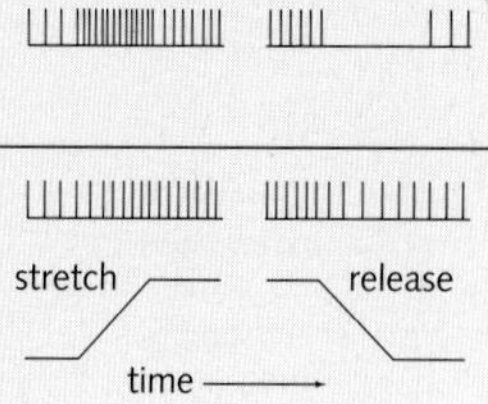	velocity of change of length, static length
II (secondary) ending	static bag, nuclear chain		static length

Fig. 5.4 Properties of the two types of sensory afferents found in the muscle spindle.

Examples of reflexes

Basic pattern

The stretch reflex is elicited when a muscle is suddenly lengthened and a reflex contraction is produced (e.g. tapping the patellar tendon causing a reflex contraction of quadriceps). Homonymous motor neurons (supplying the same muscle) and synergist motor neurons (supplying a muscle with the same action) receive an excitatory input from the spindle (Ia) afferent. The spindle afferent also inhibits antagonistic muscles via Ia inhibitory interneurons in the spinal cord.

Tendon organs form part of a reflex circuit that inhibits homonymous and synergistic motor neurons, termed the inverse myotatic reflex. The pathways for these reflexes are shown in Fig. 5.5.

Blink reflex

The blink reflex protects the cornea from foreign bodies (Fig. 5.6).

Gag reflex (Fig. 5.7)

This reflex protects the alimentary tract and upper airway from foreign bodies.

Flexion withdrawal reflex

The flexion withdrawal reflex is a more complicated motor act that protects limbs against potentially noxious stimuli detected by cutaneous structures. The flexors of the affected limb contract and the extensors are relaxed. This withdraws the limb away from the noxious stimulus.

At the same time, a crossed extensor reflex is elicited in the contralateral limb where the extensors are contracted and the flexors relaxed. This provides

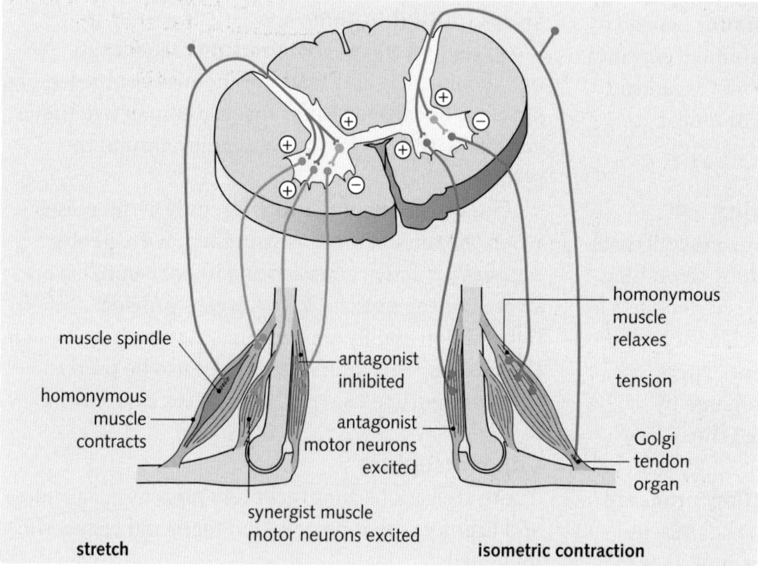

Fig. 5.5 Muscle spindle and Golgi tendon organ reflexes. Muscle spindles detect the rate of change and absolute muscle length during movement. Golgi tendon organs provide information on tension, and are particularly useful in exploratory movements as they have the protective effect of decreasing muscle force when resistance is met. They are modulated by higher centres to allow their response properties to be modified.

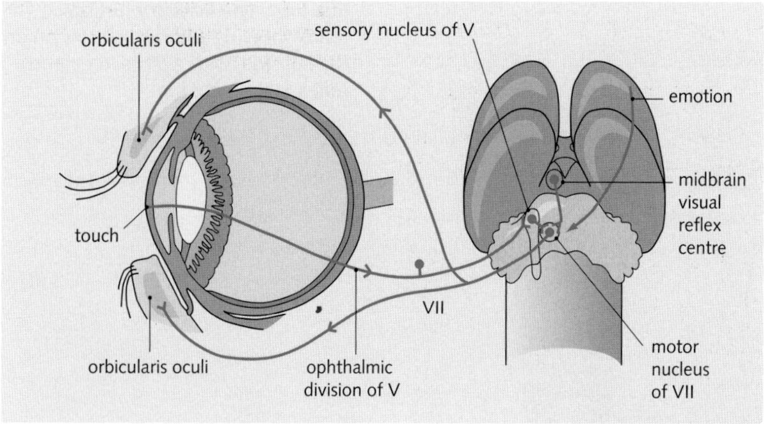

Fig. 5.6 Corneal (blink) reflex—protects the cornea from foreign bodies and other injuries.

postural support during the withdrawal of the stimulated limb.

Fig. 5.8 shows the polysynaptic pathways in the spinal cord with extensor and flexor action of stimulated and nonstimulated limbs.

Plantar reflex

The plantar reflex is elicited when the plantar surface of the foot is stroked from heel to toe, causing reflex plantar flexion of the toes in normal individuals. However, in infants (whose corticospinal tract is not yet fully myelinated) and in patients with damage to the motor cortex or corticospinal tract (an upper motor neuron lesion), dorsiflexion of the toes is elicited. This is known as a positive Babinski sign.

The motor cortex

The motor cortex lying in the frontal lobe (Fig. 5.9) is the area of the cortex that is involved in the planning and output of motor commands.

The premotor area and supplementary motor area lie immediately anterior to the primary motor area in the frontal lobe. It is thought that they plan movements because positron emission tomography scanning shows increased metabolism in the premotor area and supplementary motor area when subjects are asked to think about (but not execute) a movement. These areas are arranged according to a body plan, a motor homunculus:

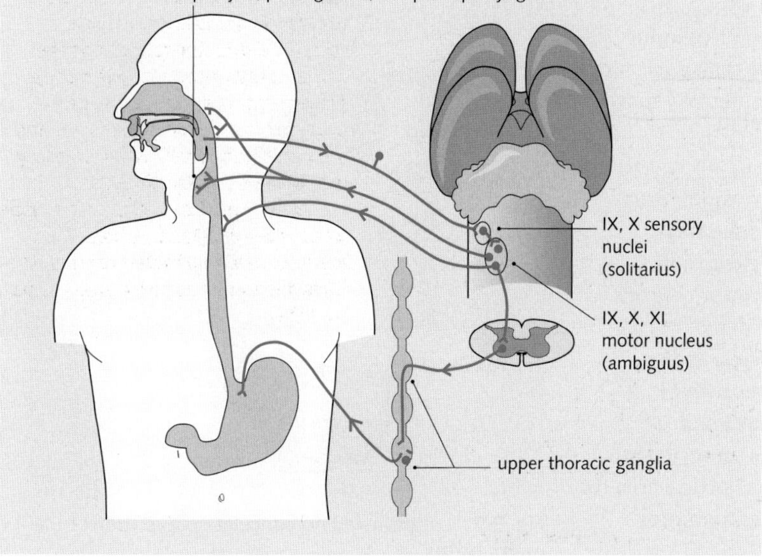

Fig. 5.7 Gag reflex showing a combination of skeletal muscle action (e.g. muscles of pharynx) and smooth muscle action (e.g. contraction of stomach).

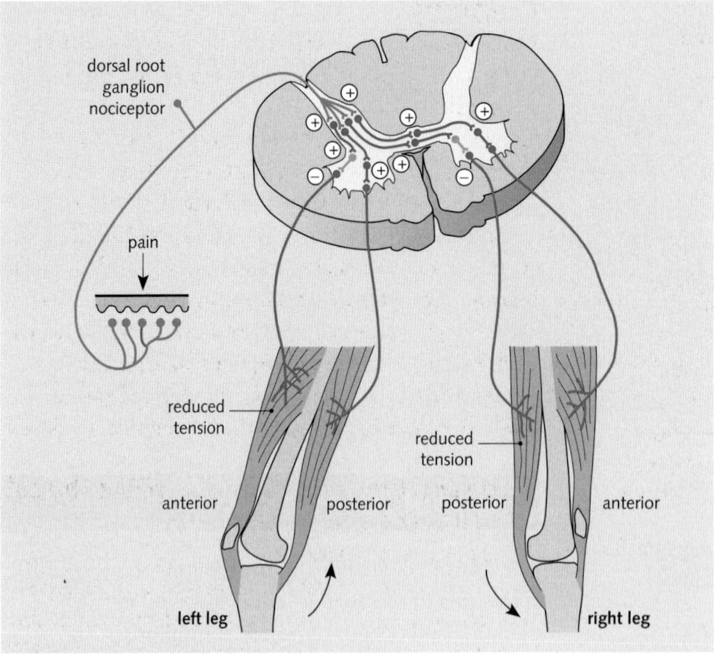

Fig. 5.8 The flexion withdrawal reflex showing withdrawal to pain on the left side, with a crossed extensor reflex in the right leg.

- The supplementary motor area projects to distal muscles and has a role in bimanual coordination.
- The premotor area projects through the reticulospinal and corticospinal tracts to proximal muscles.

Both areas receive input from motor regions that process different aspects of movement:

- The premotor area receives input from the cerebellum and basal ganglia via the thalamus, along with sensory inputs from the primary sensory and visual cortices.
- The supplementary motor area receives input from the basal ganglia through the thalamus, and also from the contralateral supplementary motor area.

Both areas also project to the primary motor area.

The primary motor area performs the final stage in cortical motor processing—execution. It projects to all contralateral body motor neurons, but principally those controlling the digits, toes and facial and vocalization muscles, and has an homuncular organization. It receives input from the rest of the motor cortex and from the cerebellum. It also receives sensory input from the somatosensory cortex—the cortical area for muscle and joint sense abuts the primary motor cortex.

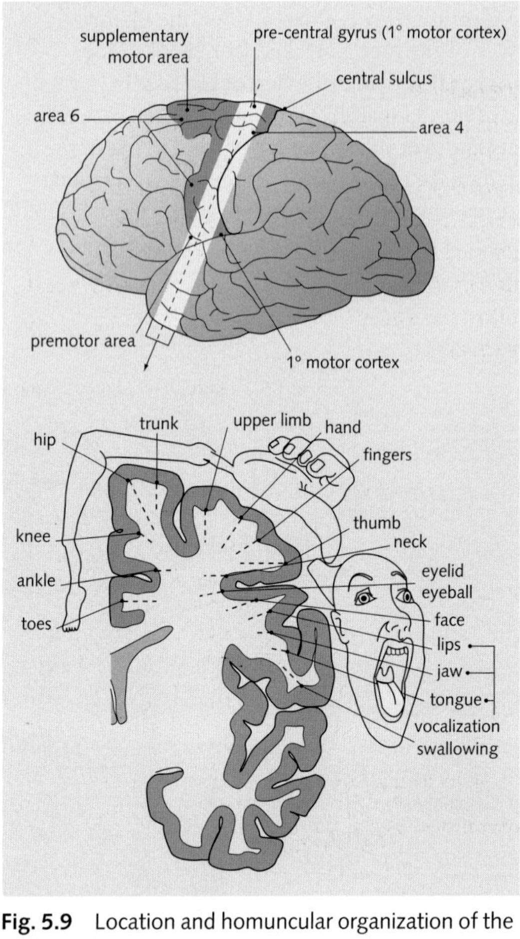

Fig. 5.9 Location and homuncular organization of the motor cortex.

Movements are represented in the motor cortex homunculi and, although the homunculus is an abstract concept, it suggests that there is a larger repertoire of movements for the hands, face and vocal muscles than for the trunk.

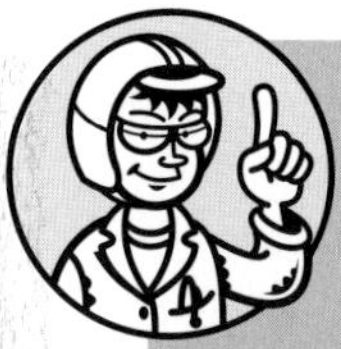

In epilepsy, disordered neuronal firing during a fit can affect the motor cortex. This produces a wave of muscle activity, termed a 'jacksonian march', that moves over the body as the disruption of function spreads over the motor cortex. This partly led to theories of homuncular organization of the motor cortex.

Basal ganglia and thalamus

Overview

The basal ganglia consist of five nuclei with extensive connections, which are involved in motor control and cognition. They are functionally inserted in a processing loop with the cortex and thalamus. Basal ganglia function is further understood by relating the signs of Parkinson's and Huntington's disease to the affected parts of the basal ganglia.

Anatomy

Fig. 1.4 (Chapter 1) shows the relationship between the putamen, caudate nucleus and all the elements of the basal ganglia.

Fig. 5.10 shows the thalamus as a rugby ball-shaped collection of cell groups with thalami on either side joined by the interthalamic connexus.

The thalamus is organized around a Y-shaped collection of white matter called the 'internal medullary lamina'. This splits the thalamus into three sections—the anterior, lateral and medial sections. Each section is composed of numerous cell groups with particular inputs and functions, and there are also cell groups inside the medullary lamina (the intralaminar nuclei).

Connections and circuits of the basal ganglia and thalamus

Caudate and putamen

The caudate and putamen contain identical cell types and together they form the main input complex of the basal ganglia, the corpus striatum (or simply 'striatum'). They receive somatotopic information from motor, sensory, association and limbic areas of the cortex, and also from the intralaminar nuclei of the thalamus.

The corticostriate projection is topographically and functionally organized so that the putamen is concerned with motor control and the caudate with eye movements and cognition. They project to the globus pallidus and the substantia nigra.

Globus pallidus

The globus pallidus is divided into internal (GP_i) and external (GP_e) segments lying lateral to the internal

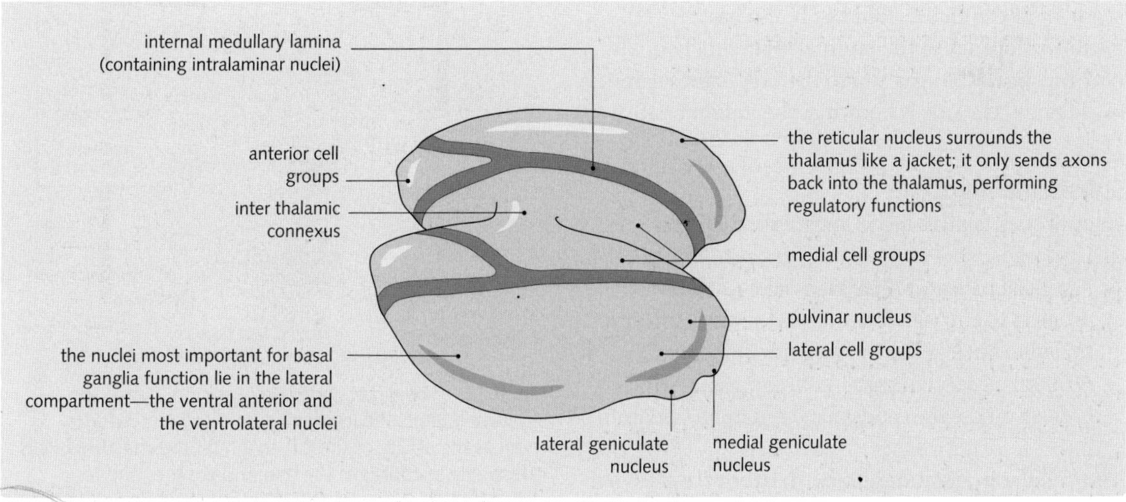

Fig. 5.10 The thalamus.

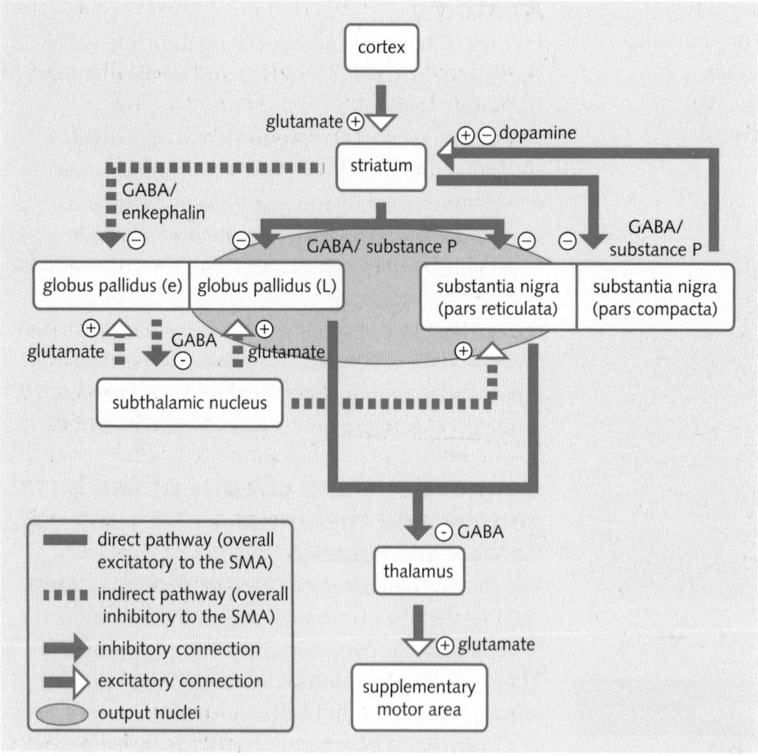

Fig. 5.11 Overview of the pathways through the basal ganglia with their neurotransmitters. Inhibitory signals from the output nuclei [GP_i and substantia nigra (pars reticulata)] cause decreased output to the supplementary motor area. The direct and indirect pathways are considered in subsequent simplified diagrams (Figs 5.13 and 5.14, respectively) (GABA, γ-aminobutyric acid).

capsule and medial to the putamen. The internal segment is the major output nucleus projecting to the ventrolateral and ventral anterior nuclei of the thalamus. The connection from the striatum to the GP_i, and thence to the thalamus, is known as the direct pathway.

Subthalamic nucleus

The subthalamic nucleus lies below the thalamus at its junction with the midbrain and receives a projection from and projects back to the external segment of the globus pallidus. It also has an excitatory output to the internal segment. The pathway from the striatum to the GP_e, subthalamic nucleus and the GP_i is known as the indirect pathway.

Substantia nigra

The substantia nigra lies in the midbrain and is divided into:

- A ventral pale part—pars reticulata, which projects to the ventrolateral and ventral anterior thalamic nuclei, and the superior colliculus.
- A dorsal pigmented part—pars compacta, which projects to the the caudate and putamen (striatum).

The cellular interactions in the striatum are shown in Fig. 5.11.

Re-entrant processing loops

Figs 5.12 and 5.13 show the direct and indirect processing loops that run through the basal ganglia. By working through each loop looking at the patterns of excitation and inhibition, it can be seen that the direct loop excites the cortex via the thalamus and the indirect loop inhibits it.

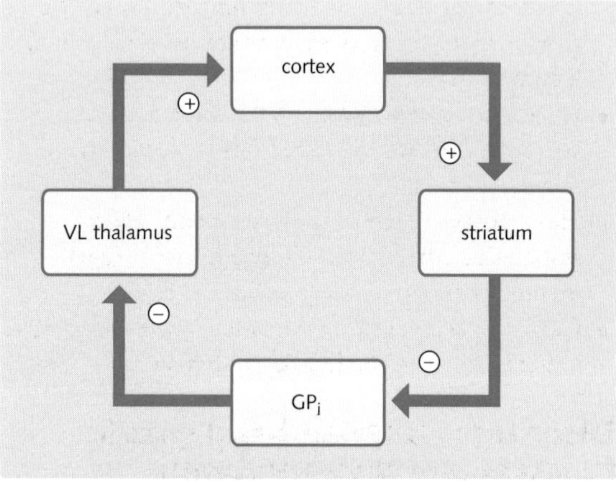

Fig. 5.12 The direct corticostriatal loop. When the striatum inhibits the internal globus pallidus (GP_i), it reduces the ability of the GP_i to inhibit the thalamus. This effectively encourages the thalamus to fire, and to stimulate the cortex (supplementary motor area) (VL, ventrolateral).

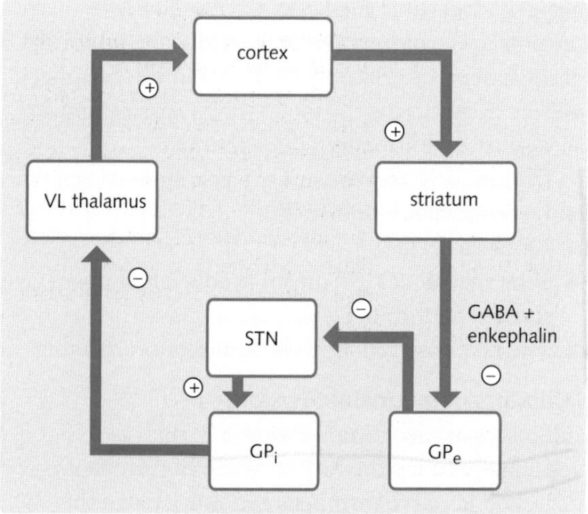

Fig. 5.13 The indirect loop. Striatal output inhibits the GP_e, reducing the inhibition of the subthalamic nucleus. The GP_i is then excited, and in turn inhibits output from the VL thalamus. The cortex therefore gets less stimulation (GABA, γ-aminobutyric acid; VL, ventrolateral; GP_e, globus pallidus external segment; GP_I, globus pallidus internal segment).

Functions of the basal ganglia

The basal ganglia select the motor programmes that are appropriate for a particular task that involves both cognitive and motor processing. They affect the pathways controlling movement and also the initiation of movement.

The basal ganglia:

- Scale the output of the motor programme so that appropriate movements are made. This is particularly important in motor programmes with fine movement (e.g. handwriting) and also where similar repetitive movements are needed (e.g. in locomotion).
- Project to the frontal eye fields via the thalamus, and have a role in the control of saccadic eye movements.
- Has a circuit with the prefrontal and other association cortices which may have a role in memory relating to body orientation.
- Connects with the orbitofrontal cortex which may indicate a role in modulating behaviour.

Disorders involving basal ganglia function and their treatment

Parkinsonism

The signs resulting from low dopaminergic input from the substantia nigra (pars compacta) to the striatum are collectively called 'parkinsonism' and are due to the basal ganglia not processing motor programmes correctly. The signs are:

- Akinesia—poverty of movement, usually noticed first by lack of blinking and producing a characteristic expressionless face.
- Bradykinesia—when movement does occur it is very slow.
- Tremor at rest—characteristically in the hands, it is called a 'pill-rolling' tremor and has a frequency of 3–6 Hz.
- Rigidity—caused by an increased tone in skeletal muscle. When passive movement is attempted, the limbs move in a series of jerks as if catching on something. This is termed 'cog-wheel' rigidity.
- Micrographia—small handwriting results from inappropriate motor scaling.
- Shuffling gait—which increases in pace as walking distance increases, termed a 'festinating' gait.
- Abnormal postural reflexes producing a stooped, flexed posture.

The causes of the reduced nigrostriatal dopaminergic projection producing parkinsonism are:

- Parkinson's disease, an idiopathic condition where cells in the compact part of the substantia nigra which project to the striatum die, and so the dopaminergic input is lost. Other cell groups are also affected—the ventral tegmental area (dopamine to ventral striatum), locus coeruleus (noradrenaline projected diffusely in central nervous system) and the raphe nuclei (5-hydroxytryptamine projected diffusely in central nervous system).
- Postencephalitic parkinsonism.
- Neuroleptic medication taken for psychosis, which antagonizes the dopamine input to the striatum.
- Neurotoxin ingestion, infamously by drug addicts taking a synthetic morphine analogue contaminated with MPTP (1-methyl-4-phenyl-1,2,3,6-tetrahydropyridine). This is metabolized by monoamine oxidase B to a compound MPP^+, which inhibits NADH dehydrogenase in dopaminergic terminals, reducing ATP production and promoting cell death.

The reduction in nigral cells is partly compensated for by:

- Increasing the number of dopamine receptors in the striatum.
- The remaining synapses releasing more dopamine (shown as an increase in the levels of

dopamine metabolites compared with dopamine levels).

The signs of parkinsonism occur when the compensatory mechanisms fail, but this occurs only at 80% cell loss. Drug treatment of parkinsonism (here restricted to the treatment of Parkinson's disease) aims to increase the function of the remaining dopaminergic innervation to the striatum.

Antimuscarinics (e.g. benzhexol and benztropine)

The arrangement of striatal circuitry (Fig. 5.13) shows that dopamine inhibits striatal output cells and acetylcholine excites them. To compensate for reduced dopamine input, acetylcholine antagonists can be given. They reduce tremor and rigidity but have little effect on bradykinesia. Side-effects are drowsiness, confusion (which can exacerbate dementia in Parkinson's disease) and reduced parasympathetic function. Acetylcholine is not the only excitatory input and this therapy will not work for long.

Dopamine precursors

This approach bypasses the rate-limiting step of dopamine synthesis—tyrosine hydroxylase. L-Dopa, the drug of choice for most Parkinson's disease patients, is metabolized by dopa decarboxylase to dopamine. Dopamine itself cannot be given because it has many peripheral effects, and does not cross the blood–brain barrier well.

Side-effects of L-dopa are:

- Nausea and vomiting caused by stimulation of D_2 receptors in the chemoreceptor trigger zone in the brainstem.
- Reduction in gastric emptying due to effects on gastric dopamine receptors.
- Dyskinesias—the striatum becomes very sensitive to its dopamine input and overdose of L-dopa can occur producing involuntary movements, which can be very disabling.
- Psychiatric effects (psychosis, depression, acute confusional state) due to alteration of all dopaminergic pathways that influence cortical function (e.g. ventral tegmental area to limbic system nuclei).

Side-effects can be treated with a peripherally acting dopamine antagonist, domperidone, counteracting gastric emptying and nausea.

To increase the proportion of L-dopa reaching the central nervous system, drugs need to be given to prevent L-dopa from being utilized by peripheral nervous structures such as sympathetic nerve terminals. Carbidopa and benserazide are inhibitors of dopa decarboxylase that act only in the periphery, as they do not cross the blood–brain barrier, and are an essential addition to L-dopa therapy.

In long-term treatment (> 5 years):

- Deterioration is inevitable.
- Akinesia recurs.
- Tolerance develops, meaning equivalent doses give shorter periods of relief.
- The response to L-dopa becomes unpredictable.

Inhibitors of monoamine oxidase B

Inhibitors of monoamine oxidase B, such as selegiline, reduce the rate at which dopamine is degraded in nerve terminals and potentiates the effect of L-dopa. It is often reserved for severe disease when L-dopa is beginning to lose its efficacy.

Direct dopamine agonists

Direct dopamine agonists (e.g. bromocriptine) stimulate striatal receptors but do not mimic the normal conditions of dopamine release in the striatum. Side effects are similar to those of L-dopa—nausea and psychiatric disturbance. Again, they are reserved for severe disease.

Newer methods to treat Parkinson's disease include:

- Neurosurgery to ablate the hyperactive globus pallidus internal segment (pallidotomy).
- The placement of electrodes for deep brain stimulation in the globus pallidus internal segment and substantia nigra (pars reticulata) which depresses their function (via conduction block).
- Implantation of dopamine-rich material from foetal tissue (this remains a controversial and, as yet, unproven therapy).

Huntington's disease

This autosomal dominant condition is caused by a defect on chromosome 4. It typically presents in mid-life, but may show anticipation in subsequent generations. The symptoms are caused by selective cell death in the striatum of both acetylcholine and GABA-containing neurons. Hyperkinesia develops with squirming dance-like or 'choreic' movement. This is because initially GABAergic output cells projecting to the external globus pallidus die, releasing it from inhibition and resulting in greater inhibition at the next set of cells in the group—the subthalamic nucleus (subthalamic lesions by themselves produce contralateral involuntary movement). Cognitive functions also deteriorate as striatal cell death continues, affecting the processing loops with the frontal lobes.

The cerebellum

Anatomy

The cerebellum is divided into four functional areas—the flocculonodular lobe, the vermis and the intermediate and lateral parts of the cerebellar hemispheres.

There are three functional units:

- The flocculonodular lobe (vestibulocerebellum) involved in the control of posture and eye movements.
- The vermis with the intermediate part of the hemisphere, or paravermis (together known as the spinocerebellum), involved in the control of both postural and distal muscles.
- The lateral part of the hemisphere (cerebrocerebellum) involved in coordination and planning of limb movements (in conjunction with the basal ganglia).

Fig. 5.14 shows the divisions of the cerebellum, including the deep nuclei that integrate cerebellar cortical processing, forming an output that passes through the superior cerebellar peduncle.

Fig. 5.15 shows the folding of the cerebellar cortex into lobules and folia that give the cerebellum its furrowed appearance.

Figs 5.16 and 5.17 show the inputs to, and outputs from, the cerebellum.

The cerebellar cortex

The processing circuit in the cerebellar cortex, as shown in Fig. 5.18, can be divided into input axons, processing interneurons and output neurons.

Mossy fibres from the spinocerebellar tract, the dorsal column nuclei and the pontocerebellar tract form the inputs, terminating on granule cells. Inputs from the inferior olivary nucleus in the brainstem (carrying information from the spino-olivary tract, brainstem and cortex) enter the circuit as parallel fibres and make many contacts on Purkinje cells. Climbing fibres from the spinal cord (via the inferior olive) also synapse with the Purkinje cells. Both parallel and climbing fibres also send inputs to the deep cerebellar nuclei.

The interneurons in the circuit have different functions.

- Granule cells, which receive most of the input to the cortex from the mossy fibres, send axons up towards the cortical surface, branching in parallel and making many contacts with other cell types in the cortical circuit.
- Golgi cells, after receiving excitation from granule cells, inhibit them in a feedback loop.
- Stellate and basket cells are also inhibitory and inhibit the output cell of the circuit—the Purkinje cell.

The inhibition of the Golgi, stellate and basket cells helps to prevent submaximally stimulated Purkinje and granule cells from firing (reducing noise).

The output of the circuit is from the Purkinje cell which also receives input from climbing fibres. Purkinje cells make GABAergic (inhibitory)

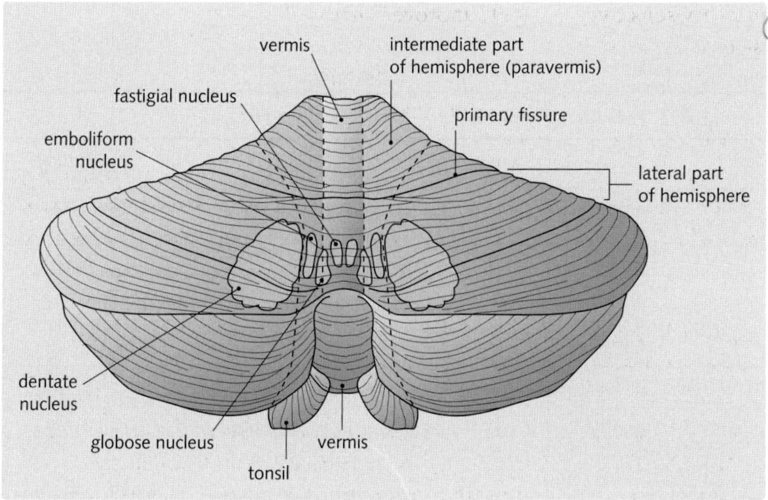

Fig. 5.14 The posterior aspect of the cerebellum, showing the deep nuclei.

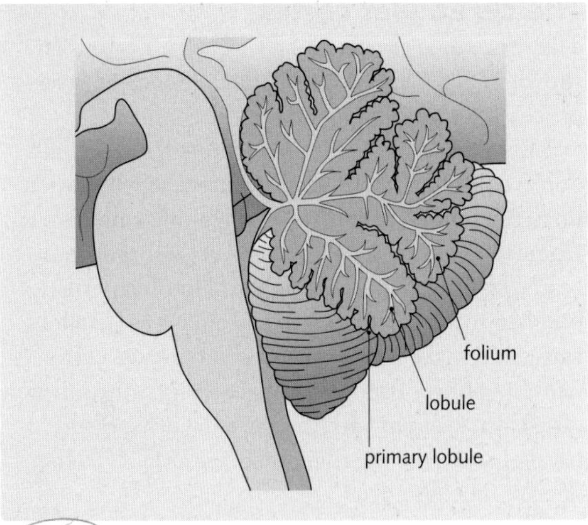

Fig. 5.15 Sagittal section through cerebellar cortex showing lobules and folia.

projections to the deep cerebellar nuclei which project to other parts of the central nervous system.

Functional units of the cerebellum

The vestibulocerebellum receives information from the vestibular nuclei (changes in head position relative to body position and gravity) and visual information from the lateral geniculate nuclei, superior colliculi and visual cortex. It projects to the vestibular nuclei, and thence to the oculomotor centres, and is involved in the control of axial muscles (balance) and the coordination of head and eye movements.

The spinocerebellum receives its main input from the spinocerebellar tract and is concerned with the control of postural muscle tone (by setting γ-motor neuron drive which affects α-motor neuron activity through the reflex loop) and movement execution.

- The vermis receives information from auditory, visual and vestibular systems, and sensory information from the proximal body. It projects to the ventromedial descending motor pathway and reticular formation.
- The intermediate hemisphere receives sensory information from the distal body and projects through the red nucleus (via the superior olive) and thence to the descending rubrospinal tract. It also projects to the contralateral motor cortex. (via the thalamus).

The cerebrocerebellum controls precision in rapid and dextrous movements, receiving information from cortical motor and sensory areas. It is inserted in a processing loop like the basal ganglia (motor cortex to pontine nuclei to cerebellar cortex to dentate nucleus to contralateral ventrolateral thalamic nucleus and red nucleus to motor cortex).

Error detection in cerebellar movement control

The Purkinje cells show an alteration in their firing pattern when errors in planned movement occur. This change consists of 'complex' spikes where, after the initial depolarization from the incoming Na^{+}, there is a smaller continued depolarization, a 'plateau' caused by incoming Ca^{2+}, and then further spikes superimposed on the plateau, again because of the opening of Ca^{2+} channels. This pattern of firing is produced by climbing fibre input and shows that the role of the olivocerebellar tract is in error detection.

Inputs to the cerebellum

Input from	Tract	Peduncle	Termination	Processing
Spinal cord	Spinocerebellar (anterior)	Superior	Vermis	Control of axial muscles, muscle tone
Medulla (gracile, cuneate + trigeminal nuclei)	Spinocerebellar (posterior)	Inferior	Paravermis	Distal limb coordination, muscle tone
Midbrain	Tectocerebellar	Inferior	Vermis	Visual + auditory
Olivary nucleus	Olivocerebellar (via medulla)	Inferior	Paravermis	Sensory
Vestibular nucleus	Vestibulocerebellar (via medulla)	Inferior	Vermis + floccus	Balance
Cerebral cortex	Pontoicerebellar (via pons)	Middle	Lateral hemispsheres	Motor planning

Fig. 5.16 Inputs to the cerebellum.

Fig. 5.17 Cerebellar outputs.

Cerebellar output			
Region	**Via deep nucleus**	**Termination**	**Function**
vermis	fastigial	motor cortex, reticular formation	control of axial muscles as movement progresses
paravermis	interposed	red nucleus—influencing fibres to thalamus and motor cortex, and those in rubrospinal tract	control of distal muscles as movement progresses
hemispheres	dentate	red nucleus and premotor cortex	movement planning, timing, and initiation
flocculonodular lobe	direct projection	lateral vestibular nucleus	control of balance and postural reflexes

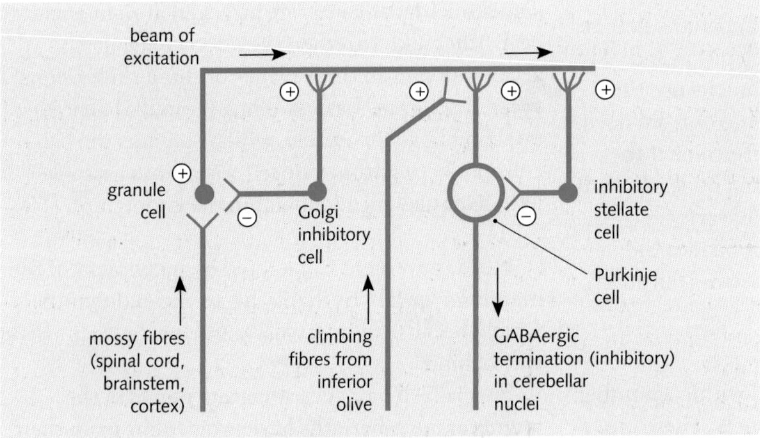

Fig. 5.18 The processing circuit in the cerebellar cortex.

When a new movement is performed, a large and long-lasting activation of Purkinje cells is seen. This corresponds to error correction signals being stored in motor memory at a special type of modifiable synapse capable of long-term depression. As the movement becomes more practised, fewer errors are made and the Purkinje activation decreases.

Effects of cerebellar lesions

Cerebellar disease produces disorders in limbs ipsilateral to the lesion; volitional movements are still present although defective.

Lesions can result from head injury, tumours, haemorrhage, ischaemia and Friedreich's ataxia. The white matter pathways carrying the connections can be damaged in multiple sclerosis.

Effects include the following:

- Disturbances of posture—wide-base standing position, ataxic gait, nystagmus in flocculonodular damage.
- Disturbances of muscle tone (hypotonia) and axial and truncal control—in vermis and intermediate hemisphere damage.
- Disturbances in control of precision movements—delays in starting and stopping movements, tremor increasing in severity through a movement, disorders in movement timing so that movements become decomposed into their components, and poor coordination of similarly acting muscle groups, making rapidly alternating movements very difficult.

The vestibular system, posture and locomotion

Control of posture

Posture

Posture is the relative position of the trunk, head and limbs in space. To keep posture stable, the body's centre of gravity needs to be maintained in position over its support base.

Postural reflexes are required to correct changes caused by displacement of the centre of gravity (by either external forces or deliberate movement). Postural change is detected by musculoskeletal proprioceptors, the vestibular apparatus and the visual system.

The vestibular system

Fig. 5.19 shows the components of the vestibular system. A more complete diagram is included in Chapter 9(Fig. 9.1). The vestibular apparatus detects changes in head position, linear acceleration and angular acceleration. The vestibular nuclei use this information together with afferent nerves from neck muscles and cervical vertebrae to determine if the head is moving alone or if the head and body are both moving. The nuclei can influence antigravity and axial musculature via a direct projection into the spinal cord. The vestibular system also has outputs which affect eye movements.

The receptor system

The inner ear apparatus is contained within a number of interconnected membranous tunnels. These are cavities within the petrous temporal bone—the bony labyrinth—which contains fluid (perilymph). Within the bony labyrinth, and bathed in perilymph, is the membranous labyrinth which is filled with endolymph. Perilymph closely resembles cerebrospinal fluid, but endolymph is much more similar to intracellular fluid in terms of ion concentration.

Two 'otolith organs'—the saccule and utricle—lie in the middle of the inner ear (the vestibule). Both of these structures contain patches of hair cells called maculae (Fig. 5.20).

- The saccular otoliths are oriented vertically, and detect changes in linear acceleration in the vertical plane and changes in head position during lateral tilt.
- The utricular otoliths are oriented horizontally, and detect changes in linear acceleration in the horizontal plane and changes in head position during flexion and extension of the neck.

The semicircular canals are arranged at right angles to each other and, together, they detect angular acceleration in all three planes of three-dimensional space. Each canal has a swelling (ampulla) near its attachment to the utricle, which contains the hair cells projecting from a ridge (crista) into a simple jelly-like substance (cupula) in the endolymph (Fig. 5.21).

Head movement is detected by movement of the membranous labyrinth relative to the endolymph which, because of its viscosity and inertia, lags a little way behind.

Specialized hair cells at certain points in the membranous labyrinths have projections from their surface into jelly-like masses floating in the endolymph.

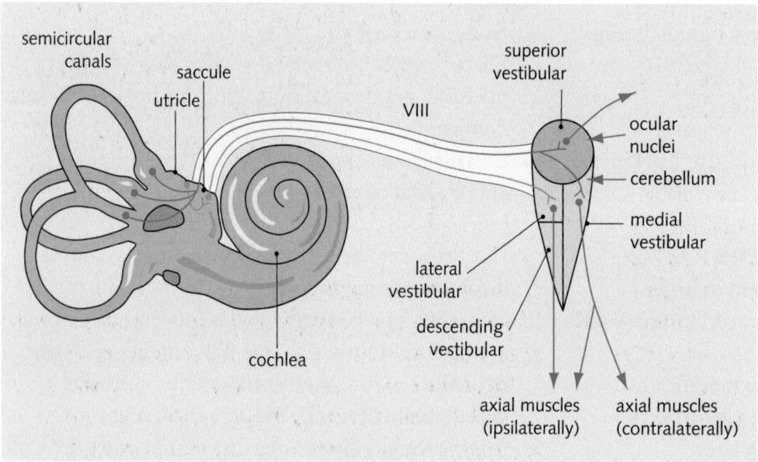

Fig. 5.19 The vestibular system.

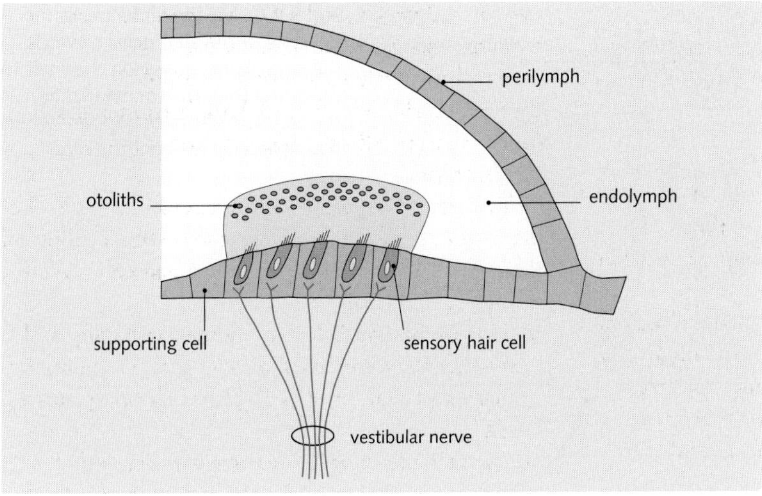

Fig. 5.20 Structure of the otolith organs.

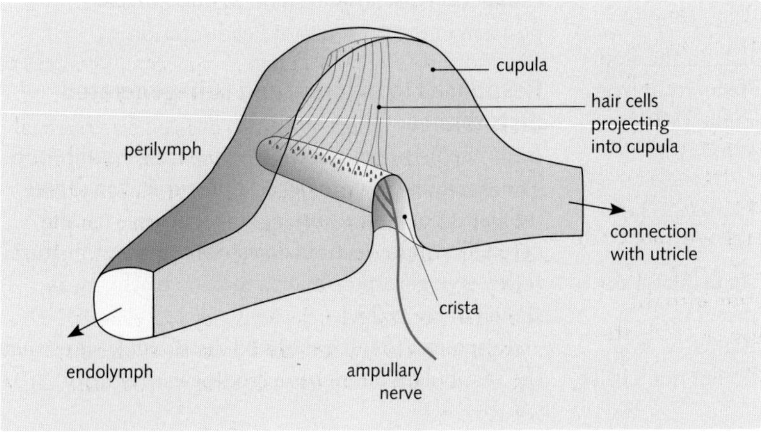

Fig. 5.21 Structure of ampullar crista.

The projections bend as the masses in the endolymph lag behind the movement of the labyrinth, as shown in Fig. 5.23. The membrane deformation produced alters the shape of cation channels. If the stereocilia bend towards the kinocilium, the cell is depolarized and releases more transmitter. Conversely, the cell will be hyperpolarized if the stereocilia are bent away and will release less transmitter.

Improving the quality of postural information

Hair cells show greatest alteration in membrane permeability when the stereocilia are moved in one direction. To detect different degrees of tilt and different degrees of flexion, the hair cells in the maculae are oriented in various planes so that they respond best to a particular head position. The vestibular nuclei can use this information to assess head position precisely.

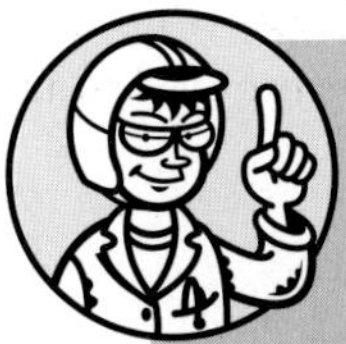

Disturbance of the vestibular system (such as might be caused by infection in the middle ear) may lead to a false sense of rotational movement (vertigo), nausea and eye movement problems. It is often caused by disruption to endolymph flow due to debris, and may be worse in particular positions.

Complementary pathways

The brain receives complementary information from the two labyrinths as they are located on opposite sides of the head. For example, as the head turns, one set of hair cells becomes depolarized, whereas the complementary set on the other side becomes

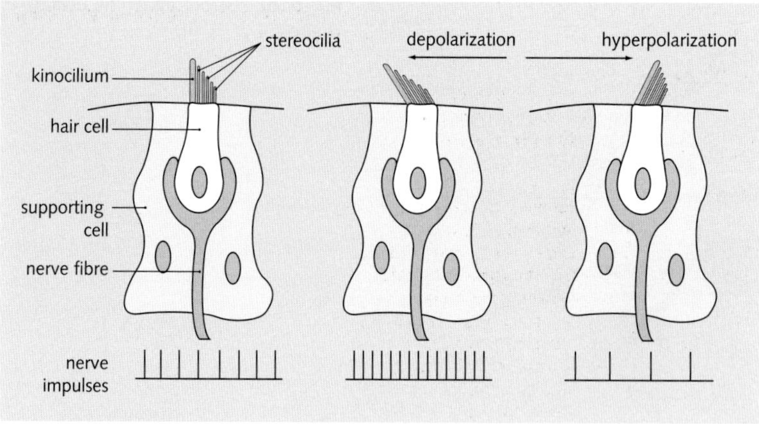

Fig. 5.22 Vestibular hair cells. Bending of the stereocilia towards the kinocilium causes ion channels to open and therefore depolarization of the cell. The opposite happens when the stereocilia are bent the other way.

hyperpolarized. This organization helps to mediate postural reflexes.

The vestibular nuclei

The vestibular nuclei lie in the medulla, on the floor of the fourth ventricle and receive information from the hair cells through the vestibular nerve (VIII).

- The semicircular canals project to the superior and medial nuclei.
- The otolith organs project to the lateral nuclei.

The medial vestibulospinal tract projects bilaterally, and the lateral vestibulospinal tract projects ipsilaterally. Both tracts influence antigravity, axial and limb extensor muscles. The vestibular nuclei also project to the thalamus, cerebellum, oculomotor nuclei and contralateral vestibular nuclei. These connections are important in maintaining eye position in the presence of head rotation.

Responses to external and self-generated disturbance

External disturbance alters the postural equilibrium. The vestibular system detects postural change and mediates postural adjustment. Together with the cerebellum, the vestibular system can adapt postural reflexes (e.g. responses on a moving platform, as shown in Fig. 5.23.).

Responses to self-generated disturbance show that the vestibular system has a feedforward control

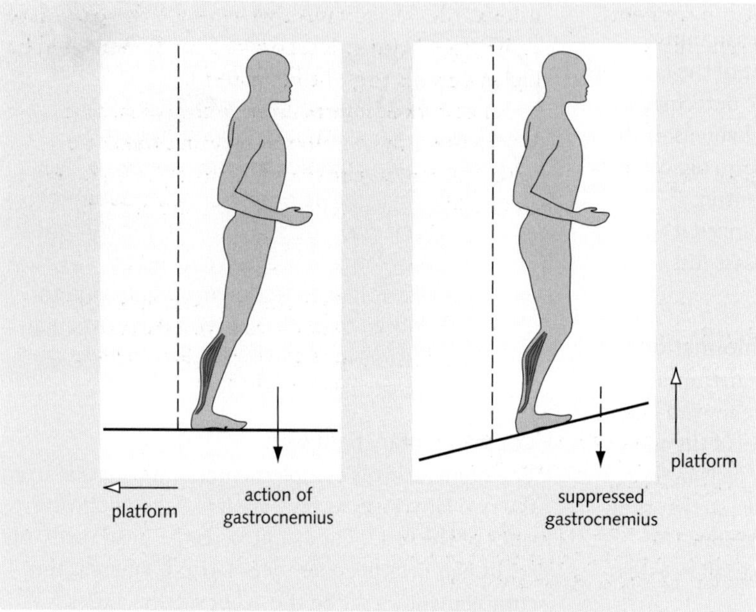

Fig. 5.23 Reflex responses to postural change can be altered.

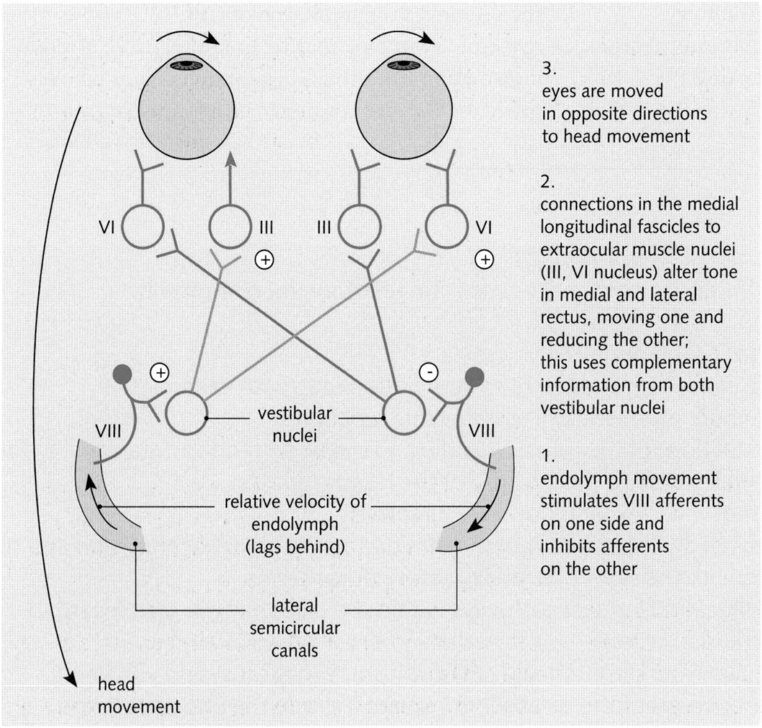
3.
eyes are moved
in opposite directions
to head movement
2.
connections in the medial longitudinal fascicles to extraocular muscle nuclei (III, VI nucleus) alter tone in medial and lateral rectus, moving one and reducing the other;
this uses complementary information from both vestibular nuclei
1.
endolymph movement stimulates VIII afferents on one side and inhibits afferents on the other
VI
III
III
VI
VIII
VIII
vestibular
nuclei
relative velocity of
endolymph
(lags behind)
lateral
semicircular
canals
head
movement

Fig. 5.24 The horizontal vestibulo-ocular reflex.

mechanism. This is important for eye movements, as a change in head position will alter the the image on the retina. To stabilize the retinal image, the vestibular system detects head movements and drives compensatory eye movements. The circuit for this is shown in Fig 5.24. The vestibulo-ocular reflex is an open loop reflex as it works without feedback. The cerebellum regulates the gain of the reflex (amount of eye movement to compensate for head movement). Eye movement control is discussed more fully in Chapter 8.

Vestibular and neck reflexes

The vestibular system mediates some of the neck reflexes (Fig. 5.25).

Control of locomotion

Locomotion requires a coordination of the systems controlling posture and the systems producing voluntary movement. This ensures that the body is supported against gravity and that the centre of gravity lies over the support base during propulsion.

A rhythm of muscle activity is needed as each limb takes its turn in supporting the body and moving it forwards. The circuits that generate this pattern of activity are in the spinal cord and can be activated by higher centres (e.g. the brainstem).

A network of interneurons in the spinal cord govern the activity of motor neurons; these are known as central pattern generators (CPGs). One CPG will activate flexor muscles, and another

Neck reflexes	
Reflex	**Action**
Vestibulocolic	Stabilises the position of the head, e.g. if the body is tilted forwards, it returns the head to the vertical position. Synergistic with the cervicocolic reflex of the neck musculature
Vestibulospinal	Tilting the head forwards (e.g. when falling) causes extension of the upper limbs, and flexion of the lower limbs. This protects from the impact of the fall. Antagonistic with the cervicospinal reflexes

Fig. 5.25 The vestibular neck reflexes. Note that these are overcome by cortical control in normal situations.

extensors, the two being mutually inhibitory. Renshaw cells in the spinal cord inhibit interneurons which are firing. Therefore activation of CPG-1 will cause its own inactivation (via Renshaw cells), which then removes the inhibition of CPG-2. This rhythmic switching may be modified by 1b afferent information from the Golgi tendon organs which prevent excessive tension in either muscle group.

- Explain the difference between feedback and feedforward control with examples.
- What is a motor programme? How is it learnt?
- What is a motor unit? Explain the term innervation ratio with examples.
- Relate the structure of the muscle spindle to its function.
- Contrast the functions of the muscle spindle and the Golgi tendon organ.
- Draw a diagram illustrating the circuitry of the biceps reflex.
- Where is the motor cortex, and how is it organized?
- Relate the signs of an upper motor neuron lesion to pyramidal tract function and compare these with the signs of a lower motor neuron lesion.
- Contrast the direct and indirect pathways within the basal ganglia with regard to their structure and functions.
- What are the signs and symptoms of parkinsonism. What causes do you know?
- What are the functions of the cerebellum? Relate them to the effects of lesion.
- What are the functions of the otolith organs and semicircular canals? Relate this to their structure.
- How does the vestibular system contribute to the vestibulo-ocular reflex?
- Describe the basic control of locomotion.

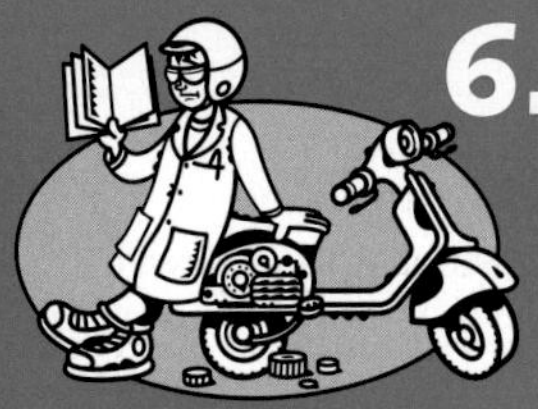

6. The Brainstem

In this chapter, you will learn about:

- The anatomy of the brainstem, including the cranial nerve nuclei.
- The functions of the reticular formation.
- How sleep affects the electroencephalograph.

The brainstem nuclei

This section describes the anatomy of the brainstem by relating cross-sectional appearance to the overall structure of the brainstem. A knowledge of the functions of the cranial nerves is essential in understanding the reasoning behind the test for brain death. The trochlear nerve (IV) is the only one to leave via the dorsal aspect of the brainstem. It has a tortuous intracranial course, and is particularly susceptible to damage in head injuries.

Fig. 6.1 shows where the cranial nerves leave the brainstem and the levels of the seven brainstem sections are shown in Figs 6.2 to 6.8.

Fig. 6.2 shows the appearance of the medulla oblongata just above its connection with the spinal cord. At this level, two 'pyramids' can be seen as enlargements of the dorsal part of the medulla. This is where the motor fibres decussate before continuing down the spinal cord in the corticospinal tracts. The gracile and cuneate sensory relay nuclei are also found at this level, along with the spinal trigeminal nucleus (cranial nerve V).

Fig. 6.3 shows a section through the middle of the medulla, illustrating the decussation of the medial lemnisci. This is the crossing of sensory (internal

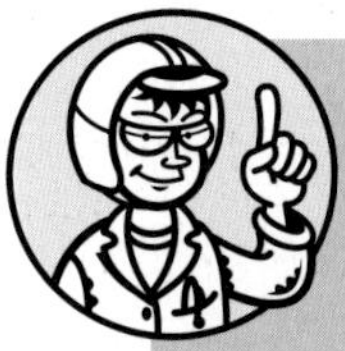

Raised intracranial pressure can cause the medulla and cerebellar tonsils to be pushed downward towards the foramen magnum. Symptoms may include headache, neck stiffness and paralysis of cranial nerves IX–XII. Lumbar puncture is very dangerous in these patients as it may lead to further herniation of the brain through the foramen magnum, and ischaemia of the compressed areas. This process is often referred to as 'coning'.

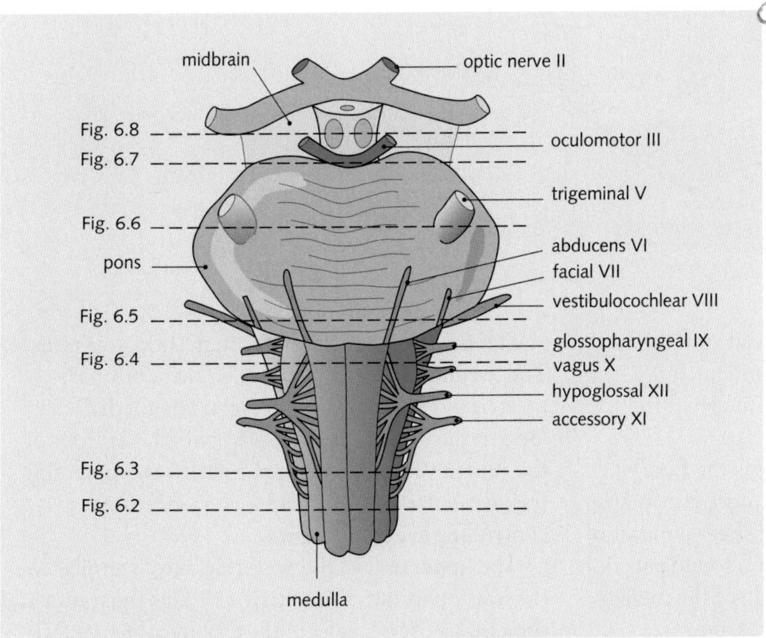

Fig. 6.1 Cranial nerves as they leave the brainstem.

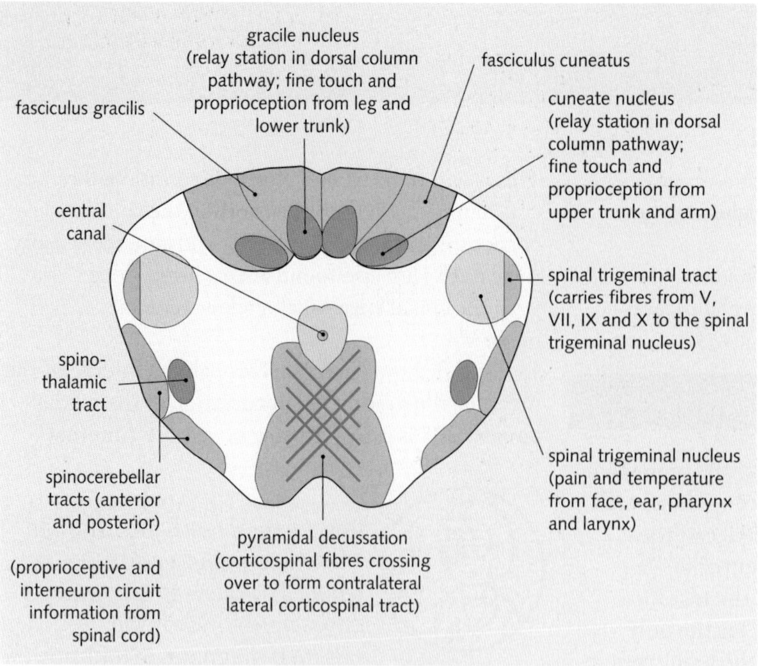

Fig. 6.2 Section through lower medulla (level of motor decussation).

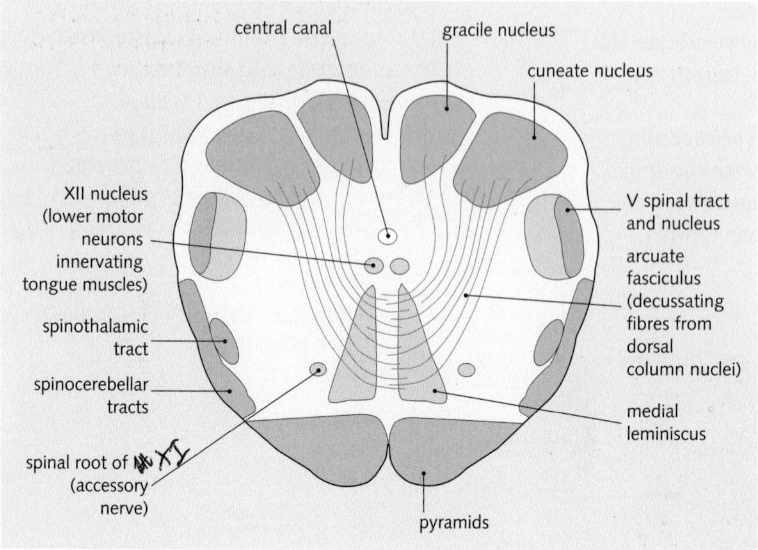

Fig. 6.3 Section through mid-medulla (level of sensory decussation).

arcuate) fibres between the gracile and cuneate nuclei. The spinal trigeminal tracts and nuclei, hypoglossal nuclei and dorsal motor nuclei of the vagus can also be seen at this level.

The upper medulla (Fig. 6.4) forms the floor of the fourth ventricle. There is much more grey matter at this level, as demonstrated by the sheer number of nuclei here. The reticular formation is found anterior to the cranial nerve nuclei, either side of the medial longitudinal fasciculus.

Fig. 6.5 shows a section through the lower pons. The medial lemniscus can still be seen, but has rotated by 90° to lie transversely. The medial longitudinal fasciculus lies just beneath the floor of the fourth ventricle, and is the pathway connecting the vestibular and cochlear nuclei with those controlling eye movements.

The upper part of the pons (Fig. 6.6) is similar to the lower part but, in addition, contains the motor and principal sensory nuclei of the trigeminal nerve (V).

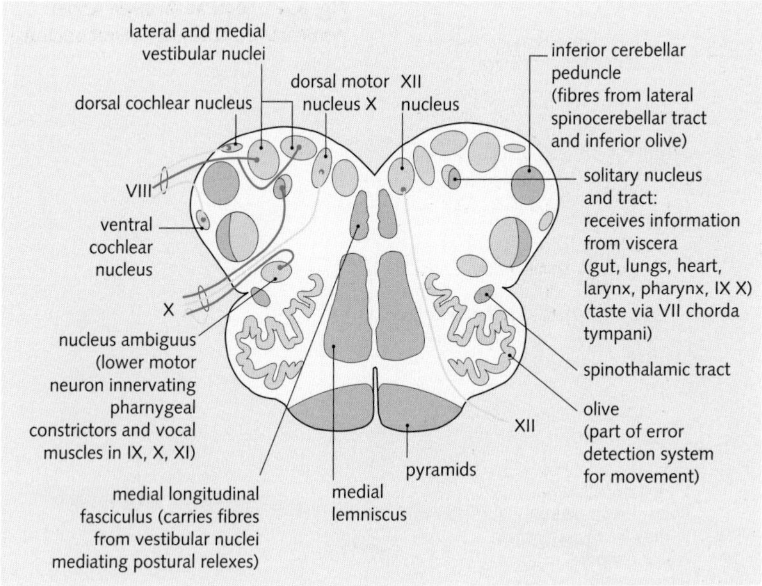

Fig. 6.4 Section through upper medulla (level of inferior olive).
Reticular formation not shown

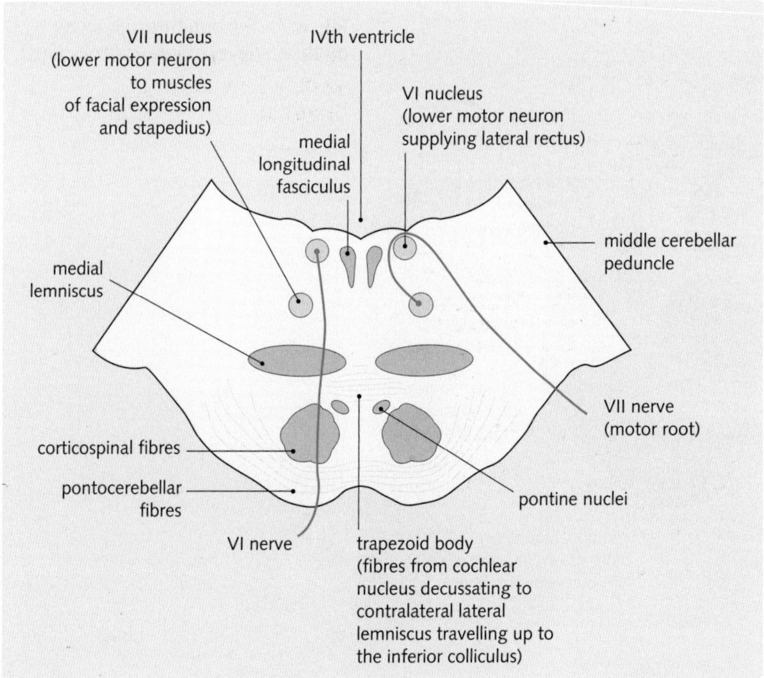

Fig. 6.5 Section through lower pons (level of the facial colliculus). Superior cerebellar peduncle and vestibular nucleus not shown (they lie on the lateral aspects of the fourth ventricle).

The anterolateral aspect of the midbrain is made up of the two cerebral peduncles (Fig. 6.7). Through each of these runs a pigmented area—the substantia nigra. The cerebral aqueduct connects the third and fourth ventricles. Just posterior (dorsal) to it, lies the tectum, which comprises the superior and inferior colliculi (Fig. 6.8).

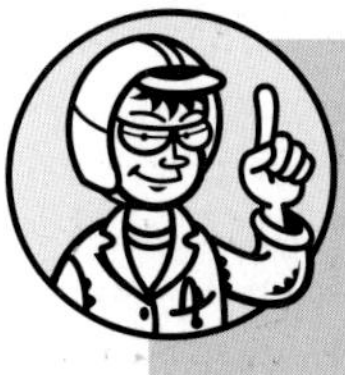

The cerebral aqueduct in the midbrain is extremely narrow and vulnerable to blockage by tumours. This can cause a non-communicating hydrocephalus.

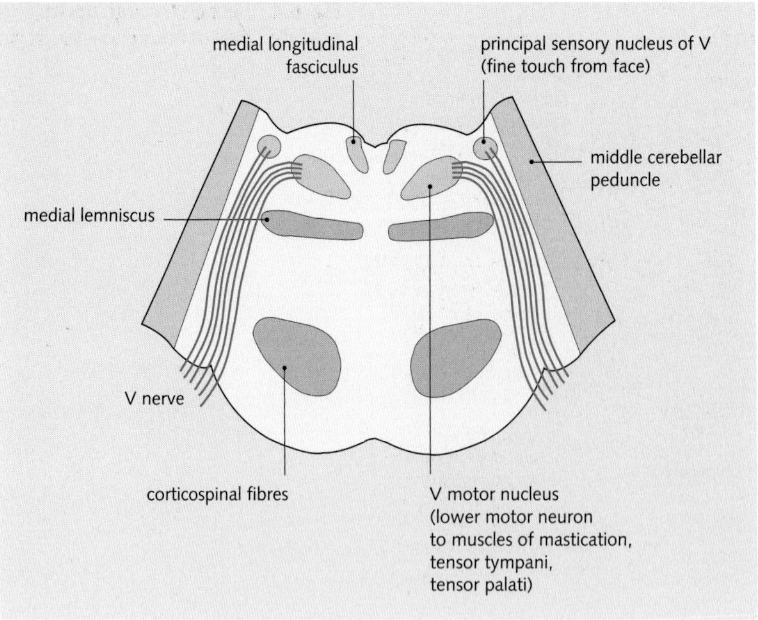

Fig. 6.6 Section through upper pons (level of the trigeminal nuclei).

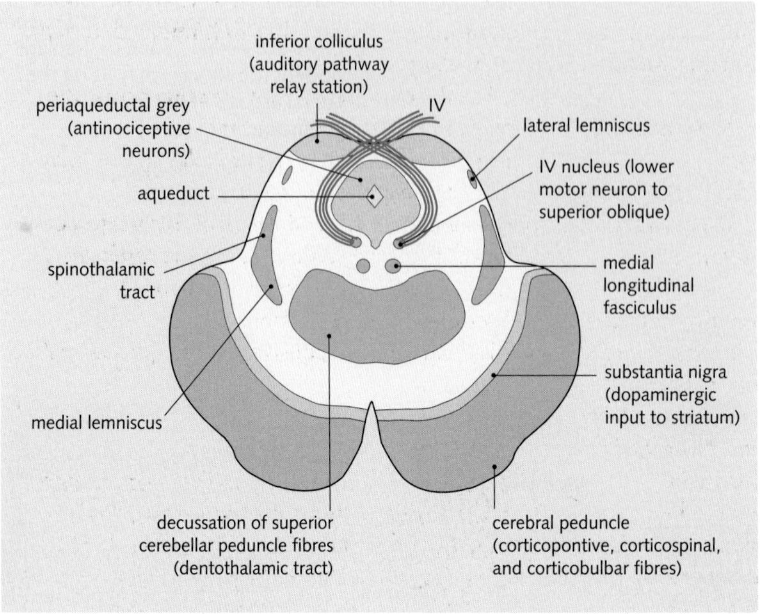

Fig. 6.7 Section through lower midbrain (level of inferior colliculus).

The reticular formation

Location and organization

If all the nuclei and tracts are identified in the brainstem (medulla, pons and midbrain), a central core of cells remains. These are loosely arranged as a network and are therefore called the brainstem reticular formation. It possibly represents a continuation of spinal cord interneurons. Closest to the midline lie the raphe nuclei, with the large-cell region adjacent to it, and the small cell region more laterally.

In this central core, cell groupings can be identified on the basis of their containing a specific neurotransmitter. These are noradrenaline, 5-hydroxytryptamine (5-HT), acetylcholine and dopamine. These projections are extensive, with the exception of the dopaminergic system which projects

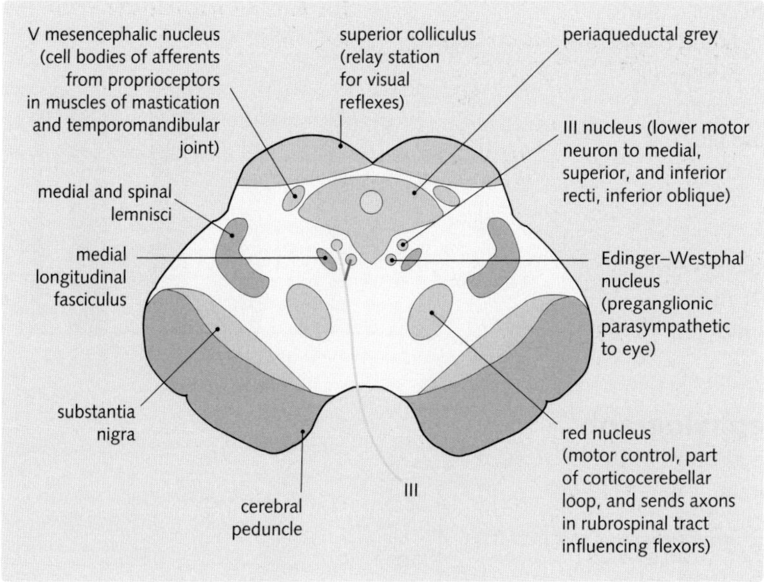

Fig. 6.8 Section through upper midbrain (level of superior colliculus).

to the striatal system, limbic areas, prefrontal cortex and anterior cingulate cortex.

The remainder of the reticular core is, as yet, not separable in terms of chemical content but can be partially defined according to function.

- A sensory portion in the lower medulla and lower pons (receiving spinoreticular fibres).
- A motor portion in the upper medulla and upper pons (receiving fibres from the corticospinal tract giving rise to the reticulospinal tracts).

The pontine and medullary neurons project into the midbrain reticular formation, which in turn projects mainly to the hypothalamus and also the thalamic reticular and intralaminar nuclei. There is also a large projection from the hypothalamus and prefrontal association cortex into the reticular formation.

The cells of the reticular formation can be histologically separated from other neurons in that:

- They have large laterally oriented dendritic trees which receive information from many sources.
- They project diffusely either to higher parts of the nervous system or to the spinal cord (most reticular cells have an upward and downward projection).

Function of the reticular formation

The functions of the reticular formation are:

- Sleeping and waking—some parts of the reticular formation are involved in producing sleep states and others in awakening mechanisms. This is related to behavioural arousal and awareness, and is thought to be mainly due to activity in the noradrenergic system). This is referred to as the reticular activating system.
- Modulation of sensory information across the thalamic relay nuclei. This includes the modulation of pain—the reticular system may have a role in the 'gating' mechanism.
- Motor control via modulation of spinal interneurons and transmitting information to the cerebellum (lateral parts of the reticular formation).
- Modulation of respiration.
- Modulation of responsiveness of hippocampal neurons.

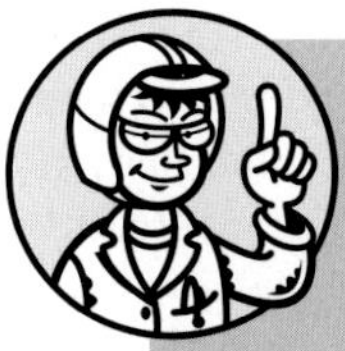

According to the monoamine theory of depression, it is a disturbance in the levels of transmitters that causes chronic states of low mood. This is based on pharmacological manipulation of the monoamine systems, which can cause an improvement in symptoms. The monoamine systems have a large number of neurons in the brainstem, and this may represent a focus for depressive dysfunction. However, this is not the whole story and research is ongoing!

- Integration of autonomic functions, particularly cardiovascular. In sleep, heart rate, blood pressure and respiration, all decline; before awakening, they are adjusted so that the transition from horizontal to vertical does not cause fainting.
- Control of endocrine functions via the hypothalamic nuclei.
- Possible role in cognition.
- Motor acts involving motivation and reward (dopaminergic system, particularly the mesolimbic projections from the midbrain to the ventral striatum).

Sleep and the electroencephalograph

The electroencephalograph (EEG) is a record of the electrical activity produced by the brain. It is obtained by attaching electrodes to the skull and connecting them to a suitable amplifier. In an awake, resting subject with the eyes open, the EEG shows a high frequency (13–30 Hz), low voltage pattern, called 'beta activity'.

As one progresses into drowsiness and then to deep sleep, the frequency content decreases below 10 Hz (i.e. the waves recorded from the skull become slower), but higher voltage. This is predominantly observed as alpha activity (8–13 Hz drowsy), theta activity (4–7 Hz sleep) or delta activity (0.5–3.5 Hz deep sleep).

Phases of paradoxical sleep or rapid eye movement (REM) sleep occur in which the EEG is of the awake pattern but the subject is difficult to arouse and has no muscle tone. This phase of sleep is important because a sleeping person woken in this phase will report dreams with a large content of visual imagery. Typically, the first REM phase occurs after about 90 minutes of sleep.

Fig. 6.9 shows that sleep can be divided into four phases according to the EEG frequency and that, during sleep, we cycle through the different stages tending to awaken just after a REM phase.

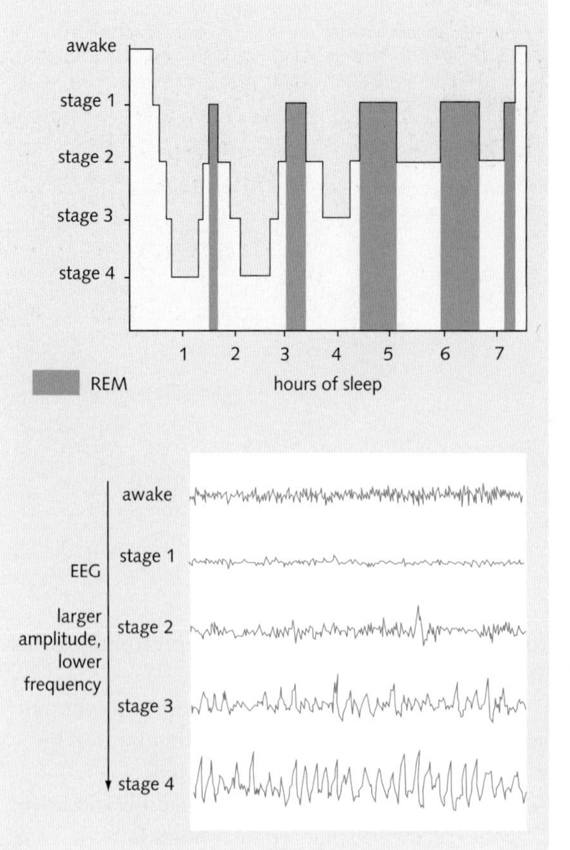

Fig. 6.9 Stages of sleep and the sleep cycle with electroencephalographs.

Brain death

Normally, death is diagnosed by the absence of a pulse, the absence of heart sounds and fixed pupils. However, if the patient is on life-support, these may not be appropriate markers. In these cases, brain death may be declared even in the presence of a heart which is still beating, according to the UK Brain Death Criteria. This requires:

- Deep coma with absent respiratory effort.
- The absence of drug intoxication and hypothermia.
- The absence of hypoglycaemia or ion imbalance.

It is diagnosed by testing brainstem function systematically or, more logically, the function of the cranial nerves:

- Fixed pupils (II/III).
- Absent corneal blink reflex (V).
- No vestibular-ocular reflexes (tested by injecting ice cold water into the external meatus, and looking for eye movement towards that ear) (VIII).
- An absence of motor responses within all cranial nerve distributions.
- Absence of a gag reflex (IX).
- No spontaneous respiration after turning off the respiratory pump, even when extreme levels of hypercapnia are reached (medulla respiratory centres).

- Summarize the cranial nerves which leave the brain in the pons, medulla and midbrain.
- What is special about the trochlear nerve which might be clinically relevant to a road traffic accident victim?
- What are the functions of the reticular formation? How might damage manifest itself?
- Name the stages of sleep. How do EEG appearances differ between sleeping and waking?
- How do you diagnose brain death (in the UK)?

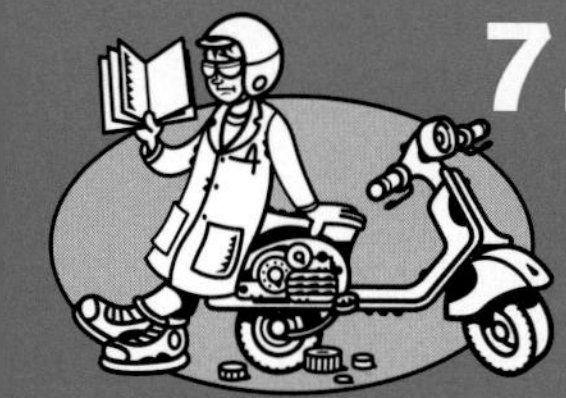

7. The Autonomic Nervous System

In this chapter, you will learn about:

- The anatomy and physiology of the sympathetic nervous system.
- The anatomy and physiology of the parasympathetic nervous system.
- Pharmacology and the autonomic nervous system.
- The enteric nervous system.
- Disorders of autonomic function.

Introduction

The autonomic nervous system controls involuntary internal processes such as digestion and the regulation of blood flow. It acts mainly on the heart, smooth muscle (such as that in blood vessel walls), metabolic processes and glandular structures. There are three branches of the autonomic nervous system:

- Sympathetic.
- Parasympathetic.
- Enteric.

The sympathetic and parasympathetic divisions are often thought of as mutually antagonistic. This is true in certain organ systems (such as the heart), but it is an oversimplification. Some parts of the body receive input only from one of the divisions, and in other areas (such as the salivary glands) their effects are similar. Their actions are coordinated and balanced by the hypothalamus and the nucleus of the solitary tract.

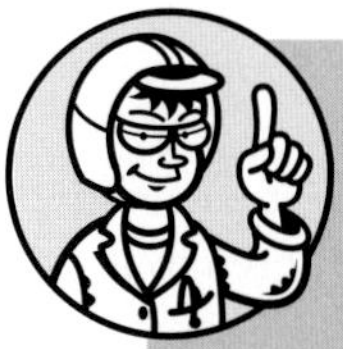

Most viscera are only innervated by autonomic nerves. Pain from these organs must therefore be signalled in some way be the autonomic nervous system. The body cannot localize to internal pain, so the pain is felt at the same level as the point of entry of the fibres to the spinal cord. This is known as referred pain (e.g. the pain of a heart attack may be referred to the shoulder and left arm).

Structure and function of the sympathetic nervous system

Physiological role of the sympathetic nervous system

The sympathetic system prepares the body for responses to stressful challenges, and causes a 'fight or flight' response, allowing sudden strenuous exercise and increased vigilance.

The sympathetic nervous system also helps control blood pressure, thermoregulation, gut function and urogenital function.

Structure of the sympathetic nervous system

There is a column of efferent cell bodies (intermediolateral column) in the lateral horn of the spinal cord, running from T1 to L2. These 'preganglionic' neurons have axons that travel through the ventral root of their segmental spinal nerve. They contact a chain of ganglia outside the central nervous system lying along the vertebral column (paravertebral ganglia), as shown in Fig. 7.1.

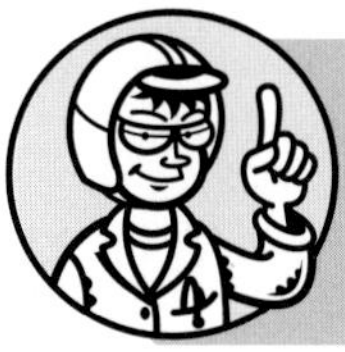

The paravertebral ganglia are sometimes referred to as the 'sympathetic chain'.

Each preganglionic neuron can influence many neurons in different ganglia by collaterals, coordinating the activation of ganglia at different spinal levels, as shown in Fig. 7.2. The postsynaptic cells in the ganglia are the 'postganglionic' neurons. Postganglionic axons are unmyelinated and pass into peripheral nerves to target sites. For the head and neck, they form a plexus around the carotid arteries and gain access to the interior of the skull by the internal carotid artery.

Afferent fibres pass through the paravertebral ganglia without synapsing, reaching their cell bodies in the dorsal root ganglia.

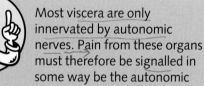

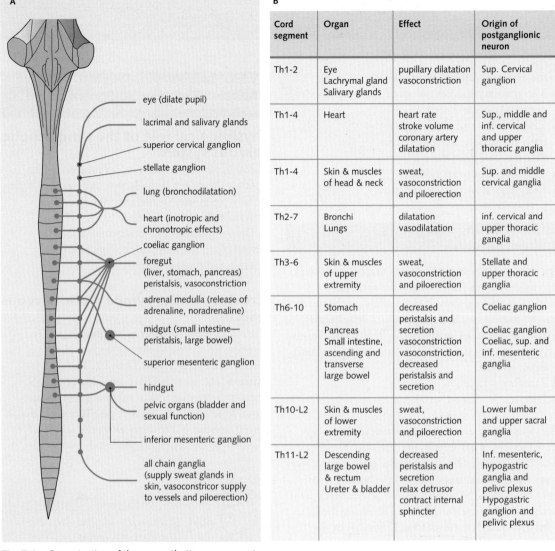

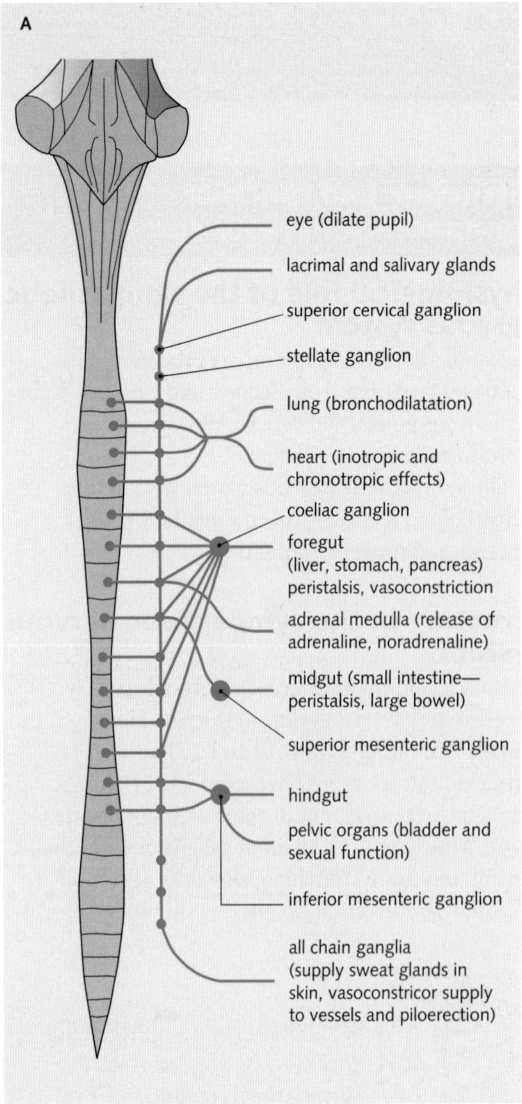

B

Cord segment	Organ	Effect	Origin of postganglionic neuron
Th1-2	Eye Lachrymal gland Salivary glands	pupillary dilatation vasoconstriction	Sup. Cervical ganglion
Th1-4	Heart	heart rate stroke volume coronary artery dilatation	Sup., middle and inf. cervical and upper thoracic ganglia
Th1-4	Skin & muscles of head & neck	sweat, vasoconstriction and piloerection	Sup. and middle cervical ganglia
Th2-7	Bronchi Lungs	dilatation vasodilatation	inf. cervical and upper thoracic ganglia
Th3-6	Skin & muscles of upper extremity	sweat, vasoconstriction and piloerection	Stellate and upper thoracic ganglia
Th6-10	Stomach Pancreas Small intestine, ascending and transverse large bowel	decreased peristalsis and secretion vasoconstriction vasoconstriction, decreased peristalsis and secretion	Coeliac ganglion Coeliac ganglion Coeliac, sup. and inf. mesenteric ganglia
Th10-L2	Skin & muscles of lower extremity	sweat, vasoconstriction and piloerection	Lower lumbar and upper sacral ganglia
Th11-L2	Descending large bowel & rectum Ureter & bladder	decreased peristalsis and secretion relax detrusor contract internal sphincter	Inf. mesenteric, hypogastric ganglia and pelivc plexus Hypogastric ganglion and pelivic plexus

Fig. 7.1 Organization of the sympathetic nervous system.

Exceptions to the general pattern of sympathetic nervous system innervation

Some preganglionic fibres do not synapse in the paravertebral ganglia, but carry on to ganglia closer to their target organs via the splanchnic nerves. The coeliac, aorticorenal, superior mesenteric and inferior mesenteric ganglia contain cell bodies providing the sympathetic nervous system innervation to the gut, kidney, liver, pancreas and urogenital organs. Some preganglionic fibres continue to the adrenal medulla. Here, they are responsible for the glandular secretion of catecholamines from cells that are functionally similar to postganglionic sympathetic neurons.

The adrenal medulla receives a direct innervation from the spinal cord that is not interrupted by a synapse in a ganglion.

Neurotransmission in the sympathetic nervous system

The transmitter released by preganglionic neurons at the ganglia (and also those synapsing in the adrenal medulla) is acetylcholine, which binds to postsynaptic nicotinic receptors. The nicotinic receptor is a cation channel which, when opened,

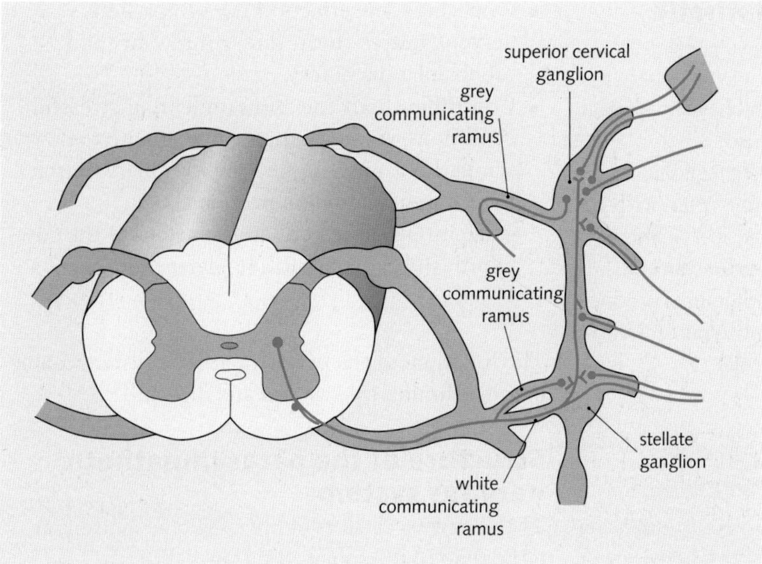

Fig. 7.2 Spinal cord efferents to the sympathetic chain.

Adrenergic receptors			
Adrenergic receptor	**Location**	**Second messenger**	**Function**
α_1	smooth muscle in blood vessels and bronchi, dilator pupillae	IP_3	contraction
α_2	smooth muscle in blood vessels, presynaptically on adrenergic synapses	decreased cAMP	contraction, reduced transmitter release
β_1	heart muscle, presynaptically on adrenergic synapses	increased cAMP	increased heart rate and force of contraction, increased transmitter release
β_2	smooth muscle in blood vessels and bronchi	decreased cAMP	relaxation

Fig. 7.3 Adrenergic receptors: location, second messenger and function.

produces a fast excitatory postsynaptic potential. The transmitter released by postganglionic neurons is noradrenaline, except in sweat glands where acetylcholine is released and binds to muscarinic receptors (which are slower metabotrophic receptors).

Transmission occurs at specialized structures along the length of the postganglionic axon called varicosities, which synthesize, release, take up and metabolize noradrenaline. This process is called 'en passage' transmission, as the action potential does not end when noradrenaline is released but carries on to the next varicosity.

Cells of the adrenal medulla release noradrenaline and adrenaline into the circulation, permitting the sympathetic nervous system to have a general humoral action on adrenergic receptors in the body.

The effect of noradrenaline release is dependent on the type of receptor that is present in the target organ, as shown in Fig. 7.3.

Other transmitters

Often, cotransmitters are released with the main transmitter in the sympathetic nervous system to give a longer-lasting and more subtle modulatory influence on postsynaptic activity (e.g. ATP is released along with noradrenaline at postganglionic sympathetic nerve endings).

Drugs acting on the sympathetic nervous system

The ganglia

Drugs affecting ganglionic transmission have no clinical use. They have complex actions because parasympathetic and sympathetic postganglionic neurons are influenced at the same time, often with opposing effects. Agonists at ganglionic acetylcholine receptors (e.g. nicotine) produce hypertension and tachycardia. Antagonists (e.g. hexamethonium) produce hypotension, but cannot be used as antihypertensive agents because of their side-effect profile.

> Although nicotine initially simulates the ganglia, it causes a depolarization block in high concentrations. This causes hypotension and decreased gut motility.

Target organs

Noradrenergic transmission can be altered by interfering with noradrenaline synthesis, release or postsynaptic interaction with different receptor subtypes. Drugs used clinically are shown in Fig. 7.4.

Structure and function of the parasympathetic nervous system

Physiological role of the parasympathetic nervous system

The parasympathetic nervous system has many actions, which can be described as:

- Opposing some effects of the sympathetic nervous system (heart rate, gut motility and bronchiolar diameter).
- Controlling body functions under non-stressful conditions, working either alone or with the sympathetic nervous system (e.g. ciliary muscle for accommodation for near objects; gastrointestinal secretions; secretions of the nose, mouth and eye; micturition; defaecation; sexual function).

The functions of the parasympathetic system can be broadly summarized as 'rest and digest'.

Structure of the parasympathetic nervous system

There are two clusters of preganglionic neurons at either end of the spinal cord (Fig. 7.5).

The cranial parasympathetic nervous system outflow comes from several nuclei in the brainstem. Structures in the head are supplied by the ciliary, pterygopalatine, otic and submandibular ganglia which receive inputs from cranial nerves III, VII and IX. Organs in the thorax and abdomen receive their parasympathetic supply via the vagus (Xth) nerve, which forms diffusely distributed collections of postganglionic neurons in the walls of, or close to, the target organs.

The sacral parasympathetic nervous system outflow comes from preganglionic neurons whose cell bodies lie in a column running from segments S2 to S4 of the spinal cord. Their axons leave the cord through the ventral root for a short distance and leave the spinal nerves as separate small pelvic nerves. The postganglionic neurons are found in the pelvic plexus located near the target organs.

Drugs acting on the sympathetic nervous system			
Drug	**Action**	**Clinical use**	**Side effects**
adrenaline	α, β agonist	anaphylaxis, cardiac arrest	hypertension, dysrhythmia
salbutamol	β_2 agonist	asthma	tachycardia, dysrhythmia, tremor
clonidine	partial α_2 agonist	hypertension	drowsiness, postural hypotension
prazosin	α_1 antagonist	hypertension	hypotension, tachycardia, impotence
atenolol	β_1 antagonist	hypertension, acute coronary syndromes, tachyarrhythmias	heart failure, fatigue, cold extremities, less bronchoconstriction than non-selective β antagonists

Fig. 7.4 Drugs acting on the sympathetic nervous system.

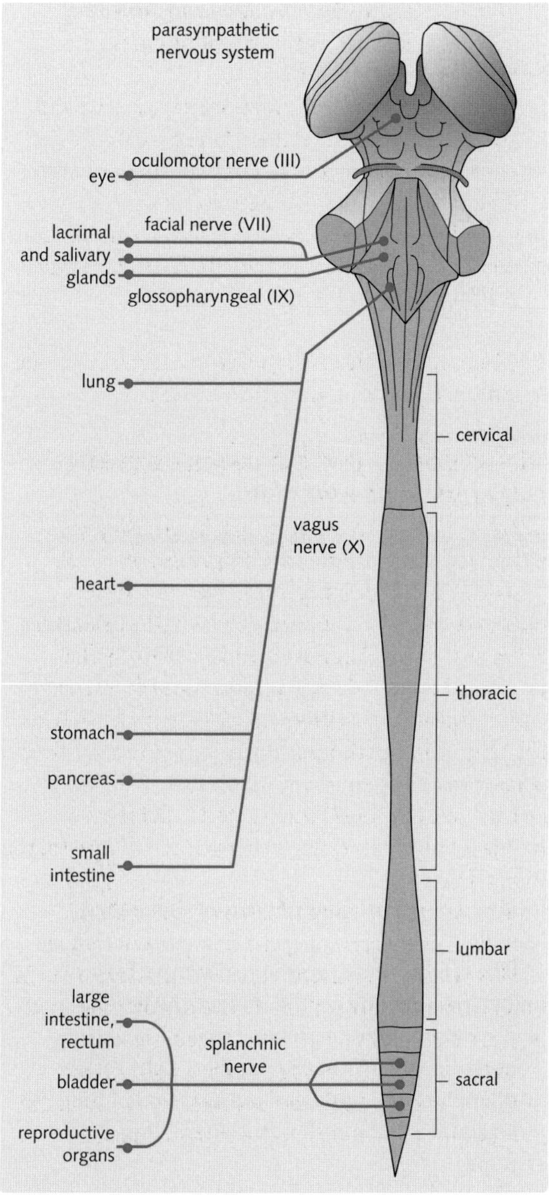

Fig. 7.5 Organization of the parasympathetic nervous system.

Neurotransmission in the parasympathetic nervous system

As in the sympathetic nervous system, parasympathetic preganglionic neurons release acetylcholine onto ganglionic nicotinic receptors.

At target organs, postganglionic neurons release acetylcholine onto muscarinic receptors, which show subtype variation localized to different target organs (Fig. 7.6).

Drugs acting on the parasympathetic nervous system

The drugs in clinical use that affect the function of the parasympathetic nervous system interact with the receptors on the target organs (Fig. 7.7).

The enteric nervous system

The enteric nervous system is a neural system embedded in the wall of the gastrointestinal tract, pancreas and gall bladder. It consists of two tubular systems:

- The submucosal (Meissner's) plexus, which lies between the mucous membrane and the circular muscle layer.
- The myenteric (Auerbach's) plexus which lies between the circular and longitudinal muscle layers.

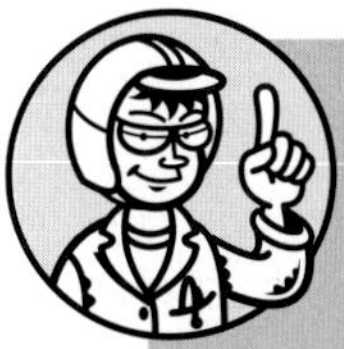

In Hirschsprung's disease, there is a congenital absence of Auerbach's plexus. This causes an absence of peristalsis and leads to distension of the colon (megacolon).

Both systems contain both sensory and motor modalities. They have inputs from other parts of the autonomic nervous system but have intrinsic activity of their own.

- The sensory neurons monitor the mechanical state of the alimentary canal, the chemical status of the stomach and intestinal contents, and the hormonal levels in the portal blood vessels.
- The output motor neurons control gut motility and secretions, as well as the diameter of local blood vessels.

The parasympathetic and sympathetic nervous systems can override the enteric division.

Disorders of the autonomic nervous system

Loss of the sympathetic innervation to the face causes Horner's syndrome. This is characterized by:

- Ptosis (drooping of the eyelid).
- Miosis (pupillary constriction).

Muscarinic receptors		
Muscarinic subtype	**Location**	**Function**
M_1	Gastric parietal cells, enteric nervous system	Slow excitation of ganglia. Gastric acid secretion, gastrointestinal motility
M_2	Cardiac atrium	Vagal inhibition of heart. Decreased heart rate and force of contraction
M_3	Smooth muscle, glands	Secretion, contraction of smooth muscle, vascular relaxation

Fig. 7.6 Muscarinic receptors.

Drugs acting on the parasympathetic nervous system			
Drug	**Action**	**Use**	**Side effects**
pilocarpine	Partial muscarinic agonist	glaucoma (increased intraocular pressure), where increased constrictor pupillae action allows greater drainage of aqueous humour	cardiac slowing, increased gastrointestinal tract activity causing abdominal pain
atropine	muscarinic antagonist	cardiac arrest, sinus bradycardia after myocardial infarction	dry mouth, dilated pupil, blurred vision, bronchodilatation, urinary retention
ipratropium	muscarinic antagonist	asthma, causing bronchodilatation and inhibiting increases in mucous secretion	inhaled and does not pass easily into the circulation, so few side effects
dicyclomine	M_1 antagonist has direct relaxant effect on smooth muscle	reduce spasmodic activity of gastrointestinal tract in irritable bowel syndrome	less severe than atropine

Fig. 7.7 Drugs acting on the parasympathetic nervous system.

- Anhydrosis (loss of sweating).
- Enophthalmos (eyes appear withdrawn into the orbit).

The innervation may be interrupted anywhere along its course—the brainstem and cervical spinal cord are rare sites of 'central Horner's syndrome'. Classically, compression of the stellate ganglion may occur in the presence of a carcinoma in the apex of the lung (Pancoast's tumour). Injury can also happen as the sympathetic fibres gain access to the head wrapped around the internal carotid artery (e.g. after dissection of the artery).

Section of the sympathetic trunk disrupts the control of structures controlled by that spinal level. Surgical section of sympathetic nerves in the cervicothoracic region has been used to treat Raynaud's syndrome (where vasoconstriction causes painfully cold hands) with little success. A poorly understood feature of peripheral sympathetic injury is 'reflex sympathetic dystrophy', which is chronic pain, accompanied by dry, shiny, red skin and poor wound healing. When this can be localized to a particular nerve root, it is called 'causalgia'.

The effects of disrupting parasympathetic innervation depend on the level of the lesion.

- A neurosyphilitic lesion in the oculomotor nerve causes loss of the pupillary light reflex, dilation of the pupil and preservation of the accommodation reflex (the Argyll Robertson pupil).
- Controlled ablation of a highly selective part of the vagal innervation to the stomach may be used as a treatment for excessive gastric acid secretion.
- Damage to the parasympathetic components in the cauda equina causes loss of bladder control and sphincter dysfunction.

Phaeochromocytomas, tumours of chromaffin tissue, are generally found in the adrenal medulla and secrete vast quantities of catecholamines. This causes hypertension (which may be extremely severe—with headaches, and even intracranial haemorrhage as presenting features). A combination of alpha and beta adrenoceptor blockade is required until surgical removal is possible.

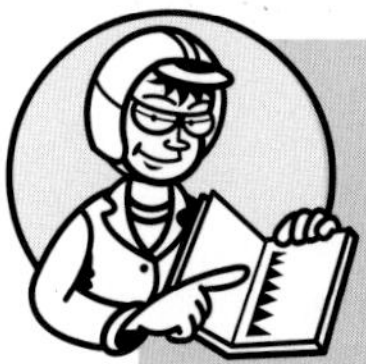

- What are the functions of the sympathetic nervous system?
- What drugs can modify sympathetic function, and how are they used?
- Relate the structure of the parasympathetic nervous system to its function.
- Compare the sympathetic and parasympathetic nervous systems. Explain why they are not exactly opposite in terms of function (give examples).
- How can drugs modulate parasympathetic function? In what clinical scenarios might they be used?
- Describe the structure and function of the enteric nervous system.

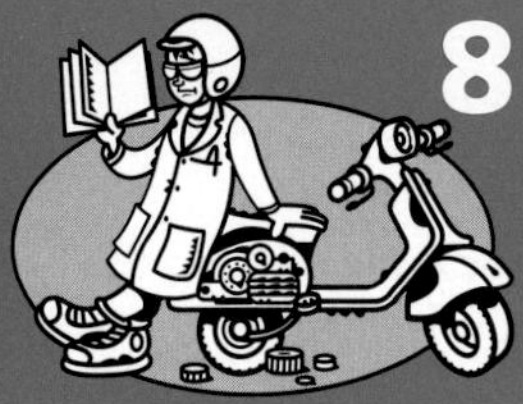

8. Vision

In this chapter, you will learn about:

- The macro- and microscopic anatomy of the eye.
- Retinal structure and function.
- Central visual pathways.
- Mechanisms of attention.
- Loss of vision.

The eye

Anatomy of the eye—transparent structures

The structures inside the eye are shown in Fig. 8.1.

The cornea is the transparent outer coat covering the pupil. It is continuous with the sclera (white of the eye) and consists of five layers. From the exterior inwards they are:

- An epithelial layer of stratified squamous cells, which is richly innervated with sensory nerves and continuously bathed in tear fluid.
- The basement membrane that gives strength to the cornea.
- The corneal stroma occupies 90% of the thickness of the cornea. It consists of thin sheets of collagen fibrils that are oriented parallel to each other in the same sheet and at right angles to fibrils in sheets either side. The spacing and arrangement of the fibrils gives the cornea its transparency.
- A basal lamina lines the inner surface of the stroma.
- The endothelial layer is a single layer of squamous cells, providing mechanisms for metabolic exchange between the aqueous humour and the cornea. It regulates the water content of the corneal stroma, preventing oedema and consequent opacity.

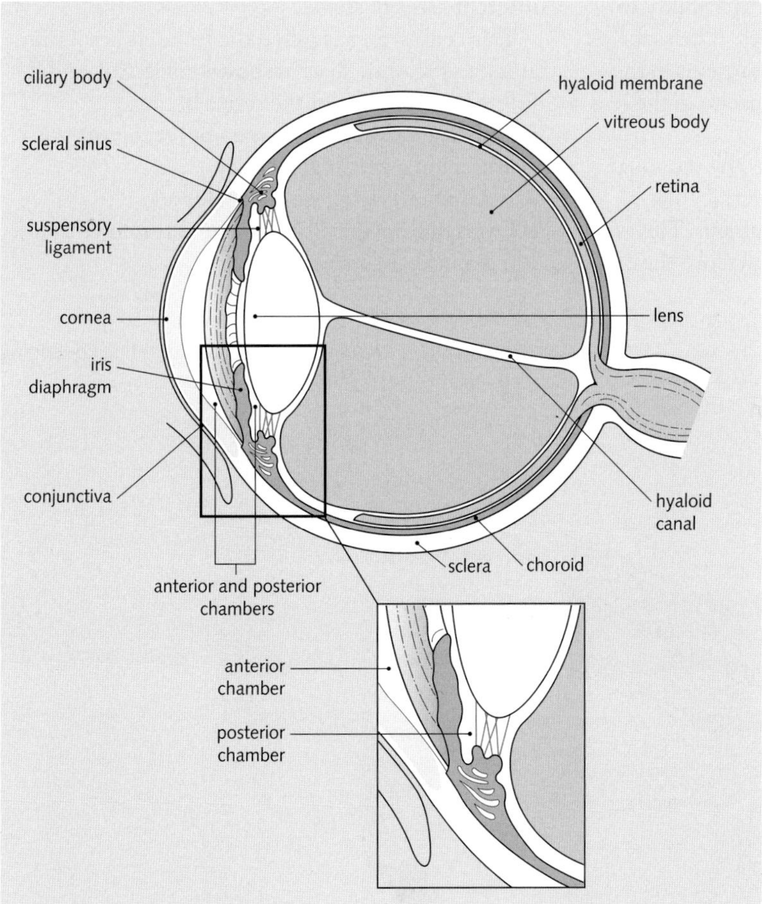

Fig. 8.1 Cross-section through the eye showing the main structures.

The iris is the part of the eye that regulates how much light enters the eyeball. It is a coloured muscular structure that overlies the lens.

The lens is seen in the central space in the iris (the pupil). It appears black as it is transparent, and the choroid is visible. The lens consists of three parts:

- It is encapsulated in a basement membrane that is elastic, and strongest at the insertion of the suspensory ligament around the equator of the lens.
- Lining the inside of the capsule on its anterior surface is a layer of cuboidal cells (subcapsular epithelium). Epithelial cells near the lateral equator differentiate into lens fibres.
- Lens fibres are thin, flattened and devoid of organelles and nuclei. They become filled with proteins (crystallins) and extend towards the centre of the lens, producing a very dense central section.

The ciliary muscle contracts to alter the curvature of the lens and change its refractive power. This is the basis of accommodation.

The lens changes with age. It loses its ability to accommodate as its elasticity reduces. It loses its transparency because of changes in proteins in the fibres or dehydration of the lens. Opacity in the lens is known as a cataract.

The shape of the eye is maintained by the tough sclera and an internal pressure (the intraocular pressure) exerted by the aqueous humour. This is produced in the ciliary body, and flows into the posterior chamber, through the pupil and into the anterior chamber. It passes out through the trabecular meshwork (a network of bands of tissue defining the edge of the anterior chamber), and via the canal of Schlemm into the episcleral veins. The normal intraocular pressure is usually 10–20 mmHg. If it exceeds 22 mmHg, the condition of glaucoma is produced, which can produce blindness by compressing the blood supply to the optic nerve. Blockages in the trabecular meshwork (e.g. by drugs which dilate the pupil, thereby pushing the iris up against the lens) can cause sharp rises in intraocular pressure. Such drugs should obviously be avoided in this condition. Glaucoma is discussed subsequently in this chapter.

The vitreous humour fills the posterior part of the eyeball. It is more viscous than the aqueous humour.

The eye is adapted for acute vision by having one small area of its sensory layer containing an extremely high density of photoreceptors (specifically for colour vision in good illumination), which it can direct accurately and quickly to different areas of space.

This central area is called the fovea. It lies 3 mm lateral to the optic disc, as shown in Fig. 8.2, and it differs from the rest of the retina because:

- Only cone (wavelength-specific) receptors are present at a very high density.
- It has no overlying vascular network.
- Overlying nerve cell bodies are displaced to allow maximal light access.

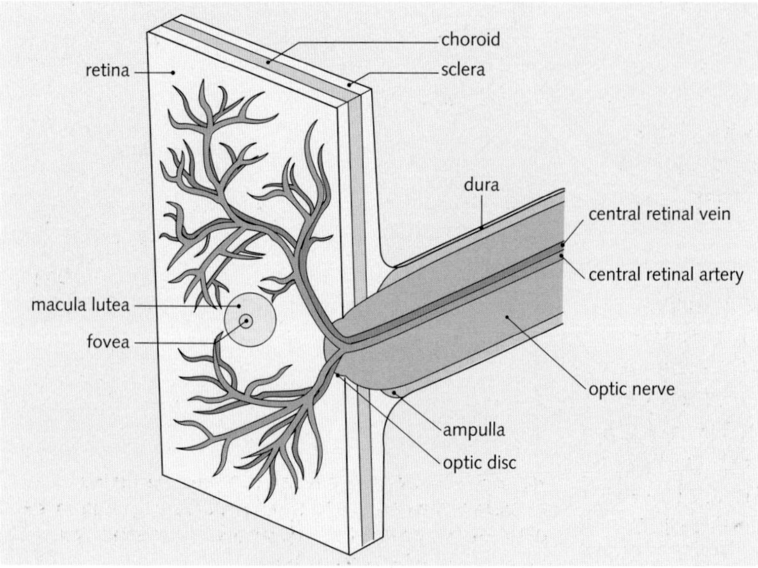

Fig. 8.2 Section of retina containing the fundus.

The fovea is the central part of a small circular region called the macula lutea. On examination with an ophthalmoscope, the pigmented epithelium underlying the macula shows through, giving it a darker appearance than the rest of the retina. The visual axis of the eye does not correspond to its geometrical axis and is displaced so that the visual axis runs through the fovea (Fig. 8.3).

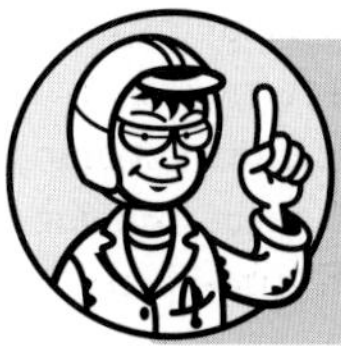

There are no photoreceptors overlying the origin of the optic nerve (optic disc). This area corresponds to the blind spot.

Optics of the eye

Light from a point of visual fixation is bent (refracted) so that a clearly focused image appears on the retina (Fig. 8.4). The lens for the visual system is a compound lens with interfaces of different refractive power (measured in dioptres, D). These occur at the cornea:

- Between the anterior chamber and the lens.
- Between the lens and the vitreous body.

The total refractive power is 58.6 D, with most of the power (42 D) at the air–cornea interface.

Accommodation

The refractive power of the lens is changed by accommodation. When the ciliary muscle contracts, it moves downwards and forwards. This reduces the tension in the suspensory ligament and allows the elastic lens to become fatter and shorter. This has the effect of focusing light from near targets (which reaches the surface of the eye as divergent rays) by convergence onto the retina. The lens is an elastic structure in young people, but it gradually hardens with age and can no longer readily change shape. Near vision therefore becomes impaired with increasing age, a phenomenon called presbyopia.

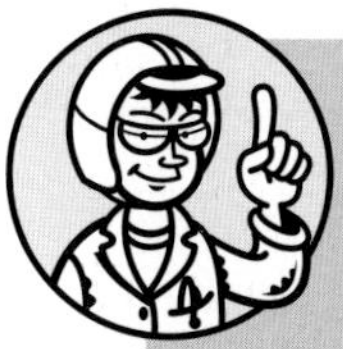

The accommodation reflex demonstrates that when the eye is focused on a distant object, the pupil is constricted. However, if the patient is asked to suddenly focus on an object close to their face, the pupil dilates. This is mediated by cranial nerve II (optic).

Retinal function and image processing

Visual pigments

Visual pigments within photoreceptors undergo chemical change as a result of absorbing the energy from photons, enabling transduction of light into a neural signal. The pigments used by the rod system and the cone system differ, reflecting their different functions.

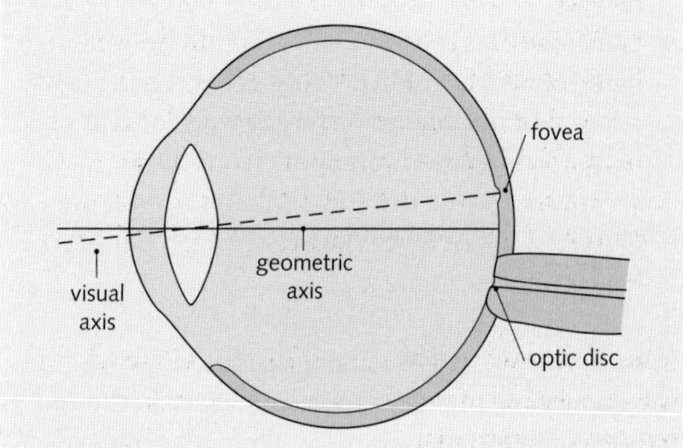

Fig. 8.3 Visual axis of the eye.

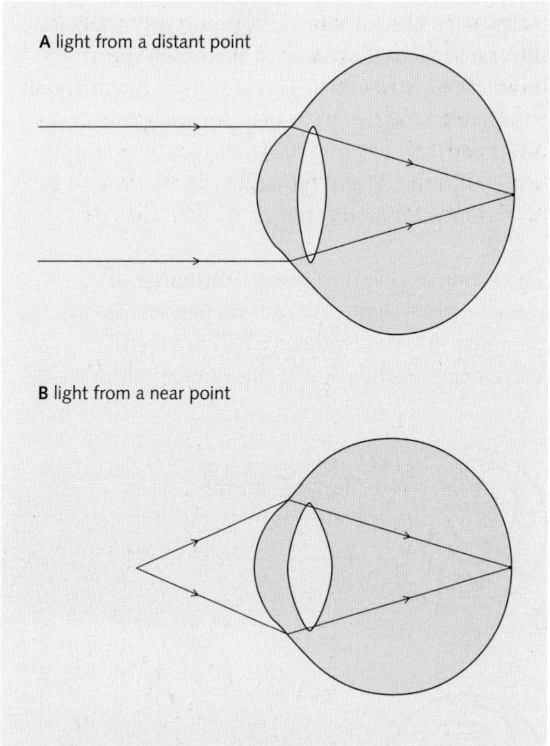

Fig. 8.4 To change from distant to near vision the refractive power of the lens has to increase by around 3.3 dioptres. For near vision the lens becomes better by a process termed accommodation.

Visual pigments have a characteristic structure consisting of the vitamin A aldehyde, retinal, covalently attached to a protein (one of the opsins). The second-messenger system that the opsins modulate involves cyclic guanosine monophosphate, cGMP (opsins resemble G-protein-coupled receptors).

The receptor function of the retina is carried out by two types of cell:

- Rods are very sensitive and respond to dim light (scotopic vision) and are found peripherally in the retina.
- Cones are less sensitive and respond best in bright light (photopic vision). There are three types of cones that respond to different wavelengths of light. Combinations of inputs from these receptors encode different colours. Cones are clustered in the fovea, where the high density leads to greater acuity.

In rods, the pigment is rhodopsin. Rhodopsin lies in the membrane of intracytoplasmic discs in the rod. It has seven membrane-spanning domains arranged around the retinal molecule, which attaches to the seventh transmembrane domain.

In cones, the variation in pigment is produced by different forms of opsin with their own specific interaction with retinal. This results in the different absorption sensitivities in the cone system:

- B cones at 420 nm (blue).
- G cones at 531 nm (green).
- R cones at 558 nm (red).

The retina responds to a restricted range of wavelengths of light. We see and perceive colours in the range 400 nm (violet) to 780 nm (red). Wavelengths either side of this range (as low as 400 nm and as high as 1400 nm) penetrate the eye, but have no receptors specialized for their detection. The activation cascade for signalling that light has reached the rod or cone outer segment, shown in Fig. 8.5, begins with the change in retinal and ends with an alteration in membrane permeability to cations.

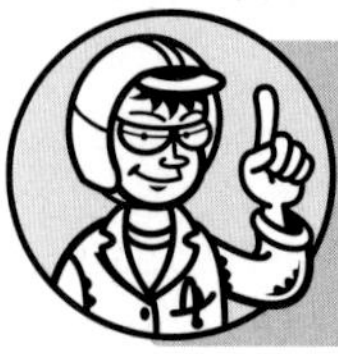

Alterations in the photopigments within cone receptors lead to colour blindness.

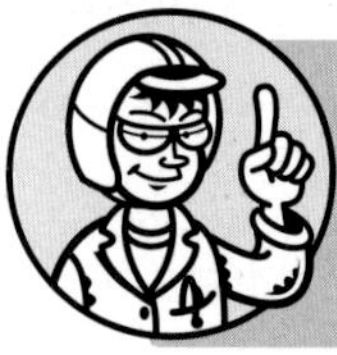

The cornea and lens become yellow with age and this filters out a lot of light in the blue wavelength band.

The photosensitive part of rhodopsin is retinal, which changes its configuration when bombarded by photons (from 11-cis retinal; with the terminal aldehyde group at an angle to the rest of the molecule to all-trans retinal; with the terminal aldehyde group in line with the rest of the molecule). This disrupts the binding of retinal to opsin, causing the two to separate, producing a conformational change in opsin.

This leads to a reduction in intracellular cGMP.

In darkness the cGMP-gated channels in the outer segment membrane are open because there has been no photon-instigated reduction in the intracellular level of cGMP. The steady inflow of Na^+ (the 'dark current') maintains the resting membrane of the receptor at –40 mV, producing a constant release of the neurotransmitter glutamate at its synapse.

After a reduction in cGMP, the channels close, hyperpolarizing the cell and reducing glutamate release at the synapse. Greater light intensities produce greater hyperpolarization (up to a maximum of –70 mV with all the Na^+ channels closed).

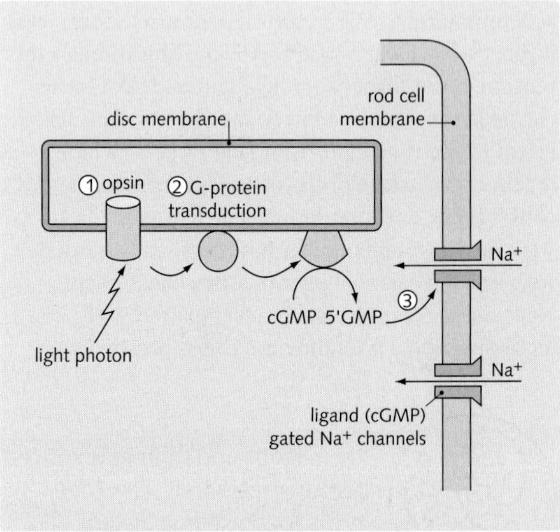

Fig. 8.5 Signal transduction of light impulses. (1) Conformational change. Afterwards, all-trans retinal no longer binds, which affects the G-protein transduction. (2) Increased activity of cGMP phosphodiesterase, which hydrolyses cGMP, reducing its intracellular level. (3) Low cGMP levels close the ligand-gated channels, and thereby hyperpolarize the rod.

Structure of the retina

The neural part of the retina responds to light, processes light signals from photoreceptors, and sends visual information to the thalamus and brainstem. The functions of different neurons in the retina depend on their connections and all the neural elements are supported with a particular type of glial cell, Müller's cell.

There is a blood–retina barrier at the endothelium of the capillary network on the anterior surface of the retina, from the central retinal artery, and at the endothelium of the capillary network in the choroid.

The photoreceptors are situated in the most posterior layer of the retina. This means that light has to travel through several cell layers before reaching them. This is particularly true in the peripheral areas of the retina.

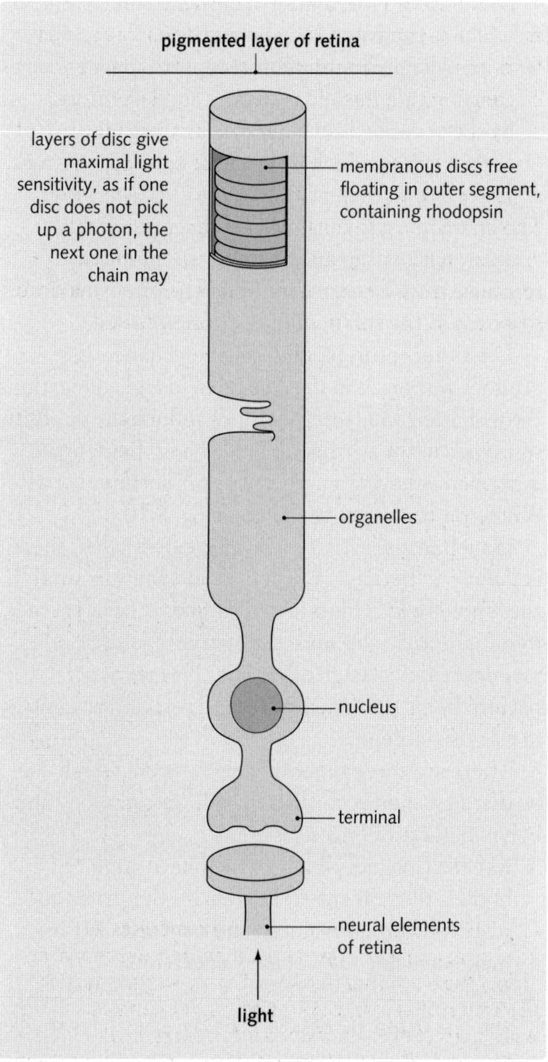

Fig. 8.6 Structure of a rod cell.

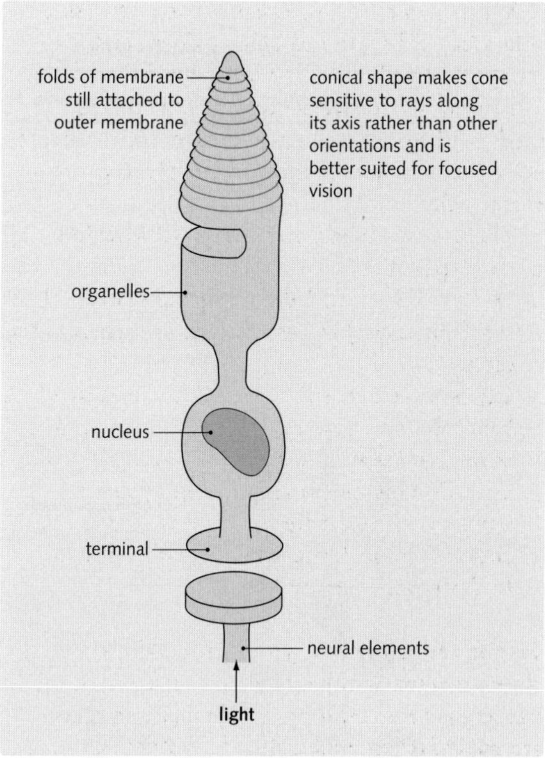

Fig. 8.7 Structure of a cone cell.

Rods and cones have different structures, as shown in Figs 8.6 and 8.7, but share the following features:

- Outer segments, which contact the pigmented epithelial layer of the retina, contain highly folded membrane structures with visual pigments.
- Inner segment contains the nucleus and organelles.
- A synaptic terminal (the most anterior structure).

Fig. 8.8 compares the connections and functions of rods and cones.

Connections in the retina

Fig. 8.9 shows the circuit in the retina. There are excitatory and inhibitory connections between photoreceptors and bipolar cells, depending on the postsynaptic glutamate receptor on the bipolar cell. Remember that light stimulation reduces glutamate release.

- For inhibitory (hyperpolarizing) synapses, reduction in glutamate release in response to illumination produces depolarization of the bipolar cell.

Comparison of rods and cones				
Receptor	**Total number**	**Location**	**Connection to output cells**	**Function**
Rod	120×10^6	peripheral retina, around the fovea	convergent pattern where many rods send information to a few output cells and this compresses information	responding to dim light with low spatial resolution and mediating visual reflexes from stimuli in the peripheral field
Cone	6×10^6	clustered in the fovea	no convergence; each cone projects to one bipolar cell, which projects to one output cell	focused, highly detailed colour vision with high spatial resolution

Fig. 8.8 Comparison of rods and cones.

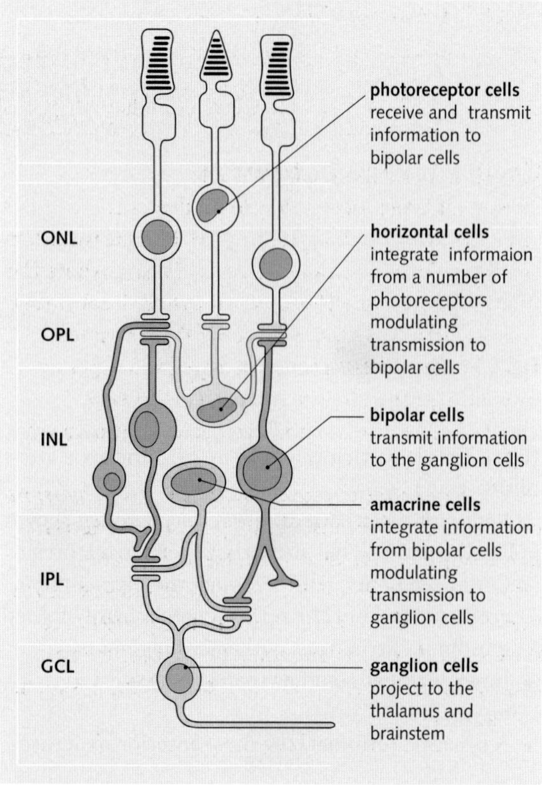

Fig. 8.9 Processing of visual information in the retinal layers (ONL, outer nuclear layer; OPL, outer plexiform layer; INL, inner nuclear layer; IPL, inner plexiform layer; GCL, ganglion cell layer).

- For excitatory (depolarizing) synapses, reduction in glutamate release will hyperpolarize the bipolar cell.

All bipolar cells excite ganglion cells.

The receptive field of a ganglion cell is the region of retina which, when stimulated, affects the firing of the ganglion cell. The size and properties of the receptive field of the ganglion cell are determined by the number of photoreceptors it is connected to via the bipolar cells and the type of connections between the photoreceptors and bipolar cells.

- If many receptors converge on a ganglion cell via bipolar cells, its receptive field will be very large, condensing a lot of information into one signal, which is typical of rod connections.
- If a small number of photoreceptors converge on a ganglion cell, its field is smaller and less information has been condensed in producing the ganglion output signal, which is typical of cone connections.

The characteristic ganglion-cell receptive field is circular, with either an excitatory or inhibitory response from a central zone and the opposite response in the surrounding peripheral zone.

Direct receptor–bipolar–ganglion connections produce responses in the central field and connections through horizontal interneurons produce the opposite responses in the peripheral field. These fields are described as having an on-centre/off-surround or off-centre/on-surround, as shown in Fig. 8.10.

Ganglion cell activity will be greatest when there is a contrast between the centre and the surround. If the whole field is illuminated or in darkness, there is minimal activity because the two antagonistic responses cancel each other out. This response pattern helps the visual system to respond to contrast in the visual scene.

There are three types of ganglion cell, which can be distinguished according to their morphology and behavioural properties.

- M cells (magnocellular) which have large cell bodies, thick axons and extensive dendrites and responding to movement and contrast. These make up some 10% of the population.
- P cells (parvocellular) which have small cell bodies and less extensive dendritic fields. They have smaller receptive fields and respond to colour. These make up approximately 80% of the population.

- The remainder have smaller cell bodies than the P cells and thinner axons. They project to the midbrain and are probably involved in reflex adjustment of head and eye position.

Their properties are summarized in Fig. 8.11.

Horizontal integration

Boundaries between light and dark (i.e. edges of objects) are enhanced by the horizontal connections provided by cells in the plexiform layers. The horizontal cells in the outer plexiform layer contact a number of photoreceptors and bipolar cells. They can cause a bipolar cell to be maximally activated when surrounding photoreceptors are not stimulated. Conversely, they inhibit the firing of the bipolar cell when there is photoreceptor activity in the 'surround' of its receptive field. This allows edges to be detected.

Amacrine cells relay signals from the rod bipolar cells (which do not directly contact the ganglion cells) to the cone bipolar cells (which do synapse with ganglion cells). This has the function of integrating rod and cone responses.

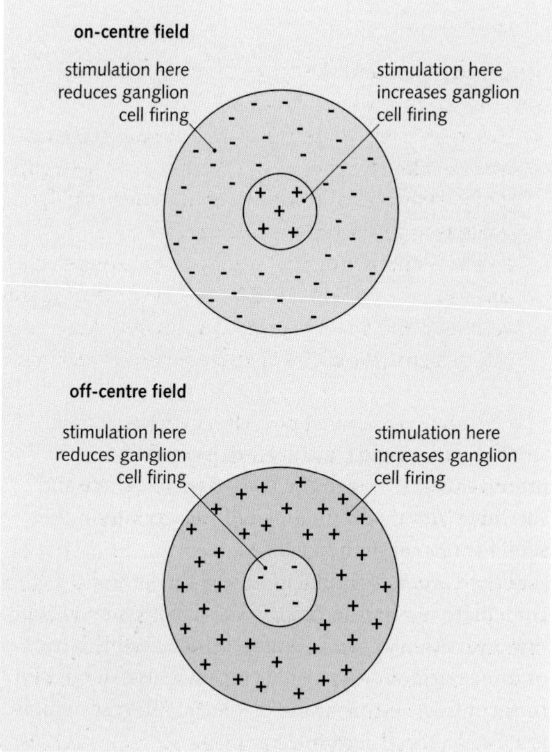

Fig. 8.10 Receptive fields of ganglion cells.

Central visual pathways and the visual cortex

Central visual pathways

The major projection from the ganglion cells (approximately 90%) passes in the optic nerve to the lateral geniculate nucleus of the thalamus, where the axons synapse on cells projecting to the visual cortex.

A smaller projection synapses (approximately 10%) in the midbrain (pretectal area and superior colliculus), controlling visual reflexes and eye movements; there is a small projection from here to higher visual processing areas.

The hemispheres process visual information from only one side of the visual axis (the contralateral), but the optic nerve leaving each eye contains information from both sides of the axis. Some fibres therefore need to cross over so that they project to the contralateral thalamus and this occurs in the optic chiasm in front of the pituitary stalk, as shown in Fig. 8.12.

Retinal ganglion cell types

Ganglion cell	Structure	Receptive field	Response properties	Projection site	Function
X	small cell, small dendritic arbor	small	wavelength specific, slowly adapting	thalamus	signals fine detail and colour
Y	large cell, large dendritic arbor	large	rapidly adapting	thalamus, midbrain	signals movement and illumination
W	large cell, large dendritic arbor	large	variable	midbrain	involved in eye movement control

Fig. 8.11 Retinal ganglion cell types.

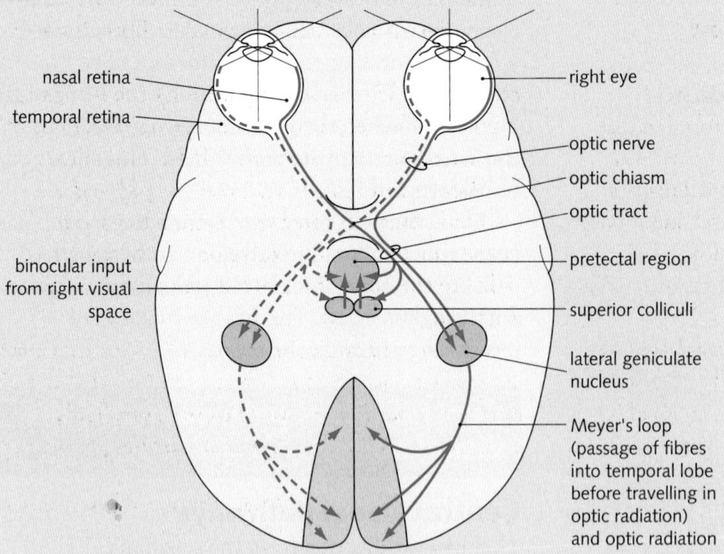

Fig. 8.12 Schematic representation of central visual pathways, showing the decussation of nasal fibres in the optic chiasm.

Thalamus and visual cortex

The lateral geniculate nucleus

The optic nerve termination in the lateral geniculate nucleus is separated by eye of origin (thus each lateral geniculate nucleus cell receives monocular information) and by ganglion cell type.

The retinal fibres terminate in six discrete layers—four parvocellular layers (dorsal laminae 4–6) and two magnocellular layers (ventral laminae 1 and 2). Each eye transmits to three of the layers with the small-field P-ganglion cells projecting to two parvocellular layers (whose cells are concerned with fine detail), and the large-field M-cells to one magnocellular layer (whose cells are concerned with movement). Laminae 1,4 and 6 receive information from the contralateral eye and 2, 3 and 5 from the ipsilateral eye. This is the first stage of segregation into parallel pathways for form, colour and movement.

The lateral geniculate nucleus has a retinotopic organization, meaning that a given area of the retina will project to only a certain part of the lateral geniculate nucleus. Cells that receive inputs from the same area of the retina are stacked in columns running perpendicular to the layers.

Cells in the lateral geniculate nucleus have the same response properties as retinal ganglion cells—small circular fields with centre/surround interactions, although the responses to centre and surround visual stimuli are much sharper than that seen for retinal ganlion cells.

There are non-retinal inputs to the lateral geniculate nucleus (from the visual cortex and the pontine reticular formation) that can alter the traffic of information to the visual cortex. This can be used to accentuate information of special interest, which is a mechanism of attention.

The visual cortex

The visual cortex lies along the calcarine sulcus on the medial aspect of the occipital lobe. The lateral geniculate nucleus projects a distorted retinotopic map onto the primary visual area (V1), Brodmann's area 17, so that information from the fovea gains access to a larger volume of cortex than information from the peripheral retina, as shown in Fig. 8.13.

Similar to other cortical areas, V1 has six layers of cells. Cells in the magnocellular and parvocellular layers in the lateral geniculate nucleus terminate in layer 4 of the V1 cortex. Interestingly, the geniculate projection is double since parvocellular cells project into the lower part of layer 4 whereas the magnocellular cells project into the upper part of layer 4. Other lateral geniculate nucleus cells (interlaminar cells) terminate in layers 2 and 3 on patches of cells termed 'blobs' (see below).

Response of V1 neurons and functional arrangement

Most V1 neurons respond to lines or edges (orientation selectivity), unlike retinal and lateral geniculate nucleus neurons, which have circular receptive fields. Cells that respond to similar line orientations are collected in columns perpendicular to the cortical surface (orientation columns).

Orientation-selective cells can be further classified:

- Simple cells respond to light/dark edges at a specific orientation in a restricted part of the visual field—imagine that they add up the input from adjacent ganglion cells so that the line is a series of small circles.
- Complex cells respond similarly but in a much larger area of the visual field, and maximally to the movement of the edge across the receptive field—imagine that they add up the input from simple cells.

For both cell types, moving stimuli produce better responses than static ones and certain directions of movement produce better responses than others.

The orientation columns are grouped together into units that are capable of responding to all orientations of lines in the same part of the visual field. These units are called hypercolumns, as shown in Fig. 8.14.

Within the hypercolumn, the orientation columns are arranged so that the inputs from the left and right eyes are kept separate, forming so-called ocular dominance columns. This enables higher processing

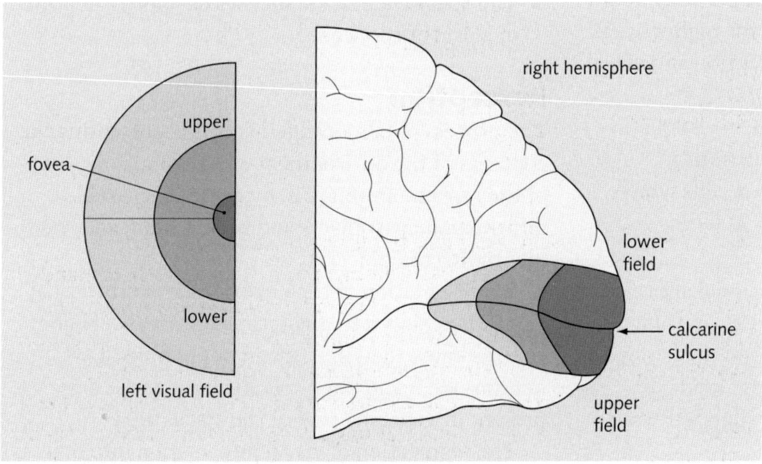

Fig. 8.13 Primary visual cortex—location and representation.

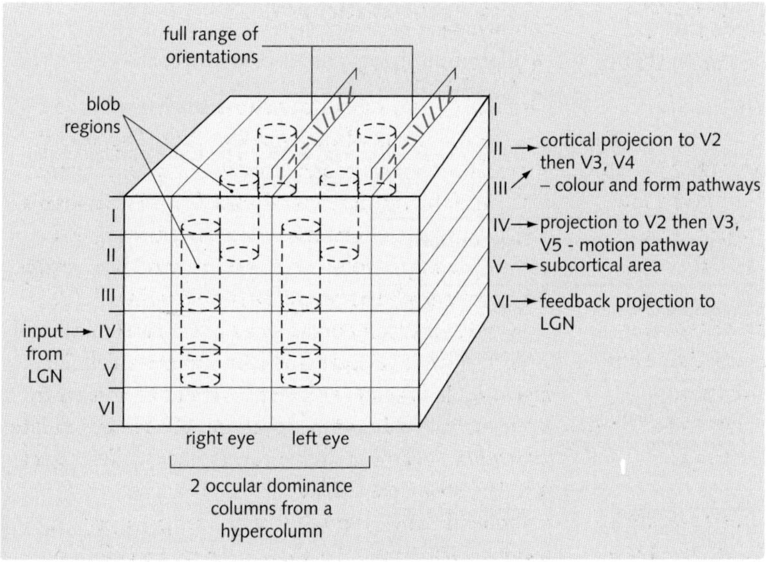

Fig. 8.14 Organization of inputs and outputs in the striate cortex. Diagram shows ocular dominance columns, blob regions and orientation selectivity (LGN, lateral geniculate nucleus).

areas to compare the information from both eyes to create depth perception.

Within the hypercolumns, there are regions between groups of orientation columns, called 'blob' regions. These are made up of groups of cells responding to colour contrast, with the centre/surround interaction response pattern to a primary colour (centre) and its complement (surround).

Progression of visual processing

The visual scene that we 'see' is built up from different processing circuits in the visual cortex. The processing circuits are formed by pathways through separate areas of the visual cortex each of which contain a retinotopic map. This allows representation of different types of activity in the visual field.

- V2 has an unknown function, but possibly acts as a processing and relay station for higher areas.
- V3 may have a role in depth perception and visual acuity.
- V4 has a role in colour perception.
- V5 is concerned with motion detection.
- Inferotemporal areas have complex cells which respond to particular stimuli such as faces.

The basis for these theoretical functional areas is the study of people with bizarre lesions in their brains, and of monkeys in which targeted lesions have been made. It was through these kinds of experiment that the concept of parallel pathways came about.

There are three pathways processing colour, motion and form. Things are not as simple as that because of the interconnections between the pathways but the major differences between them are summarized in Fig. 8.15.

Attention and perception

Attention

The process of attention is the selection of a focus from sensory information in order to process it further. A certain amount of processing of all information has to occur before attentional mechanisms select the appropriate information.

Attending to a part of our environment involves visual and motor mechanisms to orient the body in space, allowing us to scan the visual field or interact with the environment in motor tasks.

The factors that determine where attention is directed are novelty (brightness, colour and change in orientation) and relevance to current tasks.

- The pre-attentive process is a rapid scanning of a scene to detect objects/gross form.
- The attentive process focuses on specific features of a part of the scene.

Perception

The process of perception involves representing the contents of the environment and then making sense of the representation (e.g. by organizing visual information into objects and background, and then identifying the objects).

Representation of the environment in the visual cortex is achieved by the retinotopic maps. Higher centres know that, if a certain population of V1 neurons are firing, then specific boundaries are present in a specific part of the visual field.

The segregation of visual information into objects and background relies upon certain features of the visual scene. Objects are picked out using the following list of principles:

- Common shape, colour or texture.
- Continuity.

The three visual pathways

Basic function	Ganglion cell	Visual cortical regions in pathway	Responses of cells	Perceptual role
Motion	Y	V1, V2, V3, V5, then to parietal lobe	rapid responses for moving stimuli, no sensitivity to colour	detection of motion and arrangement of objects
Form	X	V1, V2, V4, then to parietal lobe and temporal lobe	slowing adapting, some colour sensitivity sensitive to orientation of edges	detection of shape of stationary objects
Colour	X	V1, V2, V4, then to temporal lobe	colour sensitive	detection of colour

Fig. 8.15 The three parallel visual pathways.

- Proximity.
- Common size.
- Closure.
- Depth, which can be worked out from:
  - Monocular information about size, texture, perspective, overlap, movement parallax.
  - Binocular information about the difference between the view from the eyes and about how the eyes move to focus on the same part of space.

The identification of objects, once picked out from the environment, relies upon comparison with memories of objects. This occurs in the visual association cortex at the occipitotemporal junction.

Eye movements

Eye movements are important in attentional mechanisms as they direct the fovea onto points of interest in the visual scene quickly and accurately. There are five types of eye movement, two of which stabilize the eye when the head moves:

- Vestibulo-ocular—uses vestibular input to hold the retinal image stable during brief or rapid head rotation. For horizontal movements, lateral rectus motor neurons (VI nucleus) are influenced by vestibular nuclei cells, medial rectus motor neurons (III nucleus) are driven by interneurons in the contralateral abducens nucleus.
- Optokinetic—uses visual input to hold the retinal image stable during sustained or slow head rotation. The underlying pathway comprises a retinal projection via the tectum to the vestibular nucleus and a cortical component from V1.

The other three eye movements keep the fovea on a visual target:

- Saccade—brings new objects of interest onto the fovea. They are very fast and occur every 300 ms. The pattern of saccadic eye movements is guided by current cognitive tasks, as shown by recordings of eye movements when pictures are scanned for details. Horizontal saccadic movements are generated in the pontine reticular formation, and vertical ones in the midbrain, under influence from a circuit involving the frontal eye fields (in the frontal lobes), the pulvinar nucleus of the thalamus and the superior colliculus.
- Smooth pursuit—holds the image of a moving target on the fovea. This type of movement is controlled by visual and frontal cortical areas, relaying information to the vestibulocerebellum.
- Vergence—adjusts the eyes for differing image distances. This movement is controlled by midbrain neurons near the oculomotor nucleus. Convergence/divergence of the eyes is induced by blur, and is important in accommodation.

Smooth pursuit movements and saccadic eye movements can alternate (e.g. when looking out of a train window) and this combination of movements is termed optokinetic nystagmus.

Strategies in visual processing

There are two strategies employed by the visual system to make sense of the visual environment.

- Bottom-up processing occurs when a visual scene is analysed purely in terms of the incoming visual information, without searching visual memory for similar scenes that might help with making sense of the scene.
- Top-down processing occurs when visual memory influences the way in which the current visual scene is processed, so that some sort of sense can be made of the way in which objects are distinguished from their background.

Disorders of attention and perception

In the condition of neglect, patients fail to turn their attention to areas in the visual scene on one-half of space, typically the side of space contralateral to a parietal lobe lesion. They will entirely ignore one side of their visual axis (e.g. eating only half the food on a plate) or describing only half of a visual scene (when looking at it and when recollecting it).

In the condition of agnosia, patients cannot recognize objects from visual examination, although they can fully describe the physical features of the object (and recognize it from tactile information). Here, there is a failure of the higher processes of perception that integrate all the visual information about an object and compare it with visual memory.

These conditions differ in important respects:

- In agnosia, there is a failure of recognition of an object wherever it is in the visual field.
- In neglect, there is a failure to attend to one-half of space, whatever the objects.

Loss of vision

Glaucoma

There are two types of glaucoma, which are both characterized by fundoscopic changes, visual field loss and raised intraocular pressure. Acute closed angle glaucoma is a sight-threatening emergency, whereas primary open angle glaucoma runs a more chronic and insidious course.

Acute closed angle glaucoma

This presents as a painful red eye, and may be associated with vomiting. Blurred vision and the appearance of light objects having a 'halo' are common in the evenings (when the pupil is dilated). The cause of the rise in intraocular pressure is shown in Fig. 8.16.

Treatment aims to lower the pressure within the eyeball—first medically (e.g. with a pupil constrictor such as pilocarpine), then flow should be restored surgically or with a laser. The other eye should be treated prophylactically.

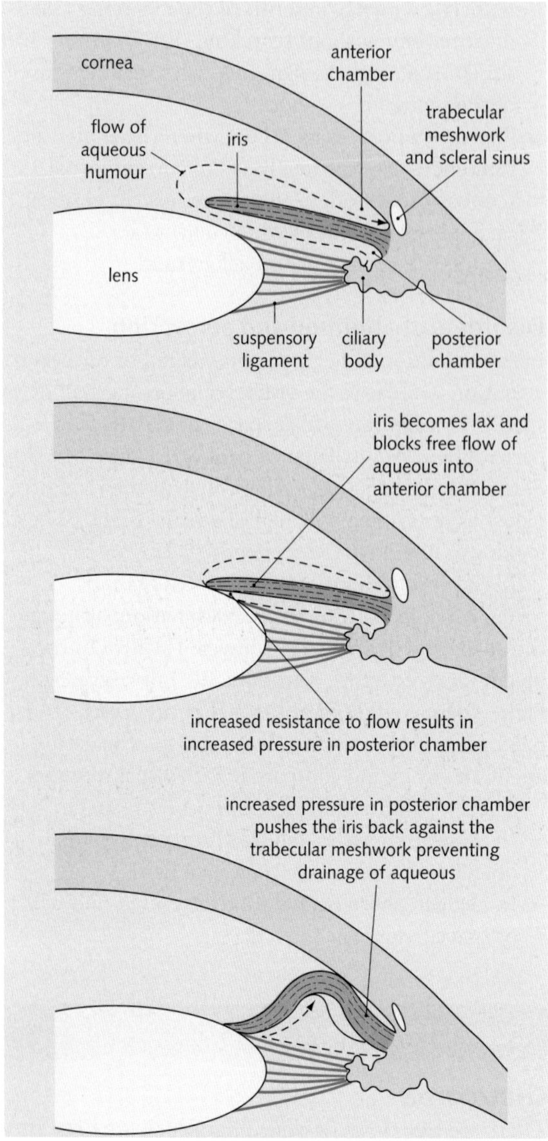

Fig. 8.16 Acute closed angle glaucoma—mechanism.

Primary open angle glaucoma

This is more common than closed angle glaucoma, and the third most common cause of blindness in the UK. The intraocular pressure rises slowly due to a blockage in the trabecular meshwork. Symptoms may not be present until severe damage has occurred, so screening programmes exist for high risk patients (elderly and those of Afro-Caribbean origin).

Signs may include:

- Visual field loss.
- 'Cupping' of the optic disc on fundoscopy.
- Haemorrhages on the optic disc.

Medical treatment includes the use of:

- β-blockers (topical)—reduces the secretion of aqueous humour.
- Parasympathomimetic agents (e.g. pilocarpine drops)—constrict the pupil.

Laser treatment and surgery may ultimately be appropriate.

Damage to the central pathways for vision

The patterns of visual loss following central lesions is dependent on the location of the lesion. These are summarized in Fig. 15.11. Three common types of visual loss are:

Monocular visual loss

Causes:

- Amaurosis fugax (optic nerve ischaemia).
- Migraine.
- Temporal arteritis leading to optic nerve infarction.
- Optic neuritis (may be part of MS).
- Rare things—methanol poisoning, hereditary optic atrophy, neurosyphilis.

Bitemporal hemianopia

Pressure on the optic chiasm caused by:

- Pituitary adenoma.
- Other tumours (e.g. meningiomas).
- Carotid artery aneurysms.

Homonymous hemianopia

Caused by:

- Posterior cerebral artery occlusion and infarction of the occipital cortex.
- May have macular (central) sparing.

Lesions affecting the optic radiations and internal capsule may cause variable degrees of visual loss (including homonymous visual impairment affecting just one quadrant).

Other causes of visual loss are summarized in Fig. 8.17.

Some causes of visual loss	
Acute	**Chronic**
Retinal detachment	Refractive error
Acute closed-angle glaucoma	Cataracts
Retinal artery occlusion (if temporary known as amaurosis fugax)	Corneal disease and oedema
Optic neuritis	Primary open angle glaucoma
Stroke affecting central visual pathways	Age-related macular degeneration
Migraine	Diabetic retinopathy
	Hereditary retinal disease
	Compression of central visual Pathways, e.g. tumour.
	Drugs: alcohol, methanol, chloroquine

Fig. 8.17 Causes of visual loss.

- Describe the functions of the different structures of the eye. What gives it its structural and nutritional support, transparency and refractive properties?
- What are the structural and functional differences between rods and cones?
- Describe the process of phototransduction.
- How do the retinal cells segregate colour information?
- Discuss the visual pathway between the retina and the visual cortex. Why is this organization advantageous?
- Discuss the functional arrangement of V1.
- What is the difference between attention and perception?
- Discuss the role of eye movements in attention.
- Discuss the difference between closed and open angle glaucoma. Which should you refer immediately as an emergency?

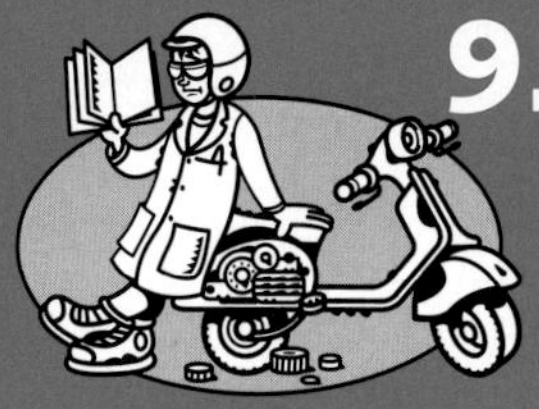

9. Hearing

In this chapter, you will learn about:

- The anatomy of the ear.
- How sound waves are transduced into neural signals.
- The central pathways of hearing.
- Special speech areas.
- Deafness and its causes.

The ear and conduction of sound

Sound waves are variations in pressure (i.e. alternating increased and decreased pressure) transmitted through the air.

Sound is principally defined in terms of its amplitude (loudness) and frequency (pitch).

- Amplitude is measured on a logarithmic scale—the decibel (dB)—as there is such a wide variation in the sound intensities the human ear can detect. For human hearing, $dB = 20 \times \log_{10}(P/P_o)$ where P = sound pressure; P_o = the average auditory threshold for frequencies from 1000 to 3000 Hz (20 mpascals or 0.002 dynes/cm^2). Thus, a 20 dB change is equal to a tenfold increase (+20 dB) or decrease (–20 dB) in loudness. Sound pressures greater than 100 dB may damage the cochlea.
- Frequency is measured on a linear scale (cycles/sec or hertz, Hz). Normal hearing occurs over the range from 20 Hz to 20 000 Hz.

The auditory system consists of the hearing apparatus (outer ear, middle ear and inner ear) and a pathway from the inner ear to the brainstem and auditory cortex.

Anatomy of the auditory apparatus

Fig. 9.1 depicts the auditory apparatus.

Outer ear

The pinna and external ear canal form a tube closed at one end by the tympanic membrane. This tube has a resonant frequency of 3 kHz. The threshold for hearing in the frequency range 2.5–4 kHz is

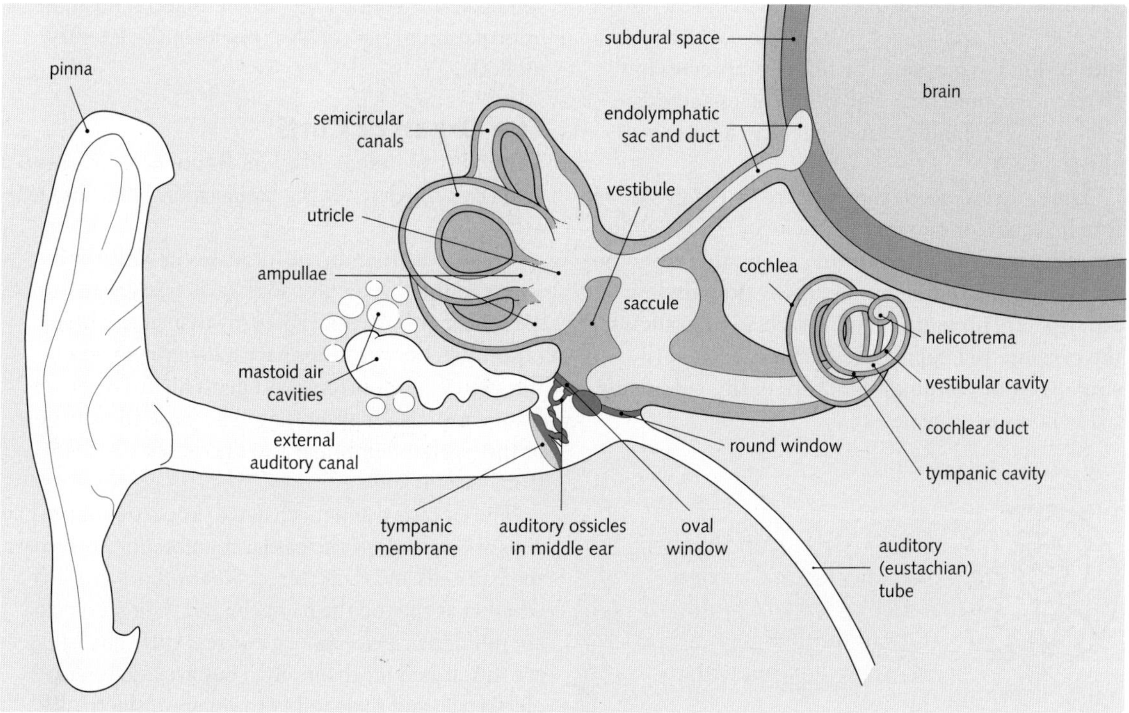

Fig. 9.1 Components and relations of the outer, middle and inner ear.

therefore decreased by –15 dB (i.e. these frequencies are easier to hear).

Middle ear

Alternating air pressure (the sound wave) makes the tympanic membrane vibrate. The ossicles vibrate along with it.

- The malleus (hammer) which is attached to the tympanic membrane itself.
- The incus (anvil) which provides a bridge across the middle ear.
- The stapes (stirrup) whose base plate sits in the oval window at the entrance to the cochlea.

The surface area of the base plate is much less (1/17th) than that of the tympanic membrane. Together with the mechanical advantage of the lever system of the incus and malleus (at frequencies near 1000 Hz), this amplifies the pressure changes by 1.3×17 or 22-fold (+28 dB). This ensures that sound waves are transmitted efficiently from air to the fluid-filled cochlea.

Vibrations of the ossicular chain are dampened down when they become extreme. Two muscles perform this function:

- The tensor tympani muscle on the malleus.
- The stapedius muscle on the stapes.

The reflex contraction of these muscles has a delay of 50–100 msec and cannot protect the cochlea from a sudden loud explosion. The reflex suppresses low frequencies more than high frequencies and may explain how we understand speech in a noisy environment.

The eardrum needs the pressure on either side of it to be equal for maximum efficiency. The middle ear mucosa constantly absorbs air, and therefore the pressure in the middle ear gradually drops below atmospheric pressure. The Eustachian tube allows the pressure to equilibrate when it is opened (by swallowing or yawning). Blockage of this tube leads to a relative hearing defect.

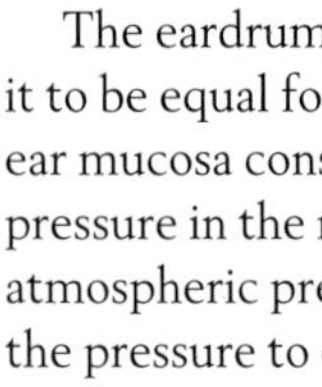

Tensor tympani and stapedius are activated milliseconds before speech, to protect the ear from the high sound intensities created within the head.

Inner ear

The cochlea is a spiral tunnel (with 2.5–3 turns, 32 mm long with a diameter of 2 mm) divided into three compartments running the whole of its length. The upper compartment (scala vestibuli) and lower compartment (scala tympani) communicate at the apex of the spiral (at the helicotrema). They contain a fluid called perilymph which resembles cerebrospinal fluid. Vibration of the base plate of the stapes causes movement in the perilymph in the scala vestibuli.

The scala media (cochlear duct) lies between the scala vestibuli and the scala tympani, and contains a fluid called endolymph. Endolymph has a high potassium concentration and therefore a positive potential (80 mV) with respect to the perilymph. The organ of Corti rests on the basilar membrane inside the cochlear duct. The cochlear duct is separated from the scala vestibuli by Reissner's membrane and from the scala tympani by the basilar membrane (Fig. 9.2).

Movement of the perilymph following displacements of the oval window makes the basilar membrane vibrate. This is then transmitted to the hair cells in the organ of Corti, which convert vibrations of their cilia into oscillating changes in their membrane potential. Cranial nerve VIII afferent neurons, whose cell bodies lie in the bony spiral lamina, contact the hair cells and send auditory information to the cochlear nuclei in the lateral medulla.

The Organ of Corti

The ability to detect different frequencies of sound is given by properties of the basilar membrane and hair cells.

The basilar membrane increases in width as it winds round the cochlea so that its transverse fibres are longer at the apex (500 μm) than at the base (100 μm). Longer fibres have a lower resonant frequency and shorter ones have a higher resonant frequency. This is accentuated because the stiffness of the basilar membrane also decreases 100-fold from base to apex.

The electrical and mechanical properties of the hair cells also vary along the basilar membrane. At the base, the hair cells and their stereocilia are short and stiff whereas at the top the hair cells and their stereocilia are more than twice as long and less stiff. The hair cells are thus tuned mechanically. They are also tuned electrically and their ability to generate electrical oscillations matches their mechanical tuning.

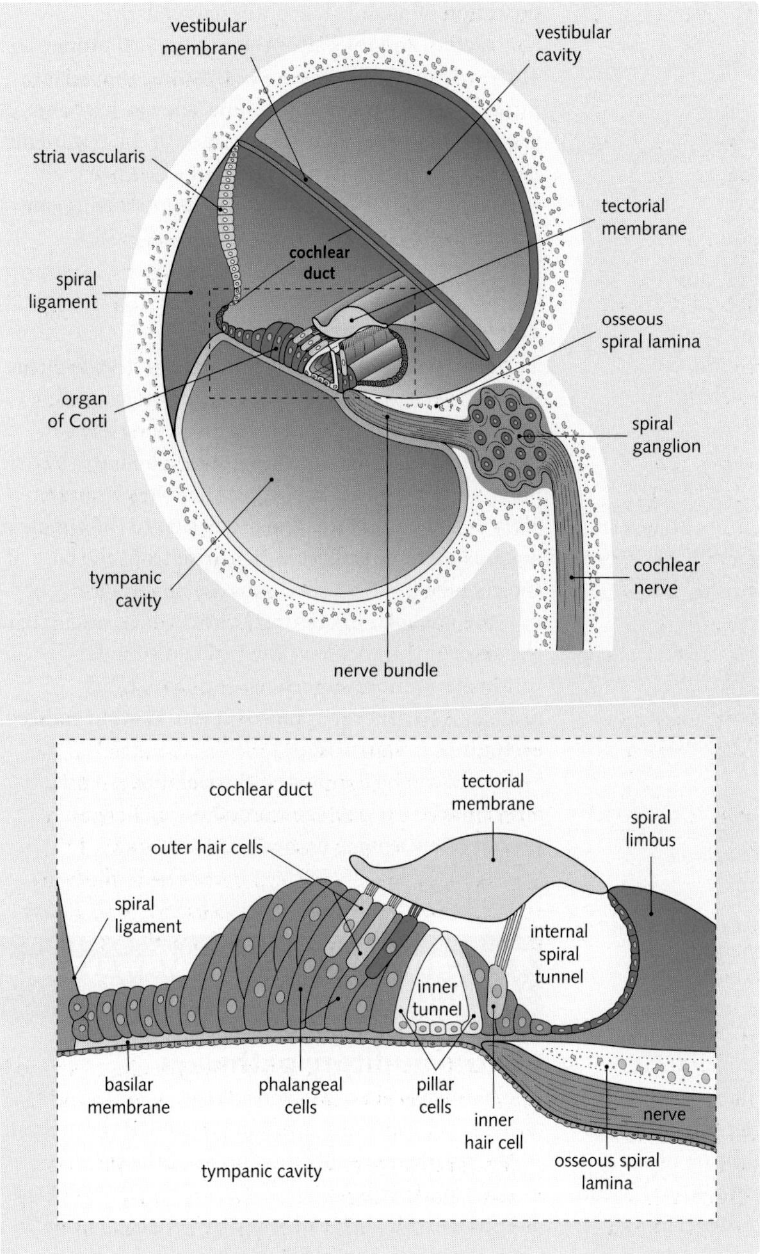

Fig. 9.2 The organ of Corti, lying in the cochlea.

The afferent fibres from the apical part of the cochlea therefore carry low-frequency sound signals, whereas those from the basal part of the cochlea carry high-frequency signals.

Transduction of vibration

The hair cells convert oscillating movements of stereocilia into neuronal signals.

Vibrations of the basilar membrane result in oscillating movement of the hair cells (Fig. 9.3). The stereocilia projecting from the upper surface of the hair cells are fixed at their extracellular end to the immobile tectorial membrane. They sway with the same frequency as the part of the basilar membrane that the hair cells rest upon.

This results in oscillating changes in the physical arrangement of the hair cell membrane and, consequently, changes in the structure of membrane ion channels. Fluctuations in ion permeability are produced, leading to oscillations of membrane potential with the same frequency as the basilar membrane (note that the maximum firing rate of a

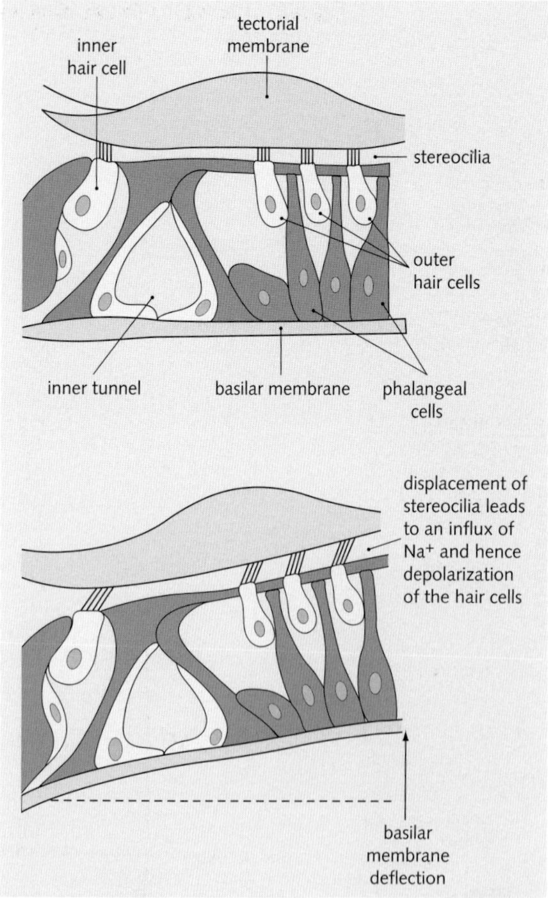

Fig. 9.3 Vibration of the organ of Corti causes bending of hair cell stereocilia, resulting in an oscillating depolarization/hyperpolarization.

nerve fibre has an upper limit of around 500 Hz so that the transduction process is not linear). Interpretation of the signals from the cochlea is probably due to the tonotopic organization of the auditory pathway for frequencies above 4000 Hz and to phase locking of the nerve action potentials for frequencies below 4000 Hz.

Control over sensitivity

Hair cells are arranged in rows on either side of the pillar cells—three rows of outer cells and one row of inner cells. The inner and outer rows have different functions based on the different proportions of output-signalling fibres and input-controlling fibres that contact them.

As a general rule, afferent neurons contact the base of the inner cells and efferents (from the superior olivary complex) contact the base of the outer cells. Inner hair cells are responsible for the detection of sound. The outer hair cells are contractile, and may alter the mechanical properties of the tectorial membrane. In this way, they may provide a mechanism for 'tuning' the ear to sounds of particular interest. The importance of the outer hair cells can be shown by the fact that excessive exposure to some antibiotics (e.g. gentamicin) can lead to deafness, even though such antibiotics exclusively damage the outer hair cells.

Tonotopic mapping

The spatial separation of frequencies in the cochlea (i.e. each auditory fibre conveys information of a restricted part of the auditory spectrum) leads to frequency selectivity of the cells to which the VIIIth nerve fibres project. Tonotopic mapping occurs as early in the pathway as the projection to the cochlear nucleus. Afferent fibres which arise from the base of the cochlea (high pitched sounds) penetrate deeply into the nucleus. In contrast, fibres which originate at the apex of the cochlea (low-pitched sounds) terminate in more superficial regions. This is analogous to other mapping systems in other sensory systems (e.g. somatotopy).

Sound can be conducted through bone. Thus, after middle ear damage, some hearing may be preserved by relying on bone conduction.

The central auditory pathways and the auditory cortex

Central auditory pathways

The pathways are organized so that:

- The tonotopic organization is retained throughout the pathways to different areas of the primary auditory cortex.
- Inputs from both ears interact with each other in the process of sound localization.

Fig. 9.4 shows that VIIIth nerve afferent fibres terminate in the dorsal and ventral cochlear nuclei, at the level of the inferior cerebellar peduncle. From here, there are two main pathways:

- Fibres from the dorsal cochlear nucleus pass in the dorsal acoustic stria, then cross to the opposite side to join the lateral lemniscus and terminate in the contralateral inferior colliculus.
- Most fibres from the ventral cochlear nucleus pass ventrally and cross to the opposite side in the trapezoid body. Some fibres end in the superior

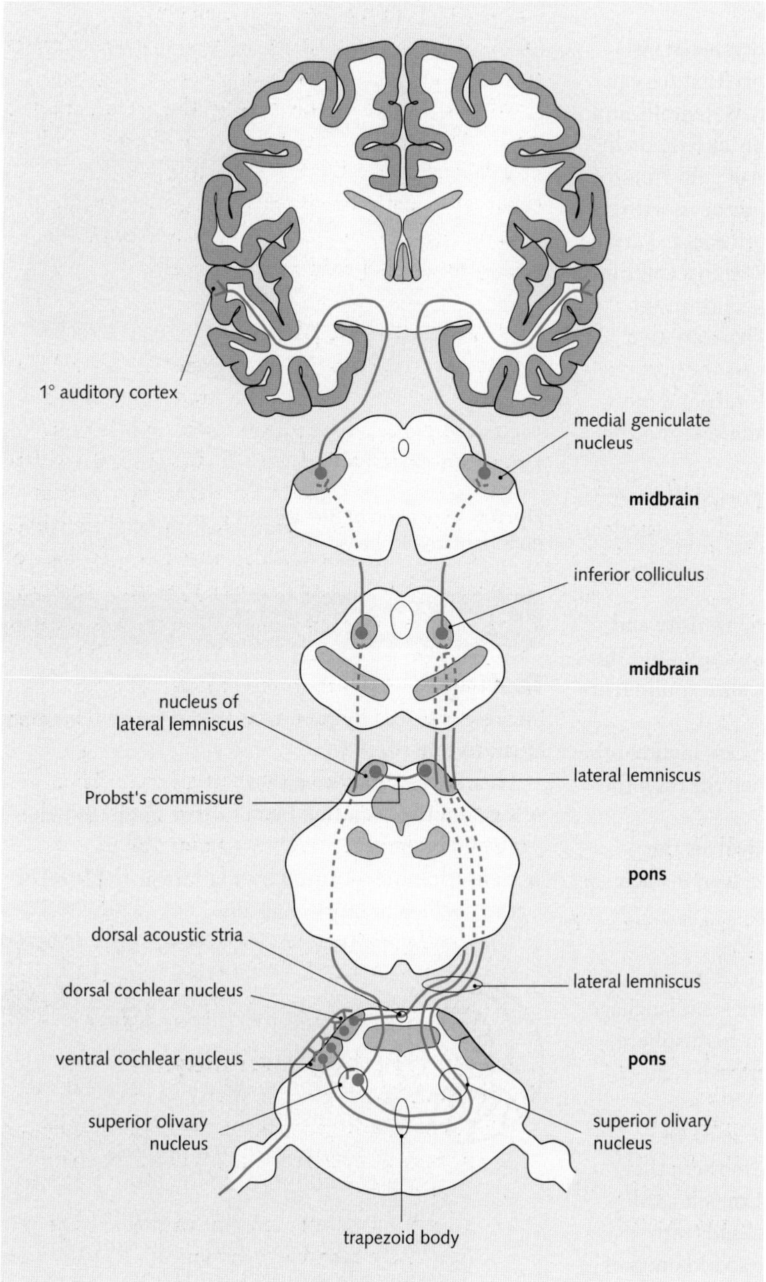

Fig. 9.4 Central auditory pathways.

olivary complex on both sides. Others continue upwards in the lateral lemniscus to the contralateral inferior colliculus. The medial part of the superior olive receives information from both ears. This is believed to be important for sound localization. Fibres from the superior olive project to the inferior colliculi, on both sides, via the lateral lemnisci.

- Fibres from the inferior colliculus project, bilaterally, to the medial geniculate nuclei of the thalamus and, from there, to the ipsilateral primary auditory cortex, on the superomedial aspect of the temporal lobe.

Damage to one side of the central auditory pathway at any level (other than the cochlear nerve) will not result in deafness in one ear. This is because of the bilateral projections to the auditory cortex, both directly and by communication between pathways.

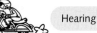

Auditory cortex

The auditory cortex is functionally organized into tonotopic maps of the frequency range that we can hear, with low frequencies represented rostrally and laterally and high frequencies caudally and medially. This gives rise to isofrequency bands of cells running mediolaterally across the primary auditory cortex.

Cells responding to input from both ears to varying degrees are arranged into columns. Within a column, the cells have a similar frequency response and the same binaural response properties. There are two types of column, which alternate across the cortex:

- Suppression columns, where cells respond more strongly to input from one ear, and these may be involved in sound localization.
- Summation columns, where cells respond more strongly to stimulation of both ears than either ear separately.

The cortex uses differences in sound intensity and time of arrival at each ear to localize sounds, and the function of each hemisphere is to localize sound from the contralateral side of space.

- From 200 Hz to 2000 Hz, the process involves the delay between a sound reaching one ear then the other (interaural delay).
- From 2000 Hz to 20 000 Hz, it involves the difference in sound intensity perceived in each ear (interaural intensity differences).

Speech processing

In most people, one hemisphere carries out language processing and is called the dominant hemisphere, usually being the left hemisphere for both right-handed and left-handed people.

Wernicke's area in the temporal lobe on the dominant side is an auditory association area that integrates sound information so that meaningful speech can be recognized. It codes sounds into phonemes, which are the most basic sound units of spoken language.

Broca's area in the frontal lobe on the dominant side processes the motor programmes that are sent to the vocal muscles, producing speech. It matches up a desired phoneme with the motor commands to produce that phoneme.

In speech production, connections between Wernicke's area and Broca's area ensure that the sounds that we wish to make are actually made.

Speech processing involves other areas, such as the frontal lobe (Fig. 9.5).

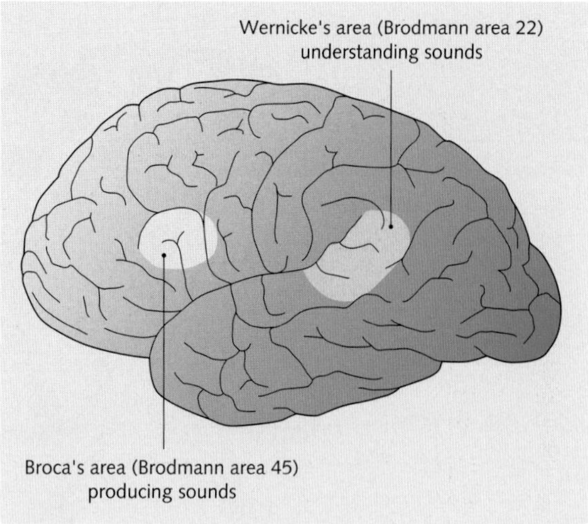

Fig. 9.5 Location of Broca's and Wernicke's areas in the dominant hemisphere.

Loss of hearing

Testing

Hearing is tested by pure-tone audiograms. These are illustrated in Fig. 9.6.

Hearing loss may be either:

- Conductive—caused by failure of sound to reach the inner ear.
- Sensorineural—caused by a failure at the level of the cochlea or more centrally.

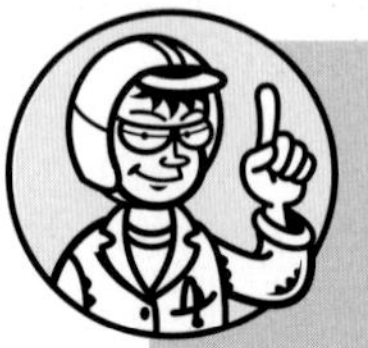

Rinne's test distinguishes between the two forms of deafness. A tuning fork is used to test each ear separately. In conductive hearing loss, sound is perceived more clearly if the base of the tuning fork is placed against the mastoid process. This overcomes the conduction deficit, and allows vibrations to reach the ossicular chain.

Sensorineural deafness

- Lesions within the cochlea itself (Fig. 9.7).
- Lesions within the petrous temporal bone (trauma, complications of middle ear infection, tumours).
- Lesions at the cerebellopontine angle (particularly acoustic neuromas, but also meningiomas and inflammatory damage such as meningitis).

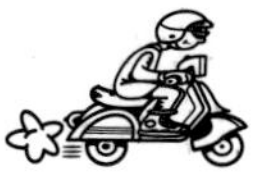

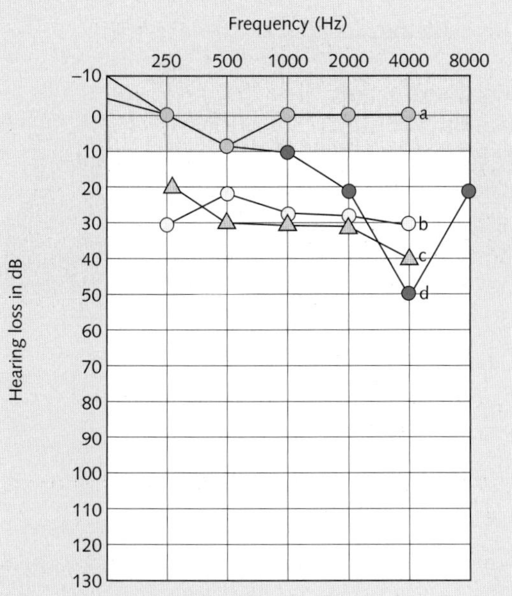

Fig. 9.6 Pure-tone audiograms—air conduction shown as circles, bone conduction as triangles. (a) Normal (b) Conductive hearing loss (c) Sensorineural hearing loss (d) Noise induced high-frequency loss.

- Cortical or pontine lesions causing deafness are rare.

Ménière's disease

This is a disease of uncertain aetiology, probably due to a build-up of endolymph. Characteristic symptoms are:

- Sensorineural deafness.
- Ringing in the ears (tinnitus).
- Vertigo with vomiting, balance disturbance and nystagmus.

It tends to be a recurrent disease and the vertigo, in particular, may be very disabling.

Management includes rest, antipsychotic drugs for the acute attack (prochlorperazine) and histamine analogues for prophylaxis (e.g. betahistine). Ultimately, surgical drainage of endolymph, destruction of the labyrinth or section of the vestibular nerve may be required.

Causes of sensorineural deafness within the inner ear

Ménière's disease
Drugs (e.g. gentamicin)
Congenital infection (rubella, syphilis)
Trauma (excessive exposure to noise, birth asphyxia)
Advancing age

Fig. 9.7 Causes of sensorineural deafness within the inner ear.

Conductive hearing loss

Causes include:

- Perforation of the tympanic membrane.
- Fluid or infection in the middle ear.
- Disorders of the ossicles.

Cochlear implants

This relatively new technique is designed to provide benefit to those people with profound deafness who do not benefit from a traditional amplification hearing aid. It comprises:

- An electrode which is surgically inserted into the cochlea.
- An external processing device (which may be sub-cutaneous).
- An external microphone.

Patients hear sounds, which are very different from what we hear. Approximately 50% will be able to discriminate speech without having to lipread. Their own speech also generally improves. It may be particularly successful in children.

- What are the auditory ossicles? Where are they located and what is their function?
- Explain the process of auditory signal transduction.
- Compare the function of inner and outer hair cells.
- How does the brain localize sound? Explain the central pathways involved.
- Explain the term 'tonotopic organization'.
- What is the difference between sensorineural deafness and conductive deafness? How might they be treated?

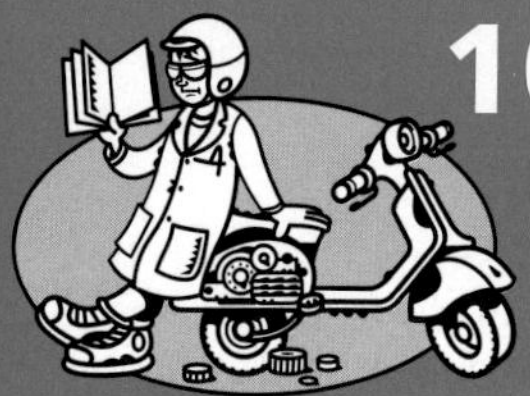

10. Olfaction and Taste

In this chapter, you will learn about:

- Receptors for smell and taste.
- The central pathways for olfaction.
- The central pathways of taste.

Receptors for smell and taste

Olfactory receptors

Olfactory receptors are located in the epithelial lining of the nasal cavity, as shown in Fig. 10.1.

Mechanisms of the sense of smell

Odours enter the mucus film of the olfactory epithelium and diffuse to the receptor cell cilia. Interaction with specific binding proteins on the ciliary surface results in changes in a second-messenger pathway. This might involve cAMP, causing Na^+ channels to open and producing depolarization in the region of the cilia.

There are many olfactory receptor proteins, which allow recognition of thousands of different odorants and at very low concentrations (parts per 10^{12}).

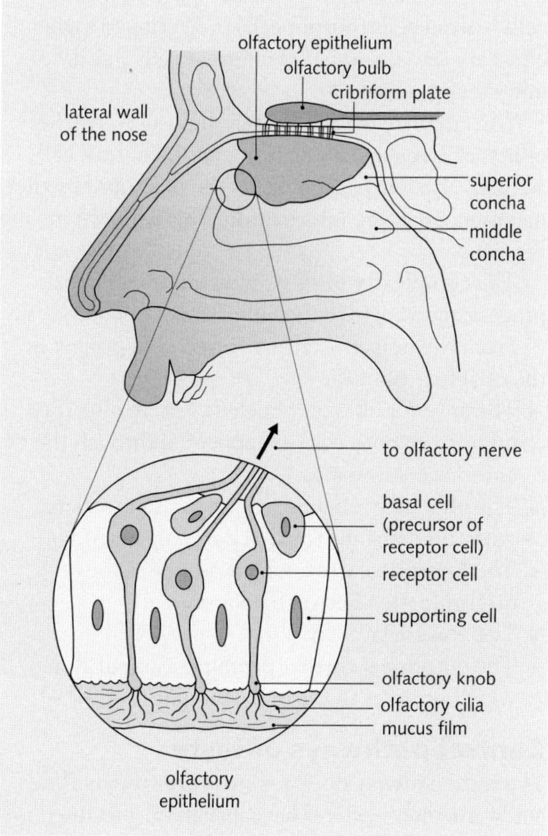

Fig. 10.1 Location and structure of the olfactory epithelium.

Taste receptors

Clusters (50–150) of taste receptors are found in the 2000–5000 taste buds in the epithelial layer of the tongue, palate and pharynx. The base of each receptor cell is innervated by a branch of a primary afferent fibre, forming a type of synapse. Their superior surface is covered in microvilli and mucus. Hydrophobic compounds can therefore reach the receptors by dissolving in the mucus, whereas hydrophilic substances dissolve in the saliva.

In the tongue, taste buds are located on different types of papillae, as shown in Fig. 10.2.

Signal transduction varies for the four taste modalities:

- Saltiness is detected by Na^+ ions passing through an amiloride-sensitive channel to depolarize the receptor cell membrane, resulting in transmitter release that activates the primary afferent fibre.
- Sourness is caused by H^+-ion production by acids. These depolarize the cell in two ways: directly by passing through amiloride-sensitive Na^+ channels, causing an inward current, and indirectly by binding to and blocking K^+ channels, which also causes depolarization.
- Sweetness is signalled when molecules bind to a specific receptor site coupled to a G-protein (gustducin). This triggers an increase in cytoplasmic cAMP, which then activates protein kinase A. This phosphorylates K^+ channels, which become blocked, leading to depolarization.
- Bitterness receptors are essentially poison detectors. Some bitter compounds (e.g. quinine) bind directly to and block K^+ channels. Other compounds bind to specific bitter membrane receptors that activate G-protein second-messenger cascades. One type of bitter receptor

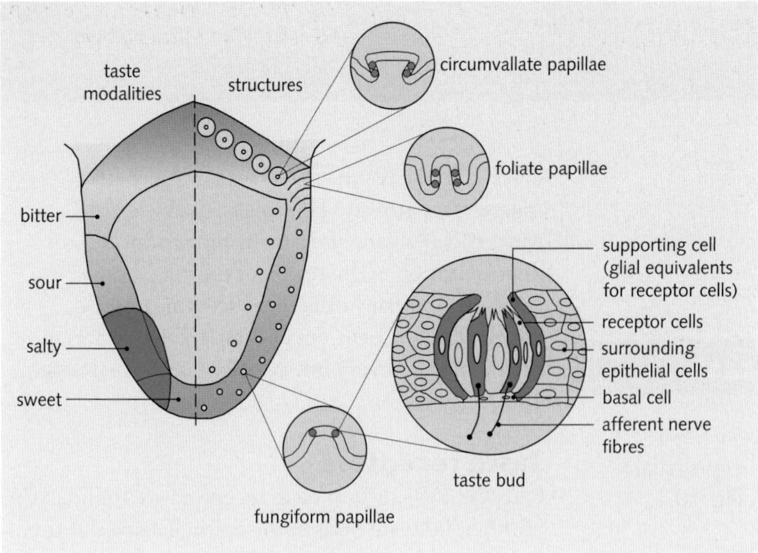

Fig. 10.2 Structure of a taste bud and location of different papillae and taste modalities on the tongue.

produces an increase in intracellular inositol triphosphate (IP_3), causing intracellular Ca^{2+} release. This leads to transmitter release and afferent nerve activation.

Taste afferent neurons are less specific than the receptors because one afferent can innervate several papillae and, in the solitary nucleus, a single cell can receive synapses from many taste afferent neurons. Taste has to be interpreted from broadly tuned input channels.

The brain may interpret taste using other inputs such as smell, temperature and texture.

Central pathways of smell and taste

Central pathways of smell

The fibres of the olfactory nerve (cranial nerve I) pass through the roof of the nose in a perforated bone called the cribriform plate. They synapse in the olfactory bulb at the base of the frontal lobe in regions called 'glomeruli'. These are made up of the diffusely branching dendritic networks of mitral cells, tufted cells (output cells projecting to higher olfactory areas) and periglomerular cells (local inhibitory neurons).

The circuitry in the olfactory bulb allows higher olfactory areas to have an influence on output cell activity; also, output inhibition can be caused by the incoming olfactory information. This is shown in Fig. 10.3.

The complexity of this circuit allows olfactory processing to begin in the bulb.

From the bulb, mitral and tufted cells project in the olfactory tract to:

- The anterior olfactory nucleus, where olfactory input from both sides is connected through the anterior commissure.
- The olfactory tubercle, which has connections with the thalamus (medial dorsal nucleus).
- The pyriform cortex, which processes the discrimination between odours.
- The amygdala.
- The entorhinal cortex (parahippocampal gyrus), which projects to the hippocampus (Fig. 10.4).

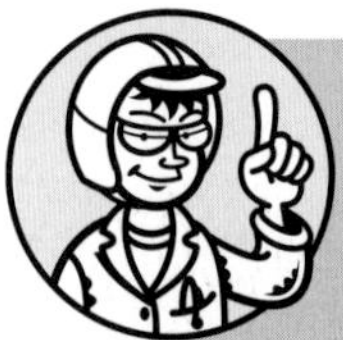

The cribriform plate is a relatively fragile part of the skull. When inserting a nasogastric tube, it should be aimed straight towards the back of the head, and not upwards. Otherwise, an inadvertent frontal lobotomy may result!

Central pathways of taste

The taste pathway does not cross over the midline and so the hemispheres have ipsilateral gustatory perception.

Taste receptors synapse on afferent neurons of cranial nerve VII, IX or X, depending on their

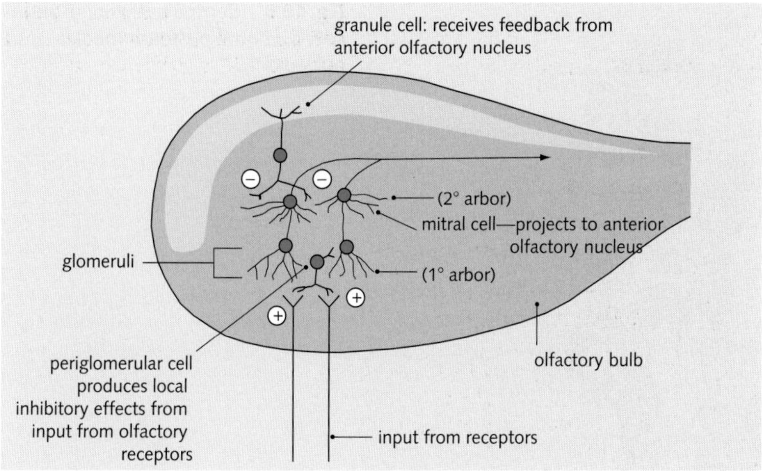

Fig. 10.3 Influences on the efferent fibres from the olfactory bulb.

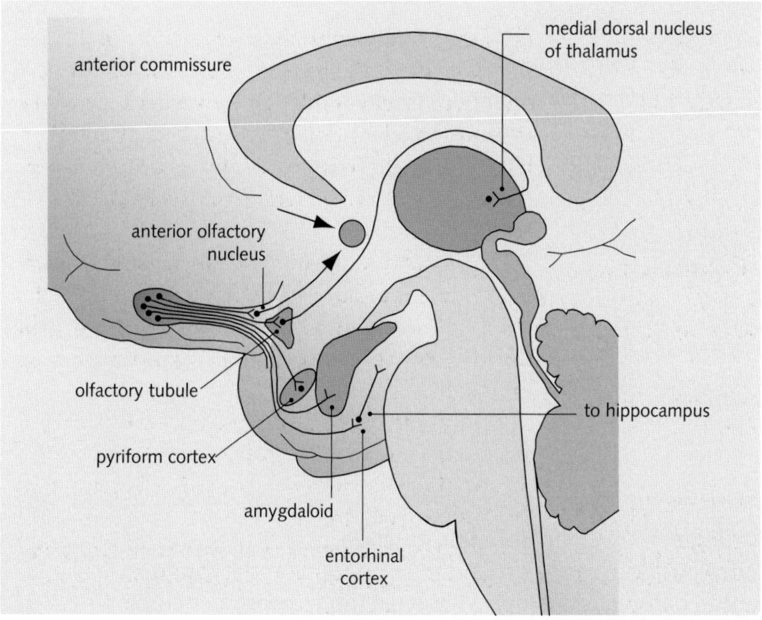

Fig. 10.4 Central pathway of smell.

location. Taste signals from the anterior two-thirds of the tongue are transmitted in the chorda tympani (VIIth cranial nerve). Taste from the posterior one-third of the tongue is relayed in the IXth nerve. The Xth nerve only sends information from the top of the pharynx. The afferent neurons pass into the medulla where they synapse in a part of the nucleus of the solitary tract, called the gustatory nucleus.

The gustatory nucleus projects to the thalamus (ventroposterior medial nucleus) and from the thalamus there are projections to the sensory cortex and the insula (Fig. 10.5).

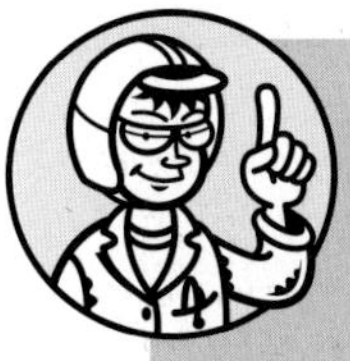

There may also be taste inputs to the hypothalamus and amygdala. Patients with temporal lobe epilepsy often experience gustatory 'auras' immediately prior to a seizure.

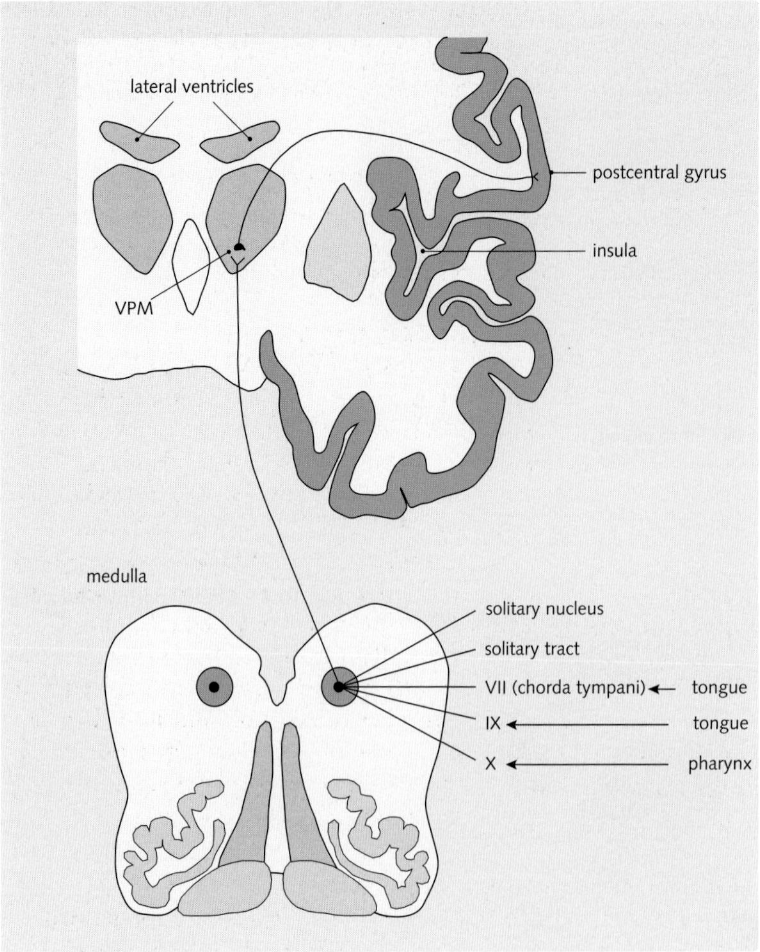

Fig. 10.5 Central pathway of taste. (VPM, ventral posterior medial nucleus).

- Explain briefly the process of olfactory transduction.
- Describe the different taste receptors and their location on the tongue.
- Outline the central pathways of smell. Where are fibres most vulnerable to injury?
- What cranial nerves are involved in the sense of taste?

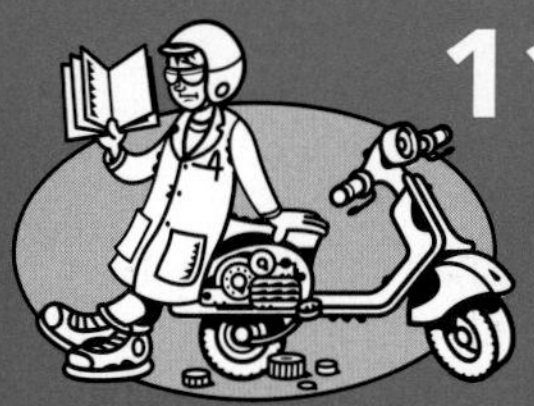

11. Basic Pathology

In this chapter, you will learn about:

- Cerebral oedema, herniation syndromes and hydrocephalus.
- Congenital diseases of the central nervous system.
- Trauma to the central nervous system.
- Cerebrovascular disease and stroke.
- Central nervous system infections.
- Demyelinating disorders.
- Degenerative disorders.
- Metabolic disorders.
- Brain tumours.
- Epilepsy.

Common pathological features of the central nervous system

Introduction

The bones of the cranium fuse in the first 2 years of life, making the skull like a rigid box, with a fixed volume.

Intracranial pressure is determined by the volume of the three contents of the skull—brain, cerebrospinal fluid and blood. None of these three contents is compressible or expandable; therefore, for the intracranial pressure to remain stable, a change in the volume of any of them must be accompanied by an equal and opposite change in the other two. This compensatory mechanism has a limited capacity in terms of speed and magnitude, and its failure results in an increase or decrease in the intracranial pressure (Fig. 11.1).

Cerebral oedema

The skull contains approximately 900–1200 mL of intracellular and 100–150 mL of extracellular fluid. An increase in the volume of either of these two components results in cerebral oedema.

The pathogenesis of cerebral oedema can be divided into three types—vasogenic oedema, cytotoxic oedema and interstitial oedema. These types of oedema usually coexist to variable degrees, depending on the primary pathology.

Vasogenic oedema is usually responsive to treatment with corticosteroids, osmotic diuretics and hyperventilation, whereas cytotoxic oedema is often resistant to these therapies. Ultimately, successful treatment relies on identifying and treating the underlying cause.

Vasogenic oedema

This is an inflammatory intercellular oedema that results from the increased permeability of the capillary endothelial cells. It is caused by either defects in the tight endothelial cell junctions or

Clinical features of raised and low intracranial pressure

	Causes	Symptoms and signs
raised intracranial pressure	space-occupying masses (e.g. tumour, haematoma, abscess) increase in brain water content (oedema) increase in cerebral blood flow volume (e.g. vasodilatation, venous outflow obstruction) increased CSF volume (excessive production, impaired absorption)	early morning headache and vomiting (often without nausea), dizziness, blurred vision, diplopia (usually caused by VI nerve palsy as a false localizing sign), papilloedema, focal sensory and motor neurological signs, depressed consciousness, coma, falling pulse rate and rising blood pressure
low intracranial pressure	decrease in cerebral blood flow volume (e.g. dehydration, blood loss) decrease in CSF volume (e.g. CSF otorrhoea and rhinorhoea, lumbar puncture, surgical CSF shunting)	headache and nausea mainly on sitting or standing

Fig. 11.1 Clinical features of raised and low intracranial pressure.

increased active transport, allowing protein-rich plasma to enter the extracellular space.

Such oedema develops around tumours, abscesses and plaques of multiple sclerosis and affects the white matter predominantly. It may also be seen in trauma, infection and ischaemic areas.

Cytotoxic oedema

This is an intracellular oedema that results from damage in the ATP-dependent sodium pump, leading to the accumulation of sodium, calcium and water within the cells (neurons and glia). It affects grey and white matter.

Such oedema is commonly seen in hypoxic brain damage and dilutional hyponatraemia.

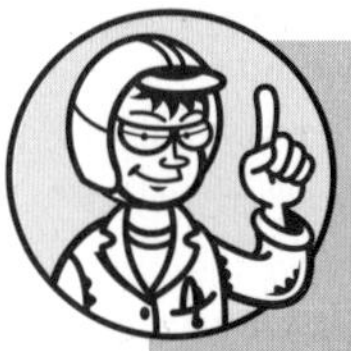

Dilutional hyponatraemia may be caused by over-enthusiastic fluid replacement or syndrome of inappropriate antidiuretic hormone secretion. In rare cases, patients may simply be drinking far too much water. This can be seen with certain psychological problems and with drug abuse (especially 'ecstasy').

Interstitial oedema

This is an extracellular oedema seen particularly in hydrocephalus. It results from the extravasation of the cerebrospinal fluid through the ependymal cells into the extracellular space of the periventricular white matter.

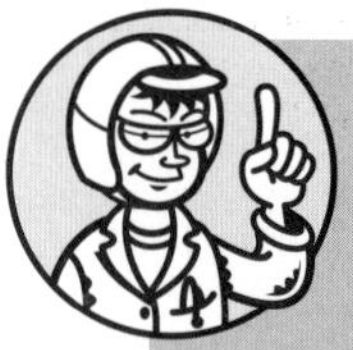

The cerebral circulation autoregulates to maintain blood flow to the brain. It follows the formula: cerebral perfusion pressure = mean arterial pressure – intracranial pressure. Therefore, in conditions such as malignant hypertension, intracranial pressure is increased, and may be very dangerous.

Cerebral herniation

The infoldings of the dura, the falx cerebri (which extends in the midline between the two cerebral hemispheres) and the cerebellar tentorium (the posterior bifurcation of the falx extending laterally over the superior face of the cerebellum with an elongated opening through which the brainstem passes) plus the foramen magnum, divides the brain into semi-separate compartments. When the intracranial volume increases, either due to an increased intracranial pressure or to a space occupying lesion in any of these compartments, the surrounding brain tissue will be pushed away and forced to herniate into an adjacent compartment, with potentially grave consequences.

Cerebral herniation is divided into four types, as shown in Figs 11.2 and 11.3.

Hydrocephalus

This is an increase in the cranial cerebrospinal fluid volume. It can be divided into three types:

- Obstructive (non-communicating) hydrocephalus: caused by a congenital or acquired obstruction in the cerebrospinal fluid pathway resulting in the accumulation of fluid proximal to the block (Fig. 11.4). It may be relieved surgically by shunting (e.g. ventriculoperitoneal shunt) or by endoscopic ventriculostomy.
- Communicating hydrocephalus: caused by either increased cerebrospinal fluid production or, more commonly, decreased cerebrospinal fluid absorption (Fig. 11.5).
- Normal pressure hydrocephalus: gross ventricular enlargement is seen without cortical atrophy on a computed tomography scan. The pathogenesis is unknown, but may be due to a partial obstruction of cerebrospinal fluid flow from the subarachnoid space. The classical clinical triad is: dementia, gait disturbance and early urinary incontinence.

Symptoms and signs of hydrocephalus are given in Fig. 11.6. Investigations that may confirm hydrocephalus include:

- Skull radiography may show changes suggestive of long-standing hydrocephalus (thinning of the skull vault, enlarged pituitary fossa, and erosions of posterior clinoids). This has become second-line now due to the advent of computed tomography.
- Head computed tomography/magnetic resonance imaging shows the pattern of ventricular dilatation and excludes the presence of space-occupying lesions.

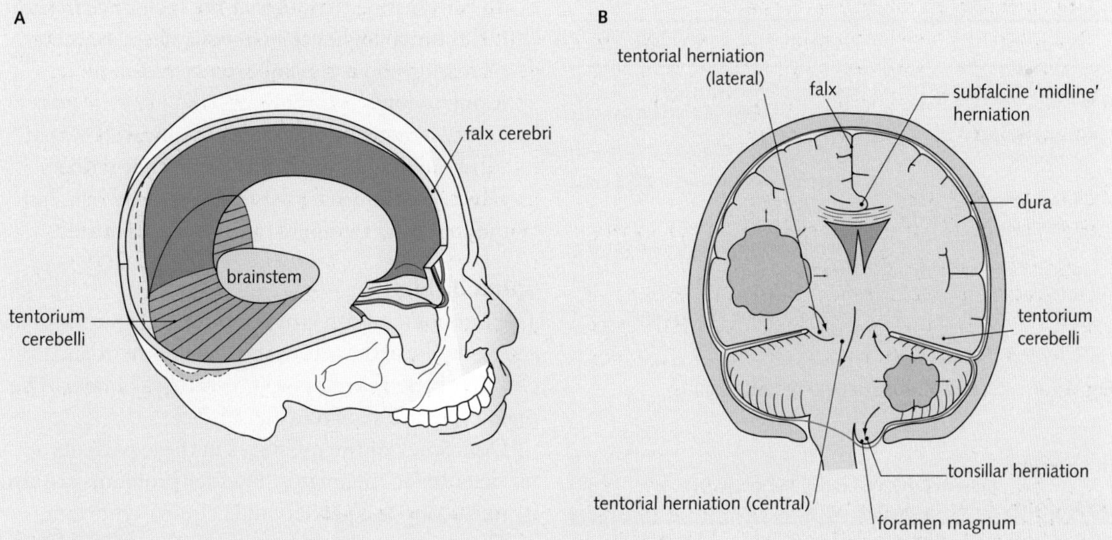

Fig. 11.2 **A.** Shows the infoldings of the dura mater which compartmentalize the brain tissue. **B.** Cerebral herniation (modified from Neurology and Neurosurgery Illustrated by Dr Lindsay *et al.*, Churchill Livingstone, 1991).

Types of cerebral herniation

Clinical type	Aetiology	Clinical signs
type 1: subfalcine herniation	unilateral hemispheric SOL causing that hemisphere to be compressed beneath the falx	frequently seen radiologically, does not usually cause any clinical signs
type 2: lateral tentorial herniation	unilateral hemispheric SOL causing the uncus of the temporal lobe to herniate through the tentorial hiatus; may progress to type 3	ipsilateral third nerve palsy, ipsilateral hemiplegia (contralateral cerebral peduncle compression)
type 3: central tentorial herniation	midline SOL, very large unilateral hemispheric SOL, or bilateral hemispheric diffuse swelling causing a vertical displacement of the diencephalon through the tentorial hiatus; may progress to type 4	impaired upward gaze (pretectum and superior colliculi compression), hemianopia (occipital lobe infarction), hemi/quadriparesis (cerebral peduncle compression), rising blood pressure and bradycardia (aqueduct compression and hydrocephalus), depressed consciousness and respiration (brainstem compression), coma
type 4: tonsillar herniation	unilateral subtentorial SOL causing herniation of the cerebellar tonsils through the foramen magnum	neck pain, tonic extension of the limbs, cardiac arrhythmia and rising blood pressure, depressed consciousness and respiration, coma

Fig. 11.3 Types of cerebral herniation (SOL, space-occupying lesion).

- Transfontanelle ultrasonography is a useful non-invasive test in neonates (which doesn't rely on them being still!).
- Intracranial pressure monitoring (a pressure transducer inserted into the lateral ventricle, brain or subdural space).

Malformations, developmental disease and perinatal injury

Neural tube defects

Neural tube defects are caused by varying degrees of failure of fusion of the neural tube and spinal canal.

Causes of obstructive hydrocephalus	
Congenital	**Acquired**
aqueduct stenosis Dandy–Walker syndrome Arnold–Chiari malformation vein of Galen aneurysm atresia of fourth ventricle foraminae	acquired aqueduct stenosis (adhesion following infection or haemorrhage) intraventricular tumours (colloid cyst, ependymoma) parenchymal tumours (pineal gland, posterior fossa) space-occupying lesion causing tentorial herniation (see Fig. 14.3)

Fig. 11.4 Causes of obstructive hydrocephalus.

Causes of communicating hydrocephalus	
Pathogenesis	**Causes**
reduced absorption by arachnoid granulations	infection (especially TB), subarachnoid haemorrhage, trauma, carcinomatous meningitis
excessive CSF production	choroid plexus papilloma
increased CSF viscosity	high protein content

Fig. 11.5 Causes of communicating hydrocephalus.

The pathogenesis of the disorders is thought to be due to a mixture of:

- Environmental factors—folic acid (folate) taken at the time of conception and in the first trimester of pregnancy reduces the incidence of neural tube defects. Other factors have not been proven, but it is interesting to note that the incidence in the UK is much higher than in Asia, despite greater education about the importance of folate supplements.
- Genetic factors—these are complicated in that subsequent children born to a mother with an affected child have a 10-fold increased risk, but monozygotic twins are rarely both affected.

Spina bifida

The lumbosacral site is most common. Spina bifida is caused by local defects in the development and closure of the neural tube and vertebral arches. The main types are shown in Fig. 11.7.

Deficiency of the meninges in these patients predisposes to meningitis. Bladder problems are also common due to a partial cauda equina syndrome.

The spinal cord may be tethered by a fibrous band or tight filum terminale, associated with increasing deficit as the child grows and the cord stretches. Surgery to release the tethered cord may therefore be indicated.

Anencephaly

Anencephaly represents failure of fusion at the cephalic end of the neural tube. Almost no forebrain structures develop, usually with absence of the skull vault. This condition is not compatible with long-term survival.

Arnold–Chiari malformation

Arnold–Chiari malformation is caused by failure of fusion at the craniocervical junction. The brainstem is displaced downwards, with the cerebellar tonsils

Symptoms and signs of hydrocephalus		
Age	**Onset**	**Symptoms and signs**
infants and young children	acute	vomiting, depressed consciousness, tense fontanelle, enlarging head, lid retraction and impaired upward gaze ('setting sun sign'), long tract signs
	chronic	mental retardation, failure to thrive, increased skull circumference
adults	acute	signs and symptoms of raised intracranial pressure (see Fig. 14.1), impaired upward gaze
	chronic: communicating hydrocephalus	headache and change in mental status
	normal-pressure hydrocephalus	usually in elderly; dementia, gait disturbance, and urninary incontinence

Fig. 11.6 Symptoms and signs of hydrocephalus.

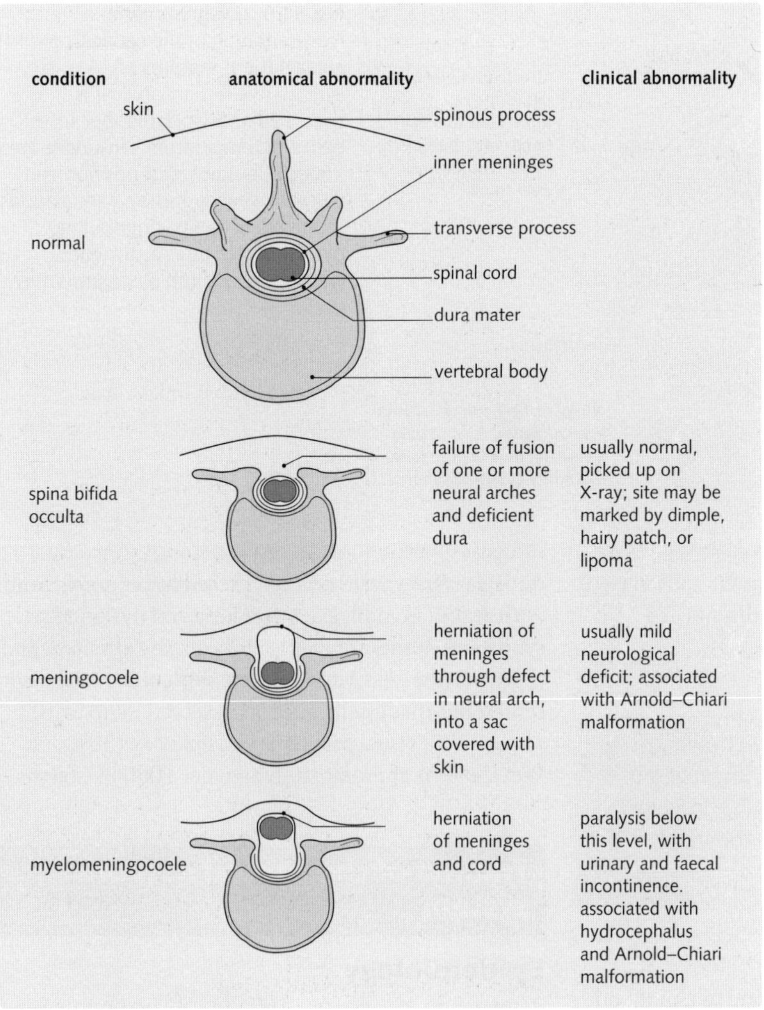

Fig. 11.7 Neural tube defects.

and medulla herniating through the foramen magnum. It is associated with hydrocephalus, especially dilatation of the third and fourth ventricles. Defects may include mental retardation, lower (ocular) cranial nerve palsies and cerebellar/brainstem signs. Complications include syringomyelia.

Prenatal diagnosis of neural tube defects

Open spina bifida and anencephaly are detectable prenatally by a raised alpha-fetoprotein (AFP). The top 3% of maternal serum AFP levels will include most neural tube defects (as well as many normal foetuses and most twin pregnancies). One in ten pregnant women with a high serum AFP level will have an abnormal baby. Confirmation is with ultrasonography and amniocentesis.

Other congenital diseases

Some other congenital diseases are listed below.

- Microcephaly—which can be developmental or caused by intrauterine infection (e.g. with maternal chickenpox in pregnancy).
- Arteriovenous malformations—these also may be associated with epilepsy or subarachnoid haemorrhage.
- Syringomyelia—a fluid-filled cavity within the cord, sometimes extending to the brainstem (syringobulbia), probably due to many different causes. It is not usually symptomatic until adulthood when it expands, sometimes provoked by a sudden increase in intracranial pressure (e.g. a fit of coughing). This is rare, but anatomically interesting. The symptoms of syringomyelia are shown in Fig. 11.8.

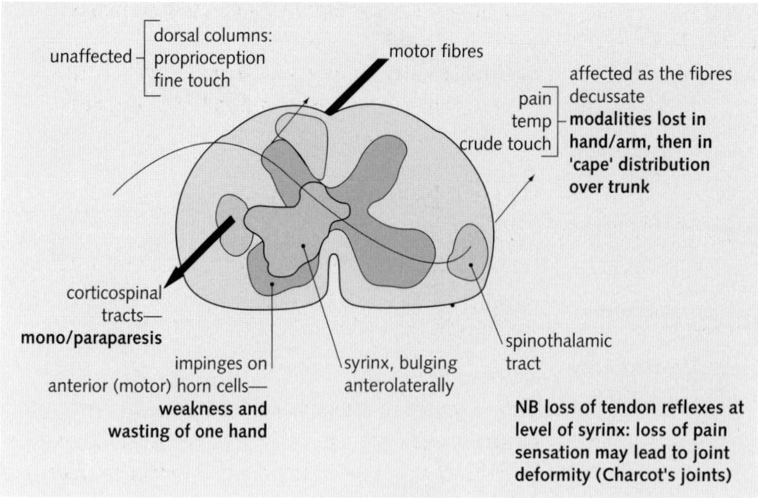

Fig. 11.8 Diagrammatic representation of the cervical cord to explain the symptoms of syringomyelia. Sensory loss is described as dissociated, because pain and temperature sensations are affected, but not joint position and vibration senses. If the cavity extends to the brainstem (syringobulbia), dysarthria, dysphagia, tongue wasting, ataxia and nystagmus may occur.

- Diastematomyelia—the spinal cord is split in two, sometimes with a bony spur. It presents as a slowly progressive cord syndrome.

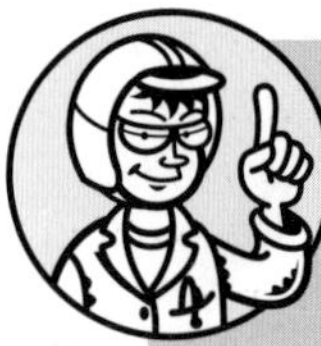

Patients who have had a spinal cord injury are at increased risk of developing syringomyelia many years after the initial injury.

Cerebral palsy

Cerebral palsy is a heterogeneous group of childhood disorders in which injury to the brain early in life results in a non-progressive neurological disorder of movement and tone (Fig. 11.9). Birth trauma, although the most widely known cause, actually only accounts for approximately 10% of cases. Spastic diplegia is the most common presentation, sometimes with ataxia, hemiplegia, tetraplegia and dyskinetic syndrome. Other modalities may also be affected, and there may be associated learning difficulties (although remember that intelligence is preserved in up to 70% of patients), visual problems and epilepsy (30%). Prevalence is approximately two per 1000 live births.

Prenatal, perinatal, and postnatal causes of cerebral palsy

Type	Cause
prenatal	intrauterine infection (especially TORCH) difficulties in pregnancy; e.g. pre-eclampsia, intracranial haemorrhage
perinatal	asphyxia kernicterus
postnatal	infection respiratory distress syndrome

Fig. 11.9 Prenatal, perinatal, and postnatal causes of cerebral palsy.

Trauma of the central nervous system

Epidemiology

Approximately 300 per 100 000 of the population require hospital admission annually for head injuries, with an annual death incidence of nine per 100 000. Approximately one-half of those admitted are under the age of 20 years. The principal causes include road traffic accidents, falls, assaults, and industrial, domestic and sports injuries. Alcohol is frequently involved. Although road traffic accidents are the cause of head injury in only 25% of all cases, they contribute to 60% of total fatalities.

Mechanisms

Trauma resulting in brain and spinal cord injuries is of three types:

- Penetrating injuries (e.g. high-velocity missile injuries, gunshot wounds).
- Crush injuries (e.g. industrial injuries).
- Acceleration/deceleration injuries (e.g. road traffic accidents).

Brain damage is a result of contusion and laceration of the cerebral cortex, often involving the frontal and temporal lobes. Deceleration injuries also cause diffuse white matter axonal damage.

Skull fractures

Fractures affecting the vault or the base of the skull are an indication that a significant head injury has occurred. They are of two types:

- Linear fractures.
- Depressed fractures—inner table is depressed by at least the thickness of the skull. The overlying scalp is either intact (simple depressed fractures) or lacerated (compound fractures).

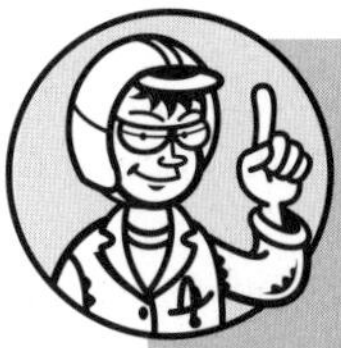

Basal skull fractures may not be immediately obvious. Signs include bilateral 'black eyes', bruising over the mastoid process (Battle's sign) and subconjunctival haemorrhage with no clear posterior margin (indicating blood tracking forward). Avoid nasogastic tubes and nasal airways in these patients.

When suspected, a skull radiograph and/or a computed tomagraphy scan should be obtained to confirm the diagnosis.

Complications of skull fractures are:

- Extradural haematoma—often caused by linear fractures crossing the middle meningeal groove and causing the rupture of the middle meningeal artery. This may be indicated by a 'lucid interval' after the injury, with a subsequently decreasing conscious level.
- Cerebrospinal fluid rhinorrhoea (cerebrospinal fluid leak from the nose)—caused by skull base fractures tearing the dura in the floor of the anterior fossa and the nasal mucosa. This might occasionally be accompanied by pneumatocoeles and fluid (visible on radiographs), particularly in the sphenoidal sinuses.
- Cerebrospinal fluid otorrhoea (cerebrospinal fluid leak from the ear) caused by fractures of the petrous temporal bone.
- Infection—particularly with compound fractures and persistent cerebrospinal fluid fistulae (cerebrospinal fluid rhinorrhoea and otorrhoea), in which case prophylactic antibiotic cover is needed.
- Post-traumatic epilepsy—particularly with compound fractures and dural tears causing cortical scarring.

Parenchymal damage

Primary effect

Loss of consciousness is the hallmark of impact brain damage. This might or might not be associated with structural cerebral damage.

Concussion

This term is often used to describe minor head injuries causing temporary loss of consciousness without macroscopic structural cerebral damage. However, microscopic neuronal damage often occurs. The effect of repeated minor head injury is cumulative (e.g. the 'punch drunk syndrome' in boxers).

Contusion/laceration

The skull and the different parts of the brain have different resistances to the movement induced by the accelerating force. When the head is hit by a moving object (or the moving head hits a static object), the brain is accelerated within the skull, and local brain contusion and laceration (coup) occur. This is particularly severe on the undersurface of the frontal and temporal lobes as the brain hits the sphenoidal wing, the petrous temporal bones and the other non-compliant dural structures. It is usually accompanied by a similar brain injury (contrecoup) at the side directly opposite the local trauma.

Diffuse axonal injury

The combination of linear and rotational acceleration of the brain and the differences in compliance between the white and the grey matter result in tearing of fibres and diffuse axonal injury. This can be identified pathologically by the presence of 'axon retraction balls' and microglial clusters, the number of which depends on the duration of survival and the severity of the head injury.

Secondary effect

Impact brain damage is unavoidable; however, head injury induces other delayed pathological processes, which may be preventable and are potentially treatable. The presenting symptoms of these complications depend on the severity of the initial head injury, but they should be suspected if further deterioration to the level of consciousness occurs or new focal neurological signs develop. Note that haemorrhage is a cause of raised intracranial pressure, and may therefore compromise cerebral perfusion. Intracranial pressure monitoring may be indicated.

Intracerebral haemorrhage

Intracerebral haemorrhage arises if arteries or veins crossing the brain tissue are torn. It occurs commonly in the frontal and temporal lobes and is often associated with overlying subdural haemorrhage. In severe head injuries, intracerebral haematoma mixed with necrotic brain tissue might rupture out into the subdural space, giving a 'burst lobe' appearance.

Acute subdural haemorrhage

This is a venous haemorrhage caused by tearing to the superficial veins. It is often associated with damage to the surface of the cerebral hemisphere. Pure subdural haemorrhage with no underlying cortical damage can also occur due to the rupture of the veins bridging from the cortical surface to the venous sinuses.

Extradural haemorrhage

This is an arterial haemorrhage caused by skull fractures tearing the middle meningeal vessels. It usually occurs in the temporal and temporoparietal regions. Such a haemorrhage can occasionally be caused by ruptured venous sinuses.

Subarachnoid haemorrhage

Traumatic subarachnoid haemorrhage occurs in most moderate to severe head injuries. Headache, restlessness and confusion are the most prominent clinical features. It is often difficult to differentiate between traumatic subarachnoid haemorrhage and aneurysmal subarachnoid haemorrhage complicated by depressed consciousness and subsequent head injury.

Cerebral swelling

Cerebral swelling is a common delayed complication of severe head injuries. It may or may not be associated with intracranial haematoma. The exact mechanism is unknown, but it is often associated with early vasodilatation or an increase in the extracellular or intracellular fluid volume.

Other complications

Other complications are:

- Cerebral ischaemia caused by hypoxia, impaired cerebral perfusion, or delayed vasospasm.
- Tentorial and tonsillar herniation caused by raised intracranial pressure.
- Infection presenting as meningitis or brain abscess in association with compound skull fractures.

Chronic subdural haematoma

Chronic subdural haematoma presents a different clinical picture compared with acute subdural haematoma. It occurs typically in middle-aged and elderly people. A history of high alcohol consumption is common, but a history of head injury is absent in approximately one-half of cases. Patients present with headache and fluctuating confusion. This should be considered in someone with a vague history of delirium (acute confusional state) or with rapidly progressing symptoms which suggest dementia.

Management

The majority of head injuries are mild and require no specific treatment. In severe head injuries, the principles of management are:

- Adequate airway and oxygenation should be ensured (ensuring that the cervical spine is protected if there is any chance of neck injury).
- Assessment of associated injuries and treatment of hypovolaemia should be initiated.

Secondary complications should be managed as follows:

- Intracranial haematomas should be treated with appropriate neurosurgical procedures.
- Cerebral swelling should be treated with mannitol, steroids, and ventilation (to maintain low arterial carbon dioxide).
- Antibiotic cover might be indicated.

Neurological sequelae of head injuries

Common neurological sequelae of head injuries are:

- Retrograde and post-traumatic amnesia.
- Focal neurological deficits.
- Post-traumatic epilepsy.
- Postconcussion syndrome.

Post-traumatic epilepsy

The factors associated with a high risk of post-traumatic epilepsy are:

- Seizures or focal neurological signs in the first week after the head injury.
- Intracranial haematoma.
- Depressed skull fractures, particularly if the dura is torn.
- Post-traumatic amnesia lasting more than 24 hours.

Injuries to the vertebral column and spinal cord

The annual incidence of injuries to the vertebral column and spinal cord is approximately two per 100 000.

In 50% of cases, spinal trauma involves the cervical spine. Injuries to the vertebral column may occur without evidence of cord or spinal nerve injuries; similarly, damage to the neural elements might present without demonstrable injuries to the bone. Neurological damage may result from any of the following four pathological processes:

- Oedema, which occurs early and subsides after a few days.
- Haemorrhage—a degree of haemorrhage into the cord (haematomyelia) is almost a constant feature following major spinal trauma. Haemorrhage into the extradural, subdural, or subarachnoid spaces may also occur and could compress the cord.
- Compression of the cord by fractured or misaligned vertebrae.
- Transection of the cord by elements of the vertebral column.

Clinical features depend on the level of injury and the extent of the lesion. The initial spinal shock (transient suppression of nervous function, including reflexes, below the level of injury) begins to subside after a few weeks, and is replaced by spastic weakness.

The principles of management of spinal injuries are:

- Immobilization to prevent further neural damage.
- Preservation of skin integrity (pressure areas).
- Preservation of bladder and bowel function.
- Management of complications (respiratory, cardiovascular, gastrointestinal).
- Long-term rehabilitation—preferably in specialist centres, which are associated with a better outcome.

Cerebrovascular disease

The risk factors for cerebrovascular disease are:

- Hypertension.
- Diabetes.
- Cardiac diseases: cardiac arrhythmias (particularly atrial fibrillation), valvular heart disease, congenital heart disease and infective endocarditis.
- Obesity, hyperlipidaemia and smoking.
- Alcohol.
- Genetic factors.
- Polycythaemia.
- Other factors: male sex, increasing age, previous cerebrovascular disease, illicit drugs (crack cocaine), antiphospholipid syndrome and homocystinuria.

Hypoxia, ischaemia and infarction

There are almost no tissue stores of oxygen or glucose in the brain. When the blood supply fails, the brain ceases to function and cerebral ischaemia/infarction occurs.

The normal cerebral blood flow rate is maintained by a number of haemostatic mechanisms at approximately 54 mL/100 g/min, which begins to fail when the mean arterial blood pressure falls below a level of 60–70 mmHg.

Progression from reversible ischaemia to infarction depends on the degree and the duration of reduced blood flow. If cerebral blood flow falls below 28 mL/100 g/min, this will result in the development of the morphological changes of infarction. The central necrotic zone of an infarct is surrounded by an 'ischaemic penumbra'—an area of tissue which is damaged, but remains viable. Restoration of blood flow may therefore give a clinical improvement.

Mechanisms of stroke

There are at least four pathological mechanisms underlying atheromatous cerebrovascular disease:

- Atheromatous changes, particularly in the internal carotid artery immediately above the common carotid bifurcation, act as a source of emboli.
- The atheromatous plaque may reach a size sufficient to stenose or occlude an internal carotid or vertebral artery, compromising the blood flow.
- Occlusion of small diameter (50–150 mm) penetrating branches of the cerebral arteries by plaques of local atheroma or lipohyalinoid degeneration (seen particularly in hypertension and diabetes) causes small 'lacunar' infarctions distal to the occlusion.
- Damage to the walls of small intracranial arteries (lipohyalinoid necrosis) and their subsequent dilatation in hypertensive patients causes small miliary aneurysms (Charcot–Bouchard aneurysms) which may rupture, causing intracerebral bleeding.

Lacunar infarctions and Charcot–Bouchard aneurysms occur most frequently in the following sites:

- The putamen and the internal capsule.
- Central white matter.
- Thalamus.
- Cerebellar hemisphere.
- Pons.

It is often very difficult to differentiate clinically between acute cerebral haemorrhage and infarction, and even pathologically between thrombotic and embolic infarctions.

Definitions

- Transient ischaemic attack is a focal neurological deficit of a presumed vascular origin from which a full clinical recovery occurs within 24 hours.
- Reversible ischaemic neurological deficit is a focal neurological deficit of a presumed vascular origin from which complete clinical recovery occurs more than 24 hours later.
- Stroke in evolution is a focal neurological deficit of a presumed vascular origin, which progresses over hours or days.
- Completed stroke is a cerebrovascular event with permanent neurological deficit.

Epidemiology

Cerebrovascular disease is the third most common cause of death after cardiovascular and malignant disease.

The annual incidence of completed stroke in the UK is approximately 1 per 500 population, with a lifetime risk of 1 in 6. The majority of these strokes are ischaemic.

Clinical features

Transient ischaemic attack

Transient ischaemic attacks are generally of thromboembolic aetiology. They should be recognized and managed promptly because they are an indication that a full stroke may be imminent.

Carotid territory transient ischaemic attacks present with:

- Transient monocular blindness (amaurosis fugax).
- Transient sensory or motor symptoms of the face, arm or leg.
- Transient aphasia.

> Amaurosis fugax is often described by patients as 'a black curtain descending over one eye'.

Vertebrobasilar transient ischaemic attacks present with a combination of:

- Dysarthria.
- Vertigo and unsteadiness.
- Diplopia.
- Circumoral paraesthesiae.
- Sensory or motor symptoms affecting the limbs singly or in combination.
- Cranial nerve palsies.

Stroke

Ischaemic stroke

Thromboembolic infarctions constitute approximately 85% of all strokes. The clinical features are extremely variable and dependent on the site and the extent of the lesion (Fig. 11.10).

Haemorrhagic stroke

Haemorrhagic strokes constitute 15% of all strokes. They are usually caused by rupture of Charcot–Bouchard aneurysms (Fig. 11.11). In the majority of cases, the symptoms develop while the patient is awake and active. Headache is a prominent feature. Clinical features depend on the site of bleeding:

- Capsular haemorrhage: hemiplegia (face, arm, and leg) and depressed consciousness.
- Pontine haemorrhage: tetraplegia, small pupils and coma.
- Cerebellar haemorrhage: severe headache, ipsilateral ataxia and depressed consciousness.

Investigations:

Investigations should be directed towards confirming the diagnosis (computed tomography, magnetic resonance imaging) and addressing the aetiological factors (electrocardiogram, carotid Doppler, echocardiogram).

Management:

In an established stroke, skilled nursing and physiotherapy are the main pillars of treatment. Specialist stroke units may have a 28% lower mortality than standard hospital care. For secondary prevention, all potentially modifiable risk factors should be addressed; aspirin or warfarin and

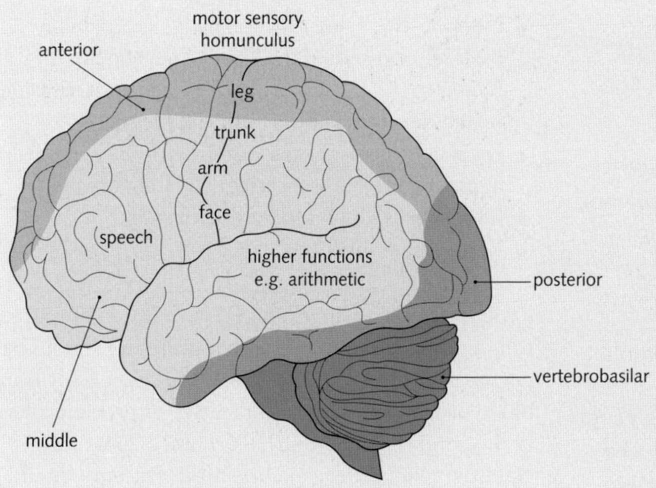

territory	typical symptoms
anterior	weakness/loss of sensation in contralateral leg
middle	dysphasia, dyslexia, dysgraphia, dyscalculia, weakness/loss of sensation in contralateral face and arm
posterior	contralateral homonymous hemianopia
vertebrobasilar	cranial nerve palsies, ataxia spinal tract symptoms, depressed consciousness

Fig. 11.10 Cerebral artery territories and symptoms of strokes in those areas.

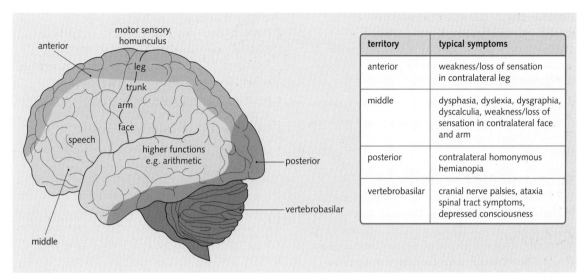

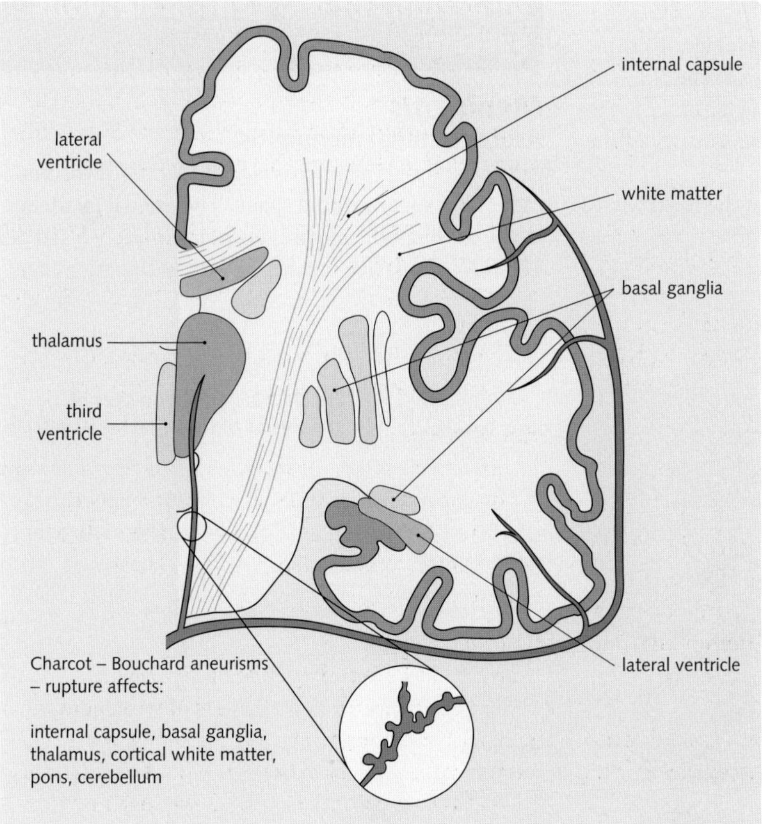

Fig. 11.11 Charcot–Bouchard aneurysms and the structures which rupture affects.

endarterectomy (for severe symptomatic carotid stenosis) should be considered.

Recent evidence suggests that all people with proven atheromatous disease should be on lifelong lipid-lowering drugs (statins).

Prognosis:
A complete recovery is achieved by 40% of patients; 20% die within 1 month, with 5–10% per year thereafter.

Subarachnoid haemorrhage

Subarachnoid haemorrhage is relatively uncommon. The annual incidence is 8 per 100 000. It is important because it typically occurs in young people between the ages of 35 and 65 years. Rupture of a cerebral berry aneurysm is the commonest cause (70%), with arteriovenous malformations accounting for 15% of cases. Berry aneurysms result from a developmental defect in the media and elastica of the cerebral arteries, causing the media to bulge outward covered only by the adventitia. Genetic factors are important, and there may be a family history of bleeds in the brain. Associations include polycystic kidney disease and coarctation of the aorta.

Berry aneurysms vary in size (on average, 1 cm) and shape, and are commonly located at the bifurcations of the cerebral arteries (Fig. 11.12). The severity of symptoms is related to the severity of the bleed with:

- Severe headache 'as if I was hit on the head with a sledge-hammer'.
- Nausea and vomiting.

The signs of subarachnoid haemorrhage are:

- Neck stiffness, positive Kernig's sign (pain on passively extending the knee when the hip is flexed to 90°) – both signs of meningeal irritation, which develop 6 hours after the bleed.
- Focal neurological signs (particularly III nerve palsy in posterior communicating artery aneurysms).
- Drowsiness, depressed consciousness.
- Retinal haemorrhages.

Patients should be investigated with head computed tomography scanning. A lumbar puncture should be performed if the scan is normal. This may show frank blood or xanthochromia (indicative of previous blood in the cerebrospinal fluid). Cerebral angiography is essential to locate the aneurysm(s). Patients should be kept in bed and given adequate analgesia. The aneurysm(s) should be clipped or coiled neurosurgically at an appropriate time.

Mortality is related to the severity of the bleeding and is particularly high in patients with depressed consciousness.

Infections of the central nervous system

Meningitis

Acute bacterial meningitis

Acute bacterial meningitis is an infection of the pia mater and subarachnoid space. The annual incidence in the developed countries is approximately 5–10 per 100 000. Causative organisms vary with patient age,

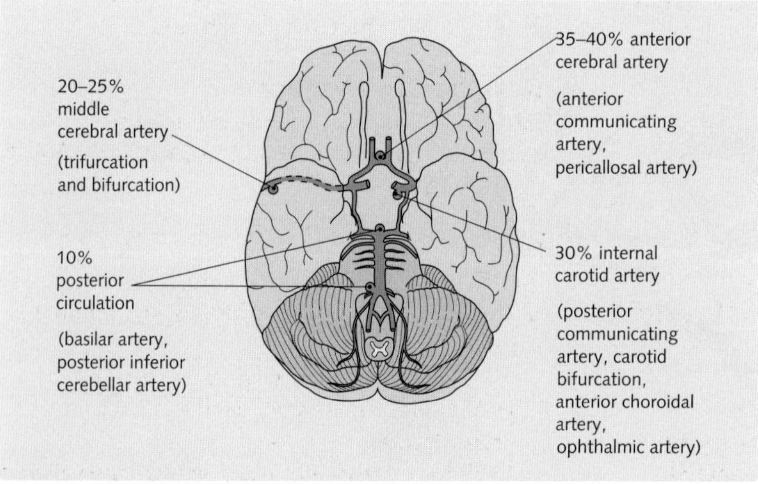

Fig. 11.12 Common sites of aneurysms of the intracranial vessels.

with three bacteria (NHS) accounting for over three-quarters of all cases:

- *Neisseria meningitidis* (meningococcus)
- *Haemophilus influenzae* (if very young and unvaccinated)
- *Streptococcus pneumoniae* (pneumococcus)

Other organisms to consider:

- Neonates: *Escherichia coli*, β-haemolytic streptococci, *Listeria monocytogenes*
- Elderly and immunocompromised: *Listeria*, tuberculosis, Gram negative bacteria
- Hospital-acquired infections: *Klebsiella*, *Escherichia coli*, *Pseudomonas*, *Staphylococcus aureus*

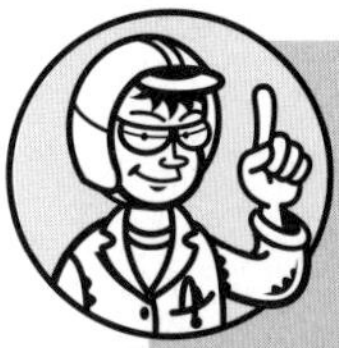

Important prenatal infections associated with neurological sequelae:
T Toxoplasmosis
O Others (Listeria, Salmonella, HIV, syphilis)
R Rubella
C Cytomegalovirus
H Herpes, hepatitis

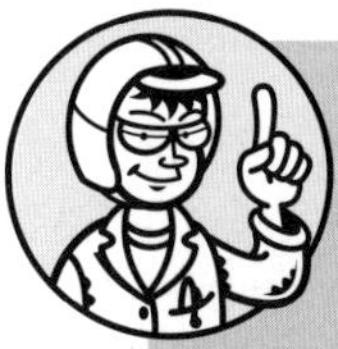

All children should now be vaccinated against haemophilus (B) and meningococcus type C, which were previously the commonest causes of meningitis in children. A good history of vaccinations is important in deciding on appropriate empirical treatment.

Clinical features are those of:

- Fever, headache, photophobia, painful eye movements. Impaired consciousness is a late and ominous feature.
- Neck stiffness, positive Kernig's sign.
- Occasionally: petechial skin rash (meningococcal meningitis), focal neurological signs, particularly cranial nerve palsies.

Investigations:

- In the presence of impaired consciousness, or focal neurological signs, a head computed tomography scan should be performed first to exclude a space-occupying lesion.
- Lumbar puncture is the key investigation. Cerebrospinal fluid will be turbid with a very high polymorphonuclear count and low glucose. An immediate Gram stain should be performed and the cerebrospinal fluid should be sent for culture.

Treatment:

- Meningitis is a very serious but potentially treatable condition.
- If the lumbar puncture cannot be performed immediately, prompt 'blind' treatment with a broad-spectrum antibiotic could be life saving. General practitioners who suspect meningitis in the community should give benzylpenicillin (1.2 g i.m./i.v.) without delay.
- Prophylactic antibiotics for close contacts (family, school, college, etc.) should be considered.

Prognosis:

- Mortality remains high.
- Overall mortality in the developed countries ranges between 5% and 30%, depending on the causative organism.

Aseptic meningitis

A large number of viruses (mumps, enteroviruses, coxsackie A and B, Epstein–Barr virus) produce an acute self-limiting aseptic meningitis. Patients are moderately ill with fever, malaise, headache, vomiting and mild neck stiffness. Impaired consciousness is suggestive of an encephalic component.

Cerebrospinal fluid examination shows moderate lymphocytosis. The protein is only slightly elevated, and glucose is normal. There is no specific treatment, and recovery after a few days is the rule.

Note that an aseptic picture is also seen in partially treated bacterial meningitis.

Intracranial abscess

Intracranial abscesses are rare in developed countries, with an annual incidence of about 0.2–0.3 per 100 000.

Brain abscess

The routes of bacterial invasion are:

- Direct extension from middle ear, sinus or tooth infections.
- Haematogenous spread: subacute bacterial endocarditis, right-to-left heart shunts, bronchiectasis.
- Skull fracture/penetrating trauma to the skull.

Common causative organisms are:

- Streptococci (*Streptococcus milleri* commonly from sinus infections).
- *Bacillus fragilis* (from ear infections).
- Anaerobic bacteria from the oropharynx.

Clinical features:

- Febrile illness.
- Seizures.
- Focal neurological signs.
- Altered consciousness.
- Raised intracranial pressure.

Investigations:

- Brain abscesses are readily evident on computed tomography or magnetic resonance imaging. A characteristic ring enhancement is often seen.
- Evidence of systemic infection (raised white cell count, positive blood cultures).
- Look for the underlying cause (consider echocardiography, chest X-ray).
- Note that lumbar puncture is contraindicated and may be fatal.

Treatment:

- Urgent surgical aspiration or excision.
- Antibiotic therapy (broad spectrum with good central nervous system penetration).
- Lower intracranial pressure (mannitol, hyperventilation, bed tilted to 'head up' position).

Mortality is high (10–15%).

Extradural (epidural) abscess

Extradural (epidural) abscesses usually result from osteomyelitis of the cranial bone or extension of infection from the frontal or mastoid sinuses. They cause intense local pain and oedema of the scalp.

Subdural abscess

Subdural abscess is a serious complication of paranasal sinus infection or cerebral abscess. It results in cortical vein thrombosis with widespread neurological deficit. Prognosis is grave.

Spinal abscess

Spinal abscesses are epidural in two-thirds of cases. One-half of the cases result from haematogenous spread of skin or urinary tract infections, and the remainder from direct spread from vertebral osteomyelitis. Staphylococcus is the commonest causative organism, followed by *Escherichia coli* and *Proteus*. Clinical features:

- Severe localized spinal pain.
- Fever.
- Signs of spinal cord compression.

Magnetic resonance imaging is the investigation of choice for spinal imaging.

Spinal abscesses should be treated with immediate surgical decompression and antibiotics.

Chronic meningoencephalitis

Tuberculous meningitis

Tuberculous meningitis is uncommon in the developed countries, with an annual incidence of 0.2 per 100 000. It is more common in socially and economically deprived communities.

Clinical features include:

- Prolonged prodromal illness followed by slowly evolving meningeal symptoms.
- Adhesive arachnoiditis causing cranial nerve palsies and hydrocephalus.
- Localized vasculitis and caseation causing focal neurological signs and seizures.

Investigations:

- A head computed tomography scan should be performed in patients with focal neurological signs or depressed consciousness.
- Cerebrospinal fluid examination shows raised lymphocyte count, high protein and low glucose.
- Ziehl–Nielsen staining occasionally reveals the presence of acid-fast bacilli, which will be confirmed by culture.

Treatment:

- A combination of isoniazid, rifampicin and pyrazinamide.
- Pyridoxine is given to prevent isoniazid-induced neuropathy.
- Corticosteroids may also be given initially to reduce the host inflammatory response.

Mortality:

- Mortality is very high, reaching 20–30% in treated patients.
- Many survivors are left disabled.

Neurosyphilis

Treponema pallidum (a spirochaete) invades the central nervous system within 3–24 months of the

primary infection in 25% of untreated cases.
Although the incidence of neurosyphilis has declined, it is important to maintain a high diagnostic suspicion since neurosyphilis may mimic other common neurological disorders.

Clinical features include:

- Asymptomatic meningeal neurosyphilis.
- Meningovascular syphilis—acute hemiplegia and sudden individual cranial nerve palsies.
- Tabes dorsalis—proprioceptive sensory loss, with unsteady, wide-based gait.
- General paralysis (of the insane)—dementia and upper motor neuron paralysis of the limbs.
- Neurosyphilitic gummata (rubbery granulomata) themselves may cause seizures and focal neurology when they are present in brain tissue.

Abnormal pupils (Argyll–Robertson) should be looked for, along with absent knee or ankle jerks and a positive Babinski sign. A consideration of whether the patient is at high risk of being HIV positive should be made, and appropriate precautions taken.

Lyme disease

Lyme disease is a spirochaetal infection caused by *Borrelia burgdorferi*, classically after an Ixodes tick bite. It presents initially with a characteristic skin rash (erythema chronicum migrans). Fifteen per cent of patients develop neuroborreliosis, which may mimic other common neurological disorders:

- Chronic meningitis.
- Encephalitis.
- Cranial nerve palsies (particularly facial).
- Painful radiculopathy.
- Peripheral neuropathy.
- Mononeuritis multiplex.

Treatment is with a cephalosporin with good central nervous system penetration (e.g. ceftriaxone)

Viral encephalitis

Viral encephalitis is an acute febrile encephalitic illness that is often associated with a meningeal component. It can be caused by many viruses, including mumps, herpes simplex and zoster, Epstein–Barr, coxsackievirus and echoviruses. Herpes simplex encephalitis (HSE) is particularly important because it is treatable.

Clinical features include:

- Headache, fever, altered consciousness.
- Occasionally, acute psychiatric symptoms (delusions, hallucination), seizures or focal neurological signs.

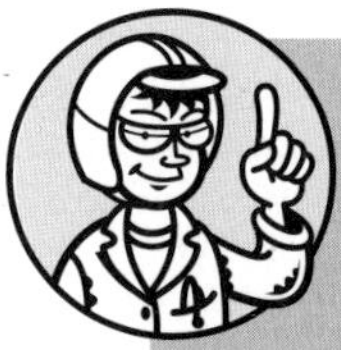

Encephalitis is inflammation of the brain parenchyma itself, without involvement of the meninges. In reality, there is generally some meningeal involvement in encephalitis and vice versa.

- Hemispheric signs (e.g. dysphasia, hemiparesis) are more likely in herpes simplex infection.

Investigations:

- A head computed tomography scan or magnetic resonance imaging excludes space-occupying lesions and may show focal abnormalities in the affected lobes (particularly the temporal lobe in HSE).
- Cerebrospinal fluid examination shows a raised lymphocyte count, with slightly raised protein and normal glucose, but may be entirely normal.
- Electroencephalogram (EEG) shows diffuse slow activity (delta waves), with focal periodic complexes (in HSE).
- Blood and cerebrospinal fluid may show rising viral antibody titres.
- Viruses may be identified in the cerebrospinal fluid (culture, polymerase chain reaction).

Treatment:

- Acyclovir is very effective in HSE. It is relatively non-toxic and should be used whenever this diagnosis is suspected.

Prognosis:

- Varies according to the causative virus.
- If untreated, the overall mortality of herpes simplex encephalitis is approximately 70%, which can be reduced to 20% with acyclovir.

Other virus-induced neurological diseases

For clinical purposes, viral illnesses are best considered by the clinical syndrome they produce (Fig. 11.13).

Fungal infections

Fungi are frequently the cause of opportunistic infections in immunocompromised patients, particularly in those with HIV. The commonest

Other virus-induced neurological diseases		
Virus	**Neurological syndrome**	**Principal symptoms**
Varicella zoster	Shingles	Painful vesicular eruption in dermatomal distribution
Retroviruses HTLV1, HIV	Tropical spastics paraparesis, AIDS	Spastic paraparesis, meningitis, myeolpathy, neuropathym dementia
Measles	Acute: meningoencephalitis Chronic: subacute sclerosing, panencephalitis (SSPE)	Deteriorating intellect, seizures, pyramidal signs
Rabies	Rabies	Psychiatric symptoms (affective disorders), hydrophobia/aerophobia, hyperreflexia and spasticity or ascending paralysis mimicking Guillan-Barré syndrome
Papoviruses (JC, SV40)	Progressive multifocal leukodystrophy	Dementia in an immuno-compromised patient
Arboviruses	Post-encephalitic Parkinsonism	Parkinsonism syndrome with dystonic movement disorders
Rubella	Progressive rubella encephalitis	Mental retardation, seizures, optic atrophy, cerbellar and pyramidal signs
Poliovirus	Poliomyelitis	Meningeal irritation, asymmetric paralysis without sensory involvement

Fig. 11.13 Other virus-induced neurological diseases.

fungi associated with central nervous system infection in the UK are *Cryptococcus*, *Nocardia*, *Candida* and *Aspergillus*. Fungal infection commonly presents with subacute meningitis complicated by cortical thrombophlebitis and cerebral abscesses. Cerebrospinal fluid examination shows moderate polymorphonuclear leucocytosis, increased protein and low glucose. The causative fungi can be demonstrated on Gram or Indian-ink staining, or by using special culture techniques.

Treatment is with antifungal agents, but mortality and morbidity are high.

Protozoan infection

Toxoplasma

Toxoplasma gondii is an intracellular protozoan parasite. Humans are occasionally infected through the ingestion of raw uncooked meat or cat faeces, or by the transplacental route. Congenital toxoplasmosis, caused by transplacental transmission, presents with hydrocephalus, hepatosplenomegaly, retinochoroiditis and thrombocytopenia.

Acquired toxoplasmosis occurs in immunocompromised patients (particularly in AIDS), with features of meningoencephalitis, seizures, focal neurological signs and depressed consciousness. Head computed tomography scanning in acquired toxoplasmosis shows characteristic contrast-enhancing lesions.

Toxoplasma immunoglobulin G antibodies are found in most patients. Brain biopsy is diagnostic.

Mortality is very high (70%).

Malaria

Cerebral malaria, causing a haemorrhagic encephalitis, is caused by *Plasmodium falciparum*. The main clinical features consist of fever and malaise, followed 2–3 weeks after initial infection by severe headache, delerium, seizures, progressive stupor leading to coma and, occasionally, focal neurological signs.

The diagnosis is established by showing malarial parasites in erythrocytes on a thick and thin blood film.

Treatment is with intravenous quinine.

Mortality is high (22%).

Prion diseases

Creutzfeld–Jakob disease (CJD) is thought to be caused by an infectious prion protein, and leads to a spongiform encephalopathy. Inherited CJD is an autosomal dominant trait, but most cases are sporadic. The 'new-variant' CJD, which has provoked such intense media interest, may have a connection with bovine spongiform encephalopathy in cattle. As yet, there is no indication of how this disease has 'jumped' species. Evidence comes from the fact that infected brain tissue from cattle can cause a spongiform encephalopathy when injected into the nervous system of various species, including cats. It is interesting to note that there has been no documented increase in the number of cases of feline spongiform encephalitis. This is despite the fact that cats almost certainly have eaten more contaminated beef offal than humans.

New variant CJD tends to affect younger patients, and presents initially with psychiatric disturbance and ataxia. Dementia invariably follows, and death occurs within 1–2 years. It is still extremely rare.

Demyelination and degeneration

Demyelination

Multiple sclerosis

Multiple sclerosis (MS) is a chronic disorder in which episodes of inflammatory demyelination affect any part of the central nervous system, producing a variety of symptoms. It has an extremely variable course with a tendency towards progressive disability.

MS cannot be diagnosed until the patient has suffered multiple attacks at different neuroanatomical sites.

Incidence and prevalence

The incidence and the prevalence of MS vary markedly between the different geographical areas and the different population groups. In the UK, the annual incidence is about 1 per 20 000, and the prevalence is about 1 per 1000.

Aetiology

The aetiology of MS is unknown, but is likely to involve environmental factors (e.g. a viral infection) in genetically susceptible patients. There is a weak human leukocyte antigen association, leading to theories of an autoimmune basis. The pathological hallmarks are scattered demyelinating lesions in the perivenous areas of the white matter of the brain and the spinal cord, referred to as 'plaques'.

Symptoms and signs

Depending on the anatomical location of the plaques, four main groups of symptoms are recognized:

- Optic nerve: attacks of optic neuritis presenting with blurring of vision associated with periorbital and retro-orbital pain exacerbated by eye movements, reduced visual acuity, central scotoma, afferent pupillary defect and a pink and swollen optic disc (which becomes pale and atrophic at a later stage).
- Brainstem: diplopia; dysconjugate eye movements, particularly internuclear ophthalmoplegia; limb and gait ataxia, titubation, tremor, dysarthria and vertigo.
- Spinal cord: sensory symptoms including Lhermitte's phenomenon (electric-shock-like sensation extending down the spine into the limbs on neck flexion); spastic weakness; bladder, bowel and sexual dysfunction.
- Other clinical features: dementia, euphoria and emotional lability; facial pain; painful tonic spasms; Uhthoff's phenomenon (transient worsening of symptoms following a hot bath or exercise).

Investigations:

MS is a clinical diagnosis and no test is pathognomonic. Cerebrospinal fluid shows oligoclonal bands in almost all cases. Evoked potentials (visual, auditory, and somatosensory) may be prolonged. Magnetic resonance imaging is abnormal in almost all patients.

Treatment:

Acute relapses are treated with oral or intravenous steroids. Analgesia and baclofen may reduce spasticity. Bladder symptoms may require specialist referral. Interferon-β is effective in reducing relapse rate, but has no proven effect on long-term disease progression. It is not effective in all patients, and is extremely expensive. Therefore, its use should be reviewed regularly.

Prognosis:

The average duration of the illness to death is 25–30 years.

Other demyelinating conditions

Acute disseminated encephalomyelitis may follow many common viral infections, and causes focal brainstem and spinal cord demyelination that resembles MS. The prognosis is variable—from complete recovery to 25% mortality in severe cases.

Central pontine myelinosis is associated with alcoholism and hyponatraemia. It presents acutely with pontine and medullary symptoms. It is treated by correcting underlying metabolic abnormalities and with vitamins. Prognosis is poor.

Degenerative diseases

Degenerative diseases in which dementia is prominent (cortical dementia)

Alzheimer's disease

Alzheimer's disease is the commonest cause of dementia, accounting for 80% of all cases of dementia in the community. The incidence increases with age; familial cases are occasionally seen. The female : male ratio is 3 : 1.

Clinical features are those of cortical dementia:

- Memory impairment (particularly of recent events), apathy, poor reasoning and judgement.
- Behavioural disturbance (aggression is often prominent).
- Aphasia, apraxia, spatial disorientation.
- Eventually patients become mute, bedfast and incontinent.

The main pathological changes are:

- Considerable brain atrophy, most evident in the superior and middle temporal gyri.
- Neurofibrillary tangles: intracellular paired helical filaments which are particularly common in hippocampal, amygdaloid, and pyramidal neurons.
- Neuritic plaques: extracellular areas of degenerating neuronal processes surrounding a central core of β-amyloid protein.
- Loss of cholinergic neurons in the medial septal nucleus, the horizontal nucleus and nucleus of diagonal band.

The cause(s) of Alzheimer's disease is not known, although genetic predisposition is likely to be very important. Risk is increased by three times in first degree relatives. The high prevalence of Alzheimer's in Down's syndrome suggests that the gene that encodes the β-amyloid precursor, on chromosome 21, is one of the most important candidate genes. A specific isoform of the lipid transport protein, apolipoprotein E, is an independent risk factor for the development of Alzheimer's disease, its gene is located on chromosome 19.

Investigations, which are largely undertaken to exclude other, treatable, causes of dementia, include:

- Imaging (computed tomography, magnetic resonance imaging) which shows brain atrophy, flattening of the gyri, widening of the sulci and dilatation of the ventricles. This will also help to exclude vascular causes of dementia which can be prevented from progressing.
- B_{12}/folate levels and thyroid function tests.

Pick's disease

Pick's disease is another form of dementia which may be indistinguishable from Alzheimer's until autopsy. Classically, it is dominated by frontal and temporal lobe symptoms. Treatment is the same.

Treatment:

- Maintenance of general health—concurrent illnesses (including affective disorders) may exacerbate symptoms.
- Avoidance of sedative drugs.
- Treatment should be considered using an inhibitor of acetylcholinesterase (e.g. donepezil) which may slow cognitive decline in some patients.

Prognosis:

- Most patients die from the complications of immobility within 5–10 years of diagnosis.

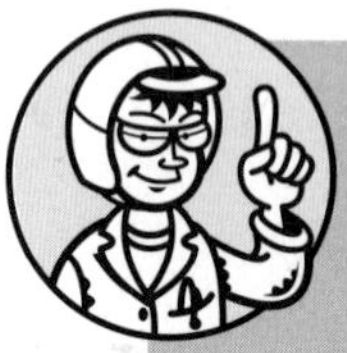

Impairment of recent memories, along with inattention leads to disorientation in time. This is a very sensitive marker for dementia.

Degenerative diseases in which extrapyramidal features are prominent (subcortical dementia)

Parkinson's disease

The annual incidence is 1 in 5000, with a prevalence of about 1 per 500. Age of onset is generally approximately 50 years onwards, but 8% of patients develop symptoms before the age of 40 years. The cause remains unclear, although genetic (particularly in early onset Parkinson's) and environmental factors are likely to be important.

The main pathological changes are:

- Loss of the pigmented cells in the substantia nigra which results in severe striatal dopamine deficiency.
- Atypical eosinophilic inclusion bodies, called 'Lewy' bodies.

Clinical features include:

- Bradykinesia as the cardinal feature. Patients present with slowness of gait, difficulties in writing and using their hands, turning in bed and reduced facial expression.
- Resting tremor classically of four or five cycles per second.
- Rigidity of lead-pipe or (with superimposed tremor) cog-wheeling type.
- Impaired postural control and loss of righting reflexes, causing flexed posture and falls in advanced cases.
- Dementia in approximately 30% of cases.
- Affective disorders are very common—particularly anxiety and depression.

Differential diagnosis:

- Benign essential tremor.
- Depression and motor retardation.
- Drug-induced parkinsonism.
- Other degenerative disorders.
  - Progressive supranuclear palsy (Steel–Richardson–Olzewski syndrome)—characterized by more tone in the neck than the limbs and falls early on in the disease.
  - Wilson's disease—a disorder of copper metabolism.
  - Diffuse Lewy body disease.
  - Alzheimer's disease.
- Diffuse cerebrovascular disease with abnormal gait.

Investigations:

- The diagnosis is usually based on the clinical features and response to treatment.
- Imaging, autonomic function tests and sphincter electromyogram are occasionally needed to exclude other parkinsonian syndromes.

Treatment:

- Anticholinergic and dopaminergic drugs are the main line of treatment. These are discussed in Chapter 5.
- Dopaminergic neuronal implantation is still a research procedure.

Prognosis:

- With treatment, life expectancy is now only slightly worse than that of the general population.

Huntington's disease

Huntington's disease is an autosomal dominantly inherited disorder. The gene is on chromosome 4. The prevalence is approximately 8 per 100 000, and onset is usually in middle age. Pathologically, there is neuronal loss in the striatum associated with deficiency of γ-aminobutyric acid (GABA), acetylcholine, enkephalin and substance-P.

Onset is insidious, with:

- Chorea (writhing, dance-like movements).
- Affective disorder and personality changes.
- Dementia of subcortical type.

Investigations:

- The clinical diagnosis is usually confirmed with genetic studies.
- Head computed tomography and magnetic resonance imaging in advanced cases show atrophy of the caudate nuclei.

Treatment:

- No specific treatment is available. Chorea is treated symptomatically with neuroleptics (e.g. haloperidol).
- Genetic counselling of the affected families is essential.

Prognosis:

- Most patients die from aspiration within 10–20 years of diagnosis.

Hereditary ataxias and related disorders

These heterogeneous disorders present with progressive ataxia as a predominant clinical feature (Fig. 11.14).

Motor neuron disease

The annual incidence of motor neuron disease is approximately 2–3 per 100 000. It usually presents between the ages of 50 and 70 years. Three major types are recognized:

- Amyotrophic lateral sclerosis: the classical form of motor neuron disease—this is a combination of upper and lower motor neuron limb and bulbar weakness.
- Progressive muscular atrophy: a lower motor neuron limb weakness.
- Progressive bulbar palsy: a combination of upper and lower motor neuron bulbar weakness.

Hereditary ataxias		
hereditary ataxia of known cause	intermittent ataxia	disorder of urea cycle disorders of lactate and pyruvate metabolism (Leigh's disease)
	progressive ataxia	abetalipoproteinuria ataxia telangiectasia xeroderma pigmentosa
hereditary ataxia of unknown cause	spinal ataxia	Friedreich's ataxia
	cerebellar ataxia	pure cerebellar degeneration

Fig. 11.14 Hereditary ataxias.

These syndromes represent a continuum, and patients progress from one syndrome to the other. Sensory symptoms and signs are usually absent. Treatment is aimed at maintaining a reasonable quality of life for as long as possible using a multidisciplinary approach. Prognosis is extremely poor and the survival is approximately 2–3 years.

Spinal muscular atrophy (SMA)

SMA is a group of hereditary conditions characterized by progressive lower motor neuron degeneration. Features include hypotonia, proximal weakness and wasting. There are four main types:

- Acute infantile SMA (Werdnig–Hoffmann disease)—presents at birth or shortly after, death is by age 3 years.
- Chronic infantile SMA—presents at 6 months, death is by 10 years.
- Juvenile onset SMA (Kugelberg–Welander disease)—presents at approximately 10 years, death is around 35 years.
- Peroneal/scapuloperoneal SMA – adult onset, survival is roughly normal.

Metabolic disorders and toxins

Vitamin deficiencies

Nutritional vitamin deficiencies are rare in developed countries and are usually seen in chronic alcoholics and socially isolated people, including elderly or mentally ill patients. Vitamin deficiency can also result from diseases (malabsorption, autoimmunity) or drugs (isoniazide), and is usually not limited to a single vitamin in isolation. Some common features and causes of vitamin deficiences are shown in Fig. 11.15.

Vitamin overdose (vitamin A) occasionally results in neurological complications (headache, papilloedema).

Toxins

Methanol

Poisoning with methanol causes headache and photophobia and, in severe cases, papilloedema, optic atrophy and blindness. Ethanol infusion (ethanol competes with methanol) and haemodialysis are the mainstays of treatment.

Alcohol

Neurological complications of alcoholism include:

- Acute intoxication. The effect of acute alcohol administration depends on the amount of alcohol consumed and on whether the subject is a naïve or chronic alcohol user. The symptoms range in severity from euphoria and mild incoordination to ataxia, dysarthria and confusion, to deep anaesthesia and respiratory suppression. Secondary effects of intoxication include head injury, hypoglycaemia and hyponatraemia. The possibility of other drugs should be considered.
- Alcohol withdrawal syndrome (tremors, hallucinations, seizures, and delirium tremens). Action tremor usually reaches a peak 24–36 hours after the cessation of drinking, and is promptly aborted by further alcohol intake. Hallucinations may be visual, auditory or tactile. Seizures occur 24–48 hours after the cessation of drinking. Delirium tremens combines the three previous features and severe autonomic overactivity (dilated pupils, pyrexia, tachycardia and sweating).
- Nutritional complications (Wernicke–Korsakoff syndrome—caused by thiamine Vitamin B_1 deficiency, and neuropathy). Early clinical features are those of ataxia, oculomotor disturbances (oculomotor palsies and nystagmus) and confusion which, if untreated, can progress to coma and death. As the patient's confusion improves following treatment, the amnesic component of the syndrome emerges in which confabulation is a prominent feature. Neuropathy is a symmetrical sensorimotor axonal neuropathy.
- Hepatic complications (acute hepatic encephalopathy and chronic portosystemic encephalopathy).
- Other syndromes: dementia/brain atrophy; alcoholic cerebellar degeneration (characterized

Clinical features and common causes of vitamin deficiencies			
Vitamin	**Function**	**Cause**	**Neurological sequelae**
A	essential for normal retinal and epithelial cell function	malnutrition	adults and children: blindness infants: mental retardation and hydrocephalus
B_1 (thiamine)	pyruvate metabolism	malnutrition, alcoholism	Wernicke's encephalopathy, Korsakoff psychosis, neuropathy
B_3 (nicotinic acid)	NAD, NADP coenzyme component	malnutrition	encephalopathy, neuropathy
B_6 (pyridioxine)	cofactor in protein metabolism	malnutrition, isoniazide treatment	neuropathy, seizures (infants)
B_{12} (cobalamine)	purine synthesis	autoimmunity, ileal disease, gastrectomy, malnutrition	dementia, myelopathy (subacute combined degeneration), neuropathy
folic acid	purine synthesis	malabsorption, malnutrition	myelopathy, neuropathy, neural tube defect
D	calcium metabolism	malabsorption, malnutrition, chronic renal failure	myopathy
E	antioxidant	malabsorption	cerebellar ataxia

Fig. 11.15 Clinical features and common causes of vitamin deficiencies.

by gait and truncal ataxia); alcoholic myopathy (acute painful proximal myopathy); central pontine myelinolysis (acute syndrome of quadriparesis, pseudobulbar palsy occasionally associated with abnormal eye movements and 'locked-in' syndrome).

Carbon monoxide poisoning

The high affinity of haemoglobin to carbon monoxide results in severe tissue hypoxia. Acute intoxication leads to acute encephalopathy with visual field defects, papilloedema and retinal haemorrhage. Many patients are left with chronic encephalopathy and parkinsonism. Hyperbaric oxygen may help to prevent this, even hours after exposure.

Heavy metals

Lead

Acute encephalopathy is seen largely in children. Chronic motor neuropathy typically presents with wrist drop.

Mercury

Mercury causes chronic encephalopathy with ataxia, dysarthria and tremor.

Manganese

Manganese causes chronic encephalopathy and parkinsonism.

Iatrogenic

Drugs

Drug-induced neurological disorders include:

- Encephalopathy (e.g. hypnotics, sedatives, antidepressants in large doses).
- Neuropathy (e.g. isoniazide, vincristine).
- Neuromuscular transmission blockade (e.g. penicillamine).
- Myopathy (e.g. steroids).

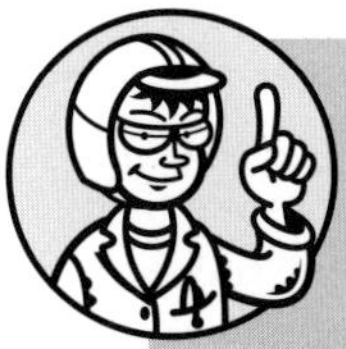

Neurological complication of opiate abuse:
- Acute intoxication.
- Withdrawal syndrome.
- Transverse myelitis.
- Neuropathy.
    - Acute painful plexopathy.
    - Acute mononeuropathies/ mononeuritis multiplex.
- Myopathy.
    - Rhabdomyolysis.
    - Chronic myopathy.
- Infection.
    - Cerebral abscess.
    - Mycotic aneurysm.

- Extrapyramidal syndrome (e.g. antipsychotic medications and antiemetics).
- Psychiatric symptoms (e.g. antiparkinsonian medications).

Radiotherapy

Neurological complications are related to the total radiation dose and the period over which it is given. Early features are related to localized oedema. Delayed features are related to necrosis, which often simulates tumour recurrence.

Neoplasms of the central nervous system

Primary brain tumours

The annual incidence of primary brain tumours is about 8.2 per 100 000, accounting for about 5% of all neoplasms in the body. However, they make up approximately 50% of all childhood malignancies.

The prevalence of the different tumour types and their anatomical location varies with age:

- Adults: gliomas, metastases, and meningiomas.
  - 80–85% supratentorial compartment.
  - 15–20% infratentorial compartment.
- Children: medulloblastomas and cerebellar astrocytomas.
  - 40% supratentorial compartment.
  - 60% infratentorial compartment.

The clinical features depend on the site of the tumour and the speed of growth, and can be divided into three main categories:

- Features of raised intracranial pressure (headache, vomiting and papilloedema).
- Focal symptoms and signs, the nature of which depends on the anatomical site of the tumour and whether the tumour effect is irritative or destructive.
- False localizing signs due to raised intracranial pressure (e.g. VIth nerve palsy).

Neuroepithelial tumours

Astrocytomas

Astrocytomas are the commonest primary tumours of the brain. They can occur at any age, but are commonest between the ages of 40 and 60 years. Male/female incidence is 2 : 1. Astrocytomas occur with equal incidence throughout the frontal, temporal and parietal lobes, but are uncommon in the occipital lobe.

There are four pathological grades (Kernohan I–IV):

- Low-grade astrocytoma (grades I and II)—commonly seen in children/young adults.
- Malignant astrocytoma (grade III).
- Glioblastoma multiformis (grade IV).

Sadly, malignant astrocytomas are far more common than benign ones.

Oligodendroglioma

Oligodendroglioma is a slow-growing tumour with low malignancy grade. It affects a younger age-group (30–50 years) and is most common in the frontal lobe. Imaging reveals a well-demarcated tumour, frequently with areas of calcification.

Medulloblastoma

Medulloblastoma is the most common malignant tumour of childhood (4–8 years). It arises from embryonic tissue in the cerebellar vermis and may seed through the cerebrospinal fluid pathways to other parts of the cranium or the spinal cord.

Ependymoma

Ependymoma is the second most common tumour of childhood, although it is also found in individuals aged in their early 20s. It occurs throughout the ventricular system or the spinal canal, but is particularly common in the fourth ventricle and in the caudal part of the spinal cord. Frequently, it infiltrates surrounding tissues. Fourth-ventricle ependymomas usually present with symptoms of intermittent hydrocephalus, ataxia, vertigo and vomiting.

Meninges

Meningioma

Meningioma is a benign tumour arising from the arachnoid that compresses rather than invades the neural tissues. Maximum incidence occurs between 40 and 60 years of age. It is most common in the sylvian region, the parasagittal surface of the parietal and frontal lobes, the olfactory grooves, the lesser wings of the sphenoid, the tuberculum sellae, the cerebellopontine angle and the thoracic spinal cord. Imaging reveals a well circumscribed lesion with occasional calcification. Surgery is a definite possibility in most of these patients.

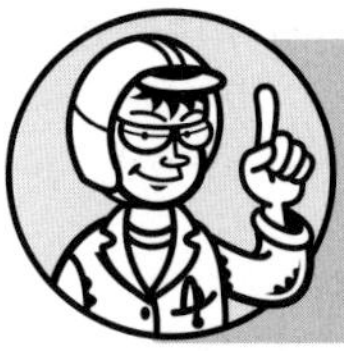

Some meningiomas contain oestrogen receptors, and may enlarge markedly in pregnancy.

Nerve sheath cells

Neurofibroma

Neurofibroma is a benign, slow-growing tumour that commonly develops on the vestibular division of cranial nerve VIII (often misleadingly called an acoustic neuroma). It tends to present in mid-life and is more common in females. Neurofibroma usually presents with sensorineural deafness, occasionally associated with tinnitus and vertigo. It may appear as part of the neurofibromatosis syndrome (most commonly type 2), when other tumours (particularly contralateral acoustic neuromas) should be sought.

Primary cerebral lymphoma (microglioma)

With the advent of HIV, and increasing numbers of immunosuppressed patients, this tumour is becoming more common. They are often periventricular, and may be multiple. Microgliomas are aggressive tumours, and account for up to 10% of central nervous system complications in AIDS patients.

Anterior pituitary gland

Pituitary adenoma

Pituitary adenoma is a benign tumour that presents with neurological or endocrinological symptoms. Large tumours usually present with headache, bitemporal hemianopia (from upward pressure on the optic chiasm), and occasionally hypopituitarism. Smaller tumours present with hyperprolactinaemia and less commonly with acromegaly/gigantism, Cushing's syndrome and thyrotoxicosis.

Other tissues

Tumours of other tissues can be summarized as:

- Blood vessels: haemangioblastoma.
- Germ cells: germinoma, teratoma.
- Microglia: primary brain lymphoma.
- Tumours of maldevelopmental origin: crangiopharyngioma, epidermoid/dermoid cyst, colloid cyst.
- Local extension from adjacent tumours: chordoma, glomus jugulare tumour.

Metastatic brain tumours

Metastatic brain tumours are around eight times commoner than primary brain malignancies. Approximately 20% of patients dying with other tumours will have intracranial metastases, 25% of which are asymptomatic. The primary tumours are:

- 44% bronchus.
- 10% breast.
- 7% genitourinary.
- 6% bowel.
- 3% skin (melanoma).
- 30% others.

Presenting features are similar to those of the primary brain tumours, but the lesions are often multiple. On computed tomography and magnetic resonance imaging, they have a round, well circumscribed appearance, often with surrounding oedema.

Investigations of brain tumours

Investigations are aimed to identify the presence of the tumour, its anatomical site, and its pathology with:

- Imaging (computed tomography, magnetic resonance imaging, angiography).
- Biopsy.

Treatment

Treatment depends on many factors, mainly the type, site and stage of the tumour, and includes:

- Symptomatic: analgesia, steroids (to reduce cerebral oedema), anticonvulsants.
- Specific: surgery, radiotherapy, chemotherapy.

Prognosis

The great majority of patients with cerebral tumours have a limited life expectancy, with a median survival of a few months. More benign tumours allow survival for many years.

Effects of systemic cancer on the central nervous system

These include:

- Direct invasion from adjacent structures.
- Metastatic disease.
- Non-metastatic 'remote effect' (paraneoplastic syndromes).
  - Immunologically mediated:
    Cerebellar dysfunction.
    Visual dysfunction.
    Sensory neuropathy.
    Opsoclonus.

- Lambert–Eaton myasthenic syndrome.
- Limbic encephalitis.
- Others (opportunistic infections, dermatomyositis, inappropriate antidiuretic hormone secretion).

Epilepsy

An epileptic seizure (fit) is a paroxysmal alteration in nervous system activity that is time limited and causes a clinically detectable event. The types of epileptic seizure are shown in Fig. 11.16.

Epilepsy is a condition in which more than one seizure has occurred, in the absence of abnormal metabolic states (most people will develop seizures if you make them sufficiently hyponatraemic!). Incidence is greatest in early and late life, with a prevalence of approximately 0.5%.

Febrile convulsions in childhood are not classed as epilepsy, although, if prolonged, these may predispose to epilepsy in later life.

Epilepsy is a clinical diagnosis and the patient is often normal on examination; therefore, a careful history is vital. It is particularly useful to obtain a history from a witness to the seizure.

A patient who has had a seizure with loss of consciousness may remember feeling odd (e.g. odd smells, metallic taste) before the event (the aura), and may remember feeling confused, disorientated and sleepy afterwards (the postictal phase), but will have no memory of the fit itself. Surprisingly, perhaps, tongue-biting, and urinary incontinence are infrequently seen.

Risk of another seizure within 1 year of the first is 40%, rising to 50% within 3 years.

Status epilepticus is defined as seizures occurring in series with no recovery of consciousness, or a seizure lasting more than 30 minutes. It constitutes a medical emergency as there is a high risk of brain damage and death.

Partial (focal) epilepsy

Focal epilepsy may arise from an intracerebral structural defect, causing motor or sensory symptoms localized to one body part, which may then spread to adjacent areas as the electrical activity spreads to contiguous regions of the cortex (e.g. jacksonian seizure). These are simple partial seizures. Sometimes, no underlying structural defect can be found.

Complex partial seizures usually arise in the temporal lobe. They are called 'complex' because they are associated with disturbance of consciousness.

Seizures arising in the medial temporal lobe may produce disturbances of smell and taste, visual hallucinations, and a sense of déjà vu. These may evolve to a tonic–clonic seizure (secondary generalization). Weakness following the event may occur for minutes or hours (Todd's paresis).

Primary generalized epilepsy

Any of the seizure types indicated in Fig. 11.16 may occur in one patient. In a generalized tonic–clonic seizure, the tonic ('increased tone') phase is a sudden tonic contraction of muscles usually with upward eye deviation. The clonic ('with clonus-type activity') phase follows. Initial EEG changes are often bilateral. This condition usually has its onset in childhood. Absence (or petit mal) attacks usually consist of a brief interruption of activity, sometimes with complex motor activity (such as fumbling with clothes), but without collapse. EEG during this event shows a three-per-second spike-and-wave activity (see Chapter 16).

Epilepsy syndromes

The International League Against Epilepsy classifies certain conditions as epilepsy syndromes, which includes clinical and EEG manifestations. These include:

- Benign childhood epilepsy with centrotemporal spikes.
- Lennox–Gastaut syndrome.
- Infantile spasms: characteristic brief episodes with shock-like flexion of arms, head and neck and drawing up of the knees (called a salaam attack). It is associated with progressive mental handicap.
- Juvenile myoclonic epilepsy: a familial late childhood onset disease, with myoclonic jerks, tonic–clonic seizures ± absence seizures, with typical interictal EEG.

Pseudoseizures

Pseudoseizures (simulated seizures) occur in up to 20% of patients referred for 'intractable epilepsy'. They may occur in association with real epilepsy or psychological disturbance.

Types of epileptic seizure	
primary generalized epilepsy	absence seizures; primary generalized tonic–clonic seizures; others: myoclonic, atypical absences; tonic, clonic and atonic seizures
partial (focal) epilepsy ± secondary generalization	simple partial seizure (without loss of consciousness), complex partial seizures (with disturbed consciousness)
secondary generalized epilepsy	due to underlying generalized cerebral abnormality
epilepsy due to underlying focal or metabolic cause	primary intracranial lesions (tumour, stroke, infections, trauma), metabolic (hypoglycaemia, hypomagnesaemia, liver failure), drugs (and most in overdose), drug withdrawal (alcohol, benzodiazepines), toxins (alcohol, carbon monoxide)

Fig. 11.16 Types of epileptic seizure.

Prolactin levels may be useful in determining whether a seizure was real or simulated. In all complex and partial seizures (except absences), prolactin levels show an immediate rise, which the patient cannot simulate!

Investigation

This includes EEG—note that approximately 50% are normal and this does not disprove the diagnosis. Computed tomography, and/or magnetic resonance imaging in adult-onset seizures, with further investigation as appropriate to the individual.

Blood tests to identify reversible causes, along with a toxic screen and electrocardiogram (to identify long Q-T syndromes) are important in all patients.

Treatment

First fits are often not treated but, unless seizures are years apart, most neurologists would treat after the second event. There are a wide range of antiepileptic medications, and choice depends mostly on seizure type. A major reason for differentiating partial from generalized seizures is that different drugs are effective for each. Some patients with suitable seizure activity may benefit considerably from surgical removal of an epileptogenic focus on a temporal lobe. Note that, in 70% of patients, epilepsy eventually remits, and trials of treatment withdrawal should be considered at an appropriate time.

Epilepsy and driving.
First fit/solitary fit.

- 1 year off driving (fit free) with medical review before restarting. If another fit occurs during this time, the patient must wait a year from that fit before review.

Loss of consciousness without known cause.

- As above.

Seizures during sleep.

- After one seizure, regulations as above. If all attacks for at least 3 years have been during sleep, and the patient has never had an awake attack, driving is allowed.

Withdrawal of antiepileptic medication.

- Advise not to drive (but not a legal obligation on the patient's part) for 6 months from time of withdrawal. Clearly, if further seizures occur, the above regulations apply.

Antiepileptic drugs

Phenytoin

Phenytoin reduces the spread of a seizure. Electroencephalogram recordings show that it does not stop the 'spiking' at a focus and so it does not prevent the onset of an epileptic discharge, but stops it from involving other areas.

It blocks voltage-gated Na^+ channels and has a higher affinity for channels in the inactivated state. This state is prolonged, preventing the channel from opening, which stops the neuron from firing rapidly. The block is use dependent as, at higher frequencies, more channels are cycling through the inactivated state. This allows selectivity of action, as the phenytoin block is more likely to occur in neurons in a seizure focus.

Oral absorption is variable and phenytoin is metabolized in the liver by an enzyme system that is saturated at therapeutic doses and, as such, shows dose-dependent kinetics. This means that, at certain doses, the serum concentration can rise rapidly to toxic levels as there is only a limited capacity to get rid of it. Because patients will vary in the doses that saturate their enzyme system, the therapeutic regime starts with low doses and then increases, with careful monitoring of serum phenytoin.

The side effects of phenytoin are:

- Vertigo and cerebellar signs—ataxia, dysarthria, nystagmus.
- At high doses, sedation and interference with cognitive functions.
- Collagen effects—gum hypertrophy and coarsening of facial features.
- Allergic reactions—rash, hepatitis, lymphadenopathy.
- Haematological effects—megaloblastic anaemia.
- Endocrine effects—hirsutism.
- Teratogenesis—may cause congenital malformations (cleft palate).

Phenytoin has many drug interactions, mainly because it induces the hepatic P_{450} oxidase system, increasing the metabolism of oral contraceptives, anticoagulants, dexamethasone and pethidine.

It is used for all types of epilepsy except absences.

Carbamazepine

The mechanism of action of carbamazepine is the same as for phenytoin:

- It is well absorbed orally, with a long half-life (25–60 hours) when first given.
- Its side-effect profile is really limited to the nervous system, with ataxia, nystagmus, dysarthria, vertigo and sedation. Similar to phenytoin, it is a strong enzyme inducer, causing similar interactions, and induces its own metabolism, which is why its half-life decreases if taken regularly.
- It is used as first line treatment for partial seizures, and second line for generalized seizures.

Sodium valproate

Sodium valproate has two mechanisms of action:

- As for phenytoin.
- It increases GABA content and GABA action, although this has no clear explanation.

It is well absorbed orally, has a half-life of 10–15 hours, and has much fewer side effects than other anticonvulsants, with the main problems being tremor, weight gain, hair thinning and ankle swelling. Rarely, it can cause hepatic failure (check liver function tests regularly) and may be teratogenic. It interacts with other central nervous system depressants (e.g. alcohol), potentiating their effects.

It is used as first line for generalized seizures.

Ethosuximide

The mechanism of action of ethosuximide is unknown. It is used only for absences, as it may make tonic–clonic attacks worse. Its side effects are nausea, loss of appetite and mood swings.

Vigabatrin (γ-vinyl-GABA)

Vigabatrin is an irreversible inhibitor of GABA transaminase and so reduces the metabolism of GABA. This means that more GABA is available for release. It is used as an adjunct to other therapies that do not adequately control a patient's epilepsy.

Its side effects are drowsiness, dizziness, depression and visual hallucinations, and it is contraindicated if patients have a history of psychiatric problems. Abrupt withdrawal leads to rebound seizures. It can be retinotoxic, causing loss of peripheral visual field.

Its use should be confined to specialist practice.

Phenobarbitone

Phenobarbitone is a barbiturate and has two anticonvulsant actions:

- It binds to the $GABA_A$ receptor, potentiating the effect of normal GABA release.
- It reduces glutamate-mediated excitation.

Its main side effect is sedation which, together with the fatal central nervous system depression that it causes in overdose, limits its use clinically. Phenobarbitone also causes cerebellar signs and is an enzyme inducer.

This is another drug to be used only in specialist practice.

Benzodiazepines

Benzodiazepines potentiate the normal effect of GABA binding.

Their side effects are sedation and may cause an increase in the requirements for anticonvulsant drugs. They are used primarily in status epilepticus.

Treatment of status epilepticus

This is a medical emergency. Always consider whether the patient is pregnant, as it may be an eclamptic fit which will only be cured by delivery of the baby. Otherwise, correct reversible causes (give a glucose infusion, and replace fluids). The initial treatment is with benzodiazepines (lorazepam or diazepam) ± phenytoin. If these therapies do not stop seizure activity, an anaesthetist is required to supervise the administration of a barbiturate such as phenobarbitone.

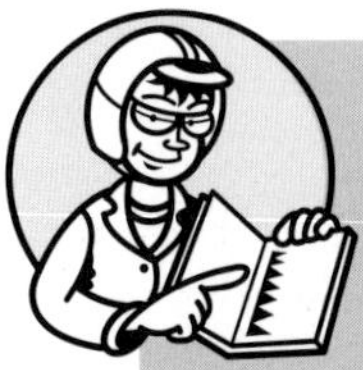

- What types of cerebral oedema do you know? How may they be treated?
- How would you diagnose hydrocephalus?
- Describe the different neural tube defects you know.
- List five complications of skull fractures.
- Explain the mechanism of ischaemic stroke. What risk factors do you know?
- What is the different pathology caused by rupture of Charcot–Bouchard and berry aneurysms?
- Name the three most common pathogens which cause acute bacterial meningitis. How would you diagnose the condition?
- Describe the classical features and symptoms of multiple scurosis.
- Name three pathological changes in the brain tissue seen in Alzheimer's disease.
- Discuss the neurological complications of alcoholism.
- Which cancers metastasize to the brain? How would you identify their presence?
- What is the threshold for treating epilepsy? What would be your first-line treatment and emergency management of status epilepticus?

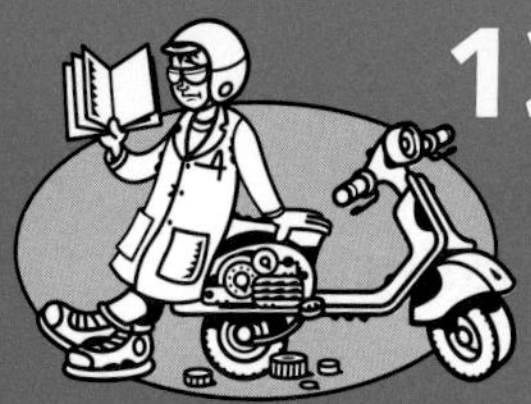

12. Pathology of the Peripheral Nerves and Muscle

In this chapter, you will learn about:
- Hereditary forms of neuropathy.
- Traumatic damage to nerves.
- Inflammatory neuropathies.
- Infectious causes of a neuropathy.
- Metabolic and toxic neuropathies.
- Neurocutaneous syndromes.
- Muscle diseases.
- Diseases of the neuromuscular junction.

Hereditary neuropathies

Hereditary motor and sensory neuropathies (HMSNs)

These include all inherited neuropathies that affect both the motor and sensory peripheral nerves. The incidence is approximately 1 : 2500. Classification is changing as molecular genetic defects are discovered. No treatments are yet available, but much can be done in terms of helping the patient overcome his or her disability. Characteristic features include:
- Distal wasting and weakness (giving 'inverted champagne-bottle legs').
- Areflexia.
- Pes cavus.
- Claw toes.
- Distal sensory loss.

HMSN I

This is also still called type 1, or hypertrophic (describing the histological appearance of the nerves) Charcot– Marie–Tooth (CMT) disease. It is usually autosomal dominant.

Because myelin genes appear to be affected, it makes sense that this is a 'demyelinating neuropathy', and nerve conduction velocities are slow. The disease usually presents in childhood or early teenage life with foot drop and leg weakness.

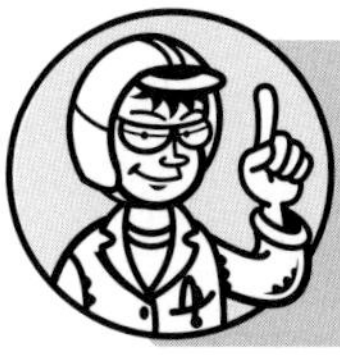

Charcot–Marie–Tooth disease is also known as peroneal muscular atrophy, referring to the wasting pattern in the legs.

Symptoms vary greatly: up to 20% of those affected are significantly disabled as adults, but a similar proportion are asymptomatic.

HMSN II

This is also still called type 2, or neuronal CMT syndrome. This is an 'axonal' neuropathy (i.e. with relatively preserved nerve conduction velocity, but small motor and sensory action potentials). It is usually autosomal dominant, in some cases linked to c1. Presentation is similar to HMSN I, but wasting may be a more prominent feature.

HMSN III

This is also called Déjérine–Sottas disease. It is more severe, presenting in infancy. Recent molecular discoveries indicate that these cases may be 'severe HMSN I'.

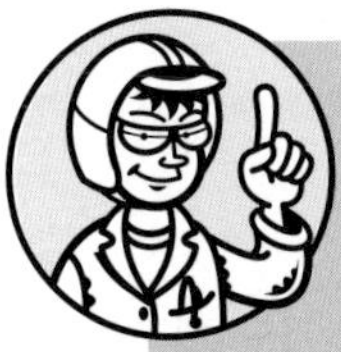

- HMSN I is a demyelinating neuropathy with slow conduction velocities.
- HMSN II is an axonal neuropathy with near-normal conduction velocities.
- HMSN III presents like an early-onset, severe HMSN I.

Hereditary sensory neuropathy

This is a rare autosomal recessive or dominant condition that usually presents in childhood. Loss of pain occurs (predominantly) in the hands and feet. Charcot joint deformities and neuropathic ulcers of the feet also appear.

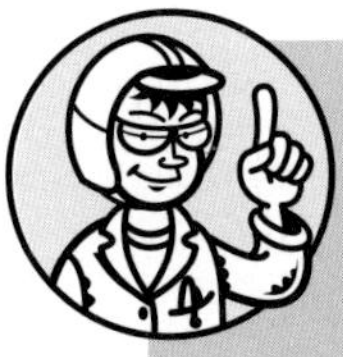

An osteoarthritic joint which has become grossly disorganized due to loss of pain sensation is known as a Charcot joint.

Hereditary sensory and autonomic neuropathy

There are five forms of hereditary sensory and autonomic neuropathies which are recognized. Their features are shown in Fig. 12.1.

Traumatic neuropathies

Trauma to a nerve causes weakness or numbness in the area supplied by that nerve, although sensory nerve injuries tend to cause symptoms and signs in an area smaller than that which the nerve supplies, owing to overlap in sensory territories. Trauma may partially or completely disrupt the nerve's function. Types of nerve injury are given in Fig. 12.2. Axons regrow at a rate of 1.0–1.5 mm/day.

Compression neuropathy

Carpal tunnel syndrome

Carpal tunnel syndrome is common, especially in women. It is caused by pressure on the median nerve as it passes deep to the flexor retinaculum at the wrist. Initial symptoms are pain and tingling in the median nerve territory (most commonly the index and middle fingers), characteristically at night, causing the patient to shake the hand over the side of the bed for relief. Sometimes the pain shoots up the arm from the wrist. Signs may be absent initially. With time, median nerve innervated muscles, especially abductor pollicis brevis, may become weak and wasted and sensory signs may be found (Fig. 12.3).

Tinel's sign (tapping over the wrist) and Phalen's test (flexing the wrist for a minute) may reproduce

Classification of HSANs

Condition	Clinical features
HSAN I	Dominant inheritance. Absence of pain and temperature sensation (particularly distal). Charcot's joints and mutilation of feet common. Autonomic involvement rare.
HSAN II	Recessive inheritance. Combination of large and small fibre loss. Sensory loss is worse distally. Anhydrosis, areflexia and mutilation of extremities occur. Blood pressure and sexual function normal.
HSAN III	'Riley-Day syndrome' – recessive. May present in neomates with hypothermia and vomiting crises. Pain and temperature insensitivity, areflexia and autonomic crises in adults (postural hypotension, hypertension, sweating, etc.)
HSAN IV	Congenital sensory neuropathy with anhydrosis. Associated with mental retardation
HSAN V	Congenital absence of pain sensation without anhydrosis. Purely affects $A\delta$ fibres

Fig. 12.1 Classification of the hereditary sensory and autonomic neuropathies (HSANs).

Types of nerve injury

Injury	Extent	Effect
Neurapraxia	Transient block. No structural damage. Usually compression of nerve is the cause	No degeneration of nerve fibres. Temporary disruption to nerve function which recovers fully
Axonotmesis	Rupture of nerve fibres within intact sheath. Prolonged pressure or crushing is a cause	Wallerian degeneration. Nerves regrow within sheath. Effects on function may be severe but complete recovery is usual
Neurotmesis	Complete seciotn a nerve	Wallerian degeneration. Paralysis/sensory lossare complete. Regeneration may be slow and incomplete.

Fig. 12.2 Types of nerve injury, their effects and potential for recovery.

symptoms, but a good history is the key to diagnosis. Predisposing factors for carpal tunnel syndrome are given in Fig. 12.4. The diagnosis may be confirmed with nerve conduction studies.

Treatment may be non-surgical (wrist splints in slight extension, or local steroid injection) or surgical (division of the flexor retinaculum leading to decompression).

'Saturday night' palsy

'Saturday night' palsy is caused by compression of the radial nerve, especially if an arm is draped over a chair for some hours. It may also occur with fractures of the humerus (as the radial nerve runs in the spiral groove). Wrist drop and weakness of finger and thumb extension occur, but not usually sensory loss. Patients generally recover spontaneously in a few months.

Ulnar nerve compression

This usually occurs at the elbow (in the groove of the medial epicondyle), particularly during general anaesthesia, with the use of crutches, and secondary to previous elbow injury. It can also occur in the cubital tunnel (the fibrous band between the heads of flexor carpi ulnaris). Symptoms include pain and paraesthesiae along the medial aspect of the forearm and numbness in the little and ring fingers, similar to that experienced when hitting your 'funny bone'. There may be wasting and weakness of ulnar-innervated small hand muscles, especially the first dorsal interosseous muscle. If the branch to flexor digitorum profundus is affected (in lesions above the cubital tunnel) there will also be weakness of flexion of the distal interphalangeal joint. The main complaint of patients is that they cannot grip objects.

Treatment involves avoiding unnecessary trauma to the nerve (no leaning on the elbows) and sometimes surgery.

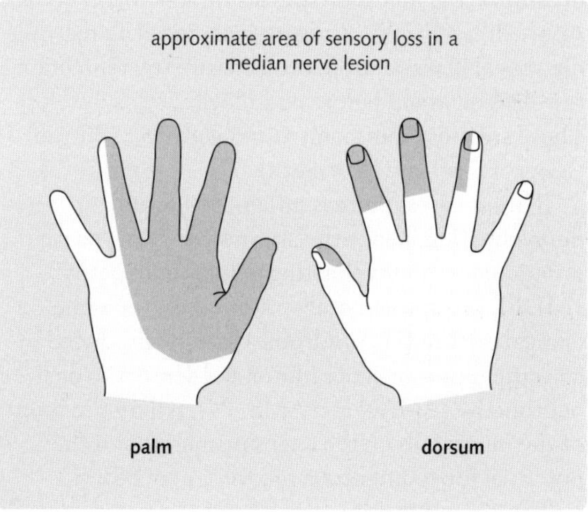

Fig. 12.3 Approximate area of sensory loss in a median nerve lesion.

Predisposing factors for carpal tunnel syndrome
arthritis of the wrist obesity pregnancy hypothyroidism and acromegaly repetitive wrist movements (washing floors, vibrating tools) hereditary neuropathy with liability to pressure palsies (HNPP)
But it is usually idiopathic!

Fig. 12.4 Predisposing factors for carpal tunnel syndrome.

Meralgia paraesthetica

This is a syndrome of tingling, pain and numbness on the anterolateral surface of the thigh caused by compression of the lateral cutaneous nerve of the thigh under the lateral end of the inguinal ligament. It is more common in the obese, in pregnancy and with very tight trousers.

Treatment, other than weight reduction and reconsideration of wardrobe, is unnecessary.

Cervical spondylosis

Cervical spondylosis is a degenerative condition of the vertebral column and intervertebral discs, which is uncommon in patients aged under 50 years. It may cause compressive injuries of cervical roots as they pass through their foramina. The roots of C5, C6 and C7 are commonly affected. The symptoms are shown in Fig. 12.5.

Avulsions

Avulsion of the spinal roots is generally caused by severe traumatic injury. The commonest area is brachial avulsions, but lumbosacral avulsions can occur. Two examples are:

- Erb's palsy: caused by avulsion of C5 and C6 roots because of pressure on the shoulder, usually after motor cycle accidents or, in babies, after forceps delivery. The shoulder cannot be abducted and the elbow cannot be flexed, therefore the arm hangs limply with the wrist flexed.
- Klumpke paralysis: avulsion of C8 and T1, usually occurring when the arm is pulled forcibly upwards (particularly due to birth trauma). Loss of function affects the small muscles of the hand and

Nerve roots damaged with cervical spondylosis			
Nerve root	**Sensory supply**	**Motor supply**	**Reflexes**
C5	Lateral arm and forearm	Shoulder abduction, elbow flexion	Biceps and supinator
C6	Lateral wrist and lateral hand	Elbow flexion	
C7	Middle finger	Elbow extension, finger flexion and extension	Triceps (with C8)

Fig. 12.5 Nerve roots commonly damaged with cervical spondylosis.

the long finger flexors and extensors. This leads to a disabling claw hand deformity and may be associated with Horner's syndrome.

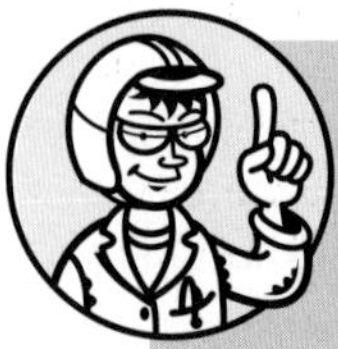

The characteristic deformity seen with Erb's palsy is known as the 'waiter's tip' position. The arm is held straight, with the hand held palm upwards, facing backwards.

Lacerations

Penetrating injury and fracture may lacerate a nerve, causing loss of function in the territory it supplies.

- Ulnar nerve: usually at the elbow, causing signs as above.
- Median nerve: with fractures in the arm, resulting in weakness of forearm flexors, flexor digitorum profundus (the patient cannot flex the distal interphalangeal joint of his forefinger) and, commonly, abductor pollicis brevis, together with sensory loss, as shown in Fig. 12.3. Note that a compression (between the two heads of pronator teres) or traumatic injury affecting the anterior interosseous nerve causes loss of flexion of the distal interphalangeal joints of the thumb, index finger, and sometimes middle finger, without sensory loss.
- Radial nerve: with fractures of the shaft of humerus, causing a similar picture to Saturday night palsy.
- Femoral nerve: femoral artery cannulation may rarely result in damage.
- Sciatic nerve: may be damaged with fractures of the femur and pelvis, misplaced intramuscular injections or penetrating injury.

Inflammatory neuropathies

Guillain–Barré syndrome (GBS)

This is a clinical syndrome caused by an acute peripheral neuropathy, affecting motor more than sensory nerves, and in most cases following infection. The incidence is approximately 1 : 50 000. Following the illness, 20% of patients remain so disabled that they are unable to work after a year, and 5% die. By definition, the illness progresses for less than 4 weeks. Approximately 70% of the patients recall a preceding diarrhoeal illness or upper respiratory tract infection a few days or weeks before neurological signs develop. These are most commonly *Campylobacter* (30% of cases) or CMV (10% of cases).

In most cases, there is inflammation and demyelination, hence the alternative name 'acute inflammatory demyelinating polyradiculopathy' (AIDP). In approximately 5% of cases, the same clinical picture (i.e. syndrome) may be produced by an acute motor or acute motor and sensory axonal neuropathy (AMAN and AMSAN), where the brunt of the injury falls on the axons primarily, and the potential for spontaneous recovery may be less.

The clinical features are:

- Development of symptoms over days or weeks.
- Bilateral flaccid weakness (and later wasting) of proximal and distal limb muscles.
- Loss of tendon reflexes.
- Progression of weakness in some cases to affect the respiratory and bulbar (speech and swallowing) muscles.
- Burning pains and numbness, but often without sensory signs.

Important complications include:

- Respiratory failure and associated respiratory infections.

- Cardiac arrhythmias.
- Labile blood pressure and postural hypotension.
- Pressure sores.
- Anxiety and depression.

Investigations:

- In AIDP, in particular, nerve conduction studies show prolonged distal motor latencies in the upper and lower limbs. Slowing of conduction velocities is a late sign, and may not be seen at all. Action potentials are often reduced.
- Cerebrospinal fluid protein is usually raised (up to 5 g/dL), but the cell count is normal.

The Miller–Fisher syndrome is a variant of GBS with:

- An eye movement disorder caused by cranial nerve III, IV or VI palsies.
- Cerebellar ataxia.
- Areflexia.

Management

Management involves avoidance of complications, by regular measurement of the vital capacity (deterioration may be rapid; the patient may require ventilation only hours after symptoms begin), constant electrocardiogram recording and careful nursing. Patients may require long stays in intensive care, with 25% requiring respiratory support. Plasma exchange and intravenous immunoglobulin are equally effective at hastening recovery. Pain may be a prominent feature—good physiotherapy and non-steroidal anti-inflammatory drugs are helpful.

The disease ultimately is self-limiting, with remyelination of axons within a matter of weeks.

Differential diagnosis of Guillain–Barré syndrome

Neuropathies:

- Porphyria.
- Acute heavy metal poisoning.
- Diphtheria.
- Vasculitis.
- HIV-related neuropathy.

Anterior horn cell:

- Poliomyelitis.

Central nervous system:

- Cord compression.
- Transverse myelopathy.
- Brainstem infarction.

Neuromuscular:

- Myasthenia gravis.
- Botulism.

Muscular:

- Periodic paralysis.
- Acute polymyositis.

Chronic inflammatory demyelinating polyradiculopathy (CIDP)

CIDP has a similar pathology to GBS, but it follows a relapsing–remitting course, with more slowly progressive onset of signs.

The condition responds in 80% of cases to steroids, intravenous immunoglobulin and plasma exchange.

Paraproteinaemic neuropathy

Paraproteinaemic neuropathy is associated with:

- Benign monoclonal gammopathy (of undetermined significance)—demyelinating neuropathy with immunoglobulin M and immunoglobulin G paraproteins.
- Multiple myeloma (especially osteosclerotic)—neuropathy in 5% cases, typically mixed sensory and motor.
- Solitary plasmacytoma—as for myeloma, often responsive to radiation or surgery to remove the primary tumour.
- Waldenström's macroglobulinaemia.

Infectious neuropathies

Postinfectious neuropathies

These include:

- Guillain–Barré syndrome.
- Diphtheria: rare in the UK due to immunization. Progressive peripheral neuropathy caused by the exotoxin, may occur a few weeks after the acute febrile illness. Supportive treatment until recovery is necessary.
- Lyme disease (Bannwarth's syndrome): rare in the UK. A Guillain–Barré-type syndrome may occur some weeks later. Treatment of the acute illness is with benzylpenicillin; the subsequent neuropathy recovers gradually.

Infectious neuropathies

These are all rare in the UK. They include:

- **Leprosy**: common in southern Asia and Africa. Causes a patchy peripheral neuropathy (primarily sensory loss) with hypopigmented, anaesthetic skin lesions and thickened nerves. Diagnosis is by skin or nerve biopsy; the acid-fast bacilli are seen within the tissue.

- **Tetanus**: caused by infection of a wound by *Clostridium tetani*. Days to weeks later, rigidity and pain in voluntary muscles occur, with difficulty opening the jaw (trismus), facial stiffness (risus sardonicus), dysphagia, back stiffness, hyperextension and respiratory difficulty. Spasms may be strong enough to cause vertebral crush fractures, and may lead to exhaustion and respiratory failure. Treatment includes debriding the initial wound, benzylpenicillin, human antitetanus immunoglobulin and good supportive care in a quiet environment (because stimulation may induce spasms). Diazepam may be used to control spasms.
- **Botulism**: caused by ingestion of *Clostridium botulinum*. A neurotoxin may cause symptoms because of cholinergic blockade. Hours to days later, lower motor neuron and autonomic symptoms may occur, generally beginning with blurred vision and diplopia. Flaccid weakness and paralysis (particularly of the laryngeal and pharyngeal muscles) spreading to include respiratory muscles. This may mimic myasthenia gravis or Guillain–Barré syndrome. Antitoxin treats the acute infection but the mainstay of management is good supportive care whilst awaiting recovery.
- **Herpes simplex** (type 2) virus: may cause lumbosacral radiculopathy.
- **Herpes zoster virus** or 'shingles': or a reactivation of latent herpes zoster which has remained dormant in the dorsal root ganglia since an attack of chickenpox in earlier life. It may occur in normal people, but is more common in the immunosuppressed (especially those with haematological malignancies and AIDS). A dermatomal vesicular rash is usually present. Symptoms caused by peripheral nerve involvement include pain, then numbness in the area of the rash, flaccid weakness in the root distribution of the rash, which may then spread (and may even progress to Guillain–Barré syndrome). Intravenous acyclovir is the treatment for all neurologically serious complications of herpes virus infections.
- **HIV**: may present with a variety of neurological manifestations. Acute complications include mild viral meningitis at the time of seroconversion, meningoencephalitis, facial palsy, peripheral neuropathy, dorsal root ganglionitis (acute ataxic neuropathy), transverse myelitis and polymyositis. Chronic neurological problems include vacuolar myelopathy, peripheral neuropathy and AIDS dementia complex. These patients are also susceptible to opportunistic infections such as: CMV radiculopathy, cryptococcal meningitis, toxoplasmosis (cerebral abscesses), progressive multifocal leucoencephalopathy and tuberculous meningitis and atypical mycobacteria. In addition, tumours such as primary central nervous system B cell lymphoma may occur.

Metabolic and toxic neuropathies

Diabetes mellitus

Diabetes is the commonest cause of neuropathy in the UK. It is more common with poorly controlled diabetics and may occur with insulin-dependant or non-insulin-dependant diabetes mellitus. The pathological cause remains uncertain (probably a combination of microangiopathy and glycosylation of nerves). The neuropathy is usually axonal. To some extent, the problems are preventable and may be improved by good diabetic control. There are five main clinical patterns of neuropathy:

- Symmetrical sensory peripheral neuropathy: most common, causing numbness, pain and tingling, usually in the feet, sometimes with weakness (a sensorimotor neuropathy). If severe, a neuropathic (Charcot) joint may result, with painless destruction and disorganization of the joint.
- Acute painful neuropathy: commonest in new diabetics, and in those with suddenly improved glycaemic control. Symptoms may make the patient's life miserable, with burning pains in the legs, particularly at night.
- Autonomic neuropathy: may affect the genitourinary system (with impotence and bladder problems), sweating (e.g. during eating), the gastrointestinal tract (with gastric atony, nocturnal diarrhoea, constipation), the cardiovascular system (especially with postural hypotension).
- Isolated nerve lesions (mononeuropathy): especially cranial nerves III (notably sparing the pupil) and VI, and the more common sites of

nerve compression in the limbs. Diabetic amyotrophy is a painful wasting and weakness in the thigh with a depressed or absent knee jerk, which may be caused by a femoral nerve neuropathy.
- Multiple mononeuropathy (affecting more than one nerve, but sparing others)—otherwise known as mononeuritis multiplex.

Careful monitoring of diabetic patients for early signs of neuropathy is therefore essential.

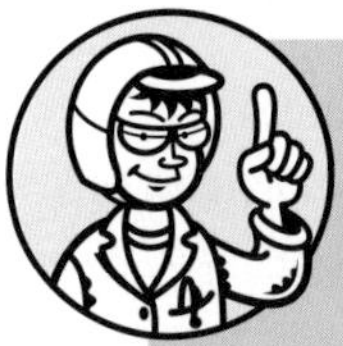

Mononeuritis multiplex is a syndrome where there are discrete focal lesions in several individual nerves. The patient may present with a series of nerve palsies or have them all at once.

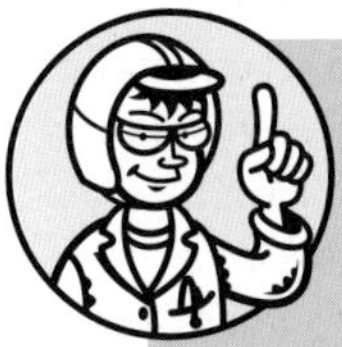

Causes of mononeuritis multiplex:
- Collagen vascular disease (e.g. systemic lupus erythematosus, rheumatoid arthritis, Sjögren's syndrome, polyarteritis nodosa).
- Diabetes mellitus.
- Sarcoidosis.
- Infections (e.g. Lyme disease, leprosy, AIDS).
- Paraneoplastic syndromes.
- Alcohol.
- Hereditary neuropathy with liability to pressure palsy.

Other metabolic and endocrine causes

Metabolic causes of neuropathy include:
- Vitamin deficiencies: B_1 (thiamine), B_6, B_{12} and E.
- Uraemia (seen in severe chronic renal failure).
- Liver failure.
- Chronic lung disease.

Endocrine causes include:
- Thyrotoxicosis.

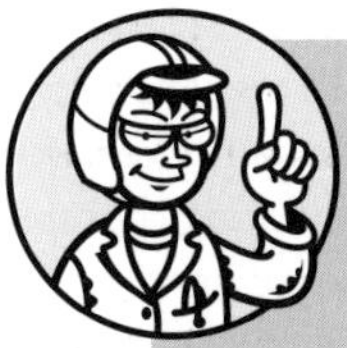

Neurological features of B_{12} deficiency:
- Sensory neuropathy (common).
- Dorsal column sensory loss.
- Subacute combined degeneration of the cord (dorsal column plus corticospinal loss).
- Dementia.
- Depression.
- Optic atrophy.

- Myxoedema.
- Acromegaly.

Toxic neuropathies

Drugs:
- Alcohol (direct effect, but may also cause thiamine deficiency).
- Antibiotics: isoniazid, nitrofurantoin, metronidazole.
- Chemotherapeutic agents: vincristine, cisplatin.
- Psychotherapeutic agents: lithium, tricyclic antidepressants.
- Amiodarone.

Industrial agents:
- Organic solvents (e.g. *n*-hexane, may affect glue-sniffers), acrylamide.
- Toluene.
- Arsenic (insecticides).
- Organophosphates (insecticides, pesticides).
- Lead (contamination of drinking water from old pipes).
- Thallium (pesticides).
- Triorthocresyl phosphate (high-temperature lubricant).

Neuropathies associated with malignancy

Although not strictly 'metabolic' or 'toxic', these are considered here for convenience. There are three main groups:
- Paraneoplastic syndromes: probably immunologically mediated distant manifestations in association with certain tumours, such as small-cell lung cancer (with subacute sensory polyneuropathy and high titres of the anti-Hu antibody). Other neurological syndromes may also

occur (e.g. cerebellar syndrome and anti-Purkinje cell antibody with breast cancer). In most cases, these are not treatable, but there are some reports of improvement with immunomodulating therapy.
- Direct infiltration: by primary or secondary tumours.
- Associated with particular malignancies: multiple myeloma, solitary plasmacytoma, Waldenström's macroglobulinaemia, and lymphoma are sometimes associated with a generalized sensorimotor neuropathy.

Neurocutaneous syndromes

Neurocutaneous syndromes are a group of disorders in which tumours and hamartomas develop in the skin, retinas and nervous system.

Tumours associated with these syndromes

Schwannoma

A Schwannoma is an abnormal (but benign) growth of Schwann cell myelin. Virtually all of these tumours affect sensory neurons, particularly the VIIIth cranial nerve.

Neurofibroma

This is a cutaneous tumour, made up of an abnormal mass of Schwann cells and fibroblasts. Although they are benign, surgical resection may be difficult as the affected nerve may have to be sacrificed.

Malignant peripheral nerve sheath tumour

This is the malignant counterpart to the Schwannoma and neurofibroma. It is commonest in deep soft tissue, close to a nerve trunk. Sites include the sciatic nerve, and the brachial and sacral plexuses. It is associated with neurofibromatosis type 1.

Neurofibromatosis

Neurofibromatosis is a common inherited (autosomal dominant) neurological condition. The incidence is 1 : 3000. Type I (von Recklinghausen's disease) and type II diseases exist. Complications (e.g. tumours of nerves or brain) may be treated, and careful monitoring of patients is therefore essential.

Type I (NF I)

Type I is caused by a mutation on c17q. Features include:

- Skin:
  - Café-au-lait patches (pale brown macules).
  - Peripheral neurofibromas; dermal (soft) and nodular (hard).
  - Axillary freckles.
  - Plexiform neuromas.
- Neurological:
  - Schwannomas of the central and peripheral nervous systems. (including VIIIth nerve tumours).
  - Meningioma.
  - Glioma (especially optic).
  - Spinal cord and nerve root neurofibromas.
- Eye:
  - Orbital haemangioma, Lisch nodules; hamartomas of the iris.
- Skeletal malformations:
  - Scoliosis.
  - Subperiosteal neurofibromas.

Diagnosis of NF I

Two or more of the following:

- Six or more café-au-lait spots > 5 mm diameter (prepubertal) (> 15 mm after puberty).
- Two or more neurofibromas or one plexiform neurofibroma.
- Axillary or inguinal freckles.
- Optic glioma.
- Two or more Lisch nodules.
- Osseous lesion.
- First-degree relative affected by the above criteria.

Type II (NF II)

Type II is caused by mutations on c22q. Features include:

- Bilateral vestibular schwannomas (acoustic neuromas).
- May also feature multiple central nervous system tumours.

Diagnosis of NF II

Bilateral VIII nerve masses on imaging, **or** first-degree relative with NF II and unilateral VIII nerve mass **or** first-degree relative and two of the following:

- Neurofibroma.
- Meningioma.
- Glioma.
- Schwannoma.
- Posterior capsular lenticular opacity.

Tuberose sclerosis

Tuberose sclerosis is a condition in which multiple hamartomas (abnormal mesodermal masses) occur, which are usually benign, but can be malignant in rare cases. The condition is autosomal dominant, but with very variable expression. Onset is in childhood. The condition is untreatable, but tumours may be removed surgically. Features are:

- Adenoma sebaceum: hamartomas of the sebaceous glands on the face.
- Fibromas: dermal and around the nail-bed (subungual and periungual).
- Shagreen patches: rough patches on the skin of the lumbar area.
- Café-au-lait spots (also on the retina—phakomata).
- Pigmented naevi.
- Neurologically, masses or tubers in the brain, especially the basal ganglia, may occur, resulting in mental retardation, behavioural disturbances, epilepsy and hydrocephalus.
- Bony changes: 'cysts' and sclerotic lesions in the phalanges.
- Hypertelorism: wide separation of the orbits.
- Lung and other organ hamartomas.

von Hippel–Lindau syndrome

von Hippel–Lindau syndrome is an autosomal dominant condition, comprising:

- Cerebellar haemangioblastomas: associated with polycythaemia.
- Retinal angiomas.
- Phaeochromocytoma.
- Renal, adrenal and pancreatic tumours.
- Sometimes other vascular tumours of the central nervous system.

Ataxia telangiectasia

Ataxia telangiectasia is an autosomal recessive condition, causing progressive cerebellar degeneration. Features include:

- Delayed motor development.
- Telangiectasiae, especially of the conjunctivae and over the ears.
- Slurred speech and ataxia.
- Ocular apraxia.
- Chorea.
- Immunoglobulin deficiencies and lymphoreticular malignancies.
- Mild mental retardation.
- Death usually before 30 years.

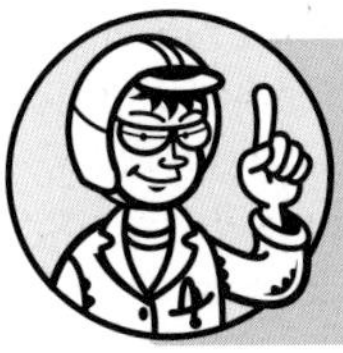

Telangiectasiae are localized areas of distended capillaries which blanche under pressure.

Diseases of the muscle and neuromuscular junction

Myopathy is a term embracing all forms of primary muscle disorder. Dystrophy refers to a group of inherited myopathies in which progressive degenerative changes occur in muscle fibres. Fig. 12.6 lists a simplified classification.

Dystrophies

Duchenne muscular dystrophy (DMD) is relatively common, with an incidence of 1 : 3500. It is caused in most cases by a mutation in the dystrophin gene, resulting in reduced levels or absence of the protein dystrophin. Becker muscular dystrophy is caused by mutations in the same gene, but these result in a truncated rather than an absent/non-functional protein, and thus a milder disease.

Dystrophies are X-linked, and therefore primarily affect boys.

In affected cases, there is progressive proximal muscle weakness and pseudohypertrophy of the calf-muscles.

Classification of muscle/neuromuscular junction disorders

Type of disorder	Examples
muscular dystrophy	Duchenne's, Becker's, facioscapulohumeral, limb-girdle, myotonic dystrophy
inflammatory myopathy	polymyositis, dermatomyositis, inclusion body myositis, infective myositis, polymyalgia rheumatica
metabolic myopathy	McArdles's disease, mitochondrial disorders, periodic paralyses
endocrine myopathy	thyroid disease, Cushing's disease
drug-induced myopathy	clofibrate, D-penicillamine, steroids, alcohol
disorders of neuromuscular transmission	myasthenia gravis, Lambert–Eaton myasthenic syndrome, stiff-man syndrome

Fig. 12.6 Classification of muscle/neuromuscular junction disorders.

Current research is very active, looking for possible methods of increasing dystrophin expression levels, but to date, therapy is aimed at physical aids to overcome disabilities and to prevent complications. Systemic corticosteroids may improve the natural history of the disease for up to 2 years, but have serious side effects. Despite treatment, most sufferers of DMD will lose the ability to walk by the age of 12 years, and die from respiratory or cardiac failure in early adult life.

Other muscular dystrophies include limb-girdle muscular dystrophy and facioscapulohumeral muscular dystrophy.

Polymyositis

Polymyositis is an acquired inflammatory myopathy, which affects women more commonly than men. The incidence of this together with dermatomyositis is approximately 1 : 100 000. It is a disorder of acute or subacute onset, with fever, muscle pain and tenderness, and proximal weakness, which may spread and be so severe as to require ventilation. Pathologically, infiltration of $CD8^+$ T cells occurs in associaion with necrosis of muscle fibres. The primary cause is unknown.

Dermatomyositis has a different pathological basis (associated with B cell and $CD4^+$ T cell infiltration of the vessels) and is associated with photosensitivity and a 'heliotrope' rash around the eyes. In adults, but not in children, it may be associated with underlying malignancy (in 40% of those aged over 40 years).

Both conditions respond to steroids.

Inclusion body myositis

This condition is the commonest cause of acquired myopathy in the elderly, especially in men. Features are similar to polymyositis, and include progressive distal and proximal weakness. It does not respond to steroids.

Polymyalgia rheumatica

This is an important disorder in the elderly, with an incidence of 1 : 1000 in those aged over 50 years. It is associated with temporal arteritis and, importantly, there is a risk of sudden blindness if it is untreated. The condition is sensitive to steroids.

Metabolic myopathies

All metabolic myopathies are rare. McArdle's disease, a glycogenosis caused by deficiency of myophosphorylase, is the commonest of this group of disorders, and is associated with painful muscle cramps and weakness during exercise. Recently, the periodic paralyses (Fig. 12.7) have been found to be caused by ion-channel mutations and are now included in the class of disorders know as 'channelopathies'.

Disorders of neuromuscular transmission

Myasthenia gravis

The prevalence of myasthenia gravis is approximately 1 : 20 000. Women are affected twice as frequently as men. The condition is characterized by fatiguable weakness of periocular, facial, and proximal muscles [i.e. it worsens with exercise, and usually gets worse as the day goes on (diurnal)].

Myasthenia gravis is associated with acetylcholine-receptor antibodies at the neuromuscular junction. Both immunological and genetic factors appear to be important in its pathogenesis.

The condition is associated with lymphoid hyperplasia and tumours of the thymus. Weakness may respond to surgical thymic removal, especially in young patients with a short history. Otherwise, treatment is with immunosuppression and with anticholinesterases.

Lambert–Eaton myasthenic syndrome

This is characterized by weakness that is initially lessened with exercise. It is a rare disorder that is more common in men. It is caused by an autoimmune destruction of presynaptic voltage-gated calcium channels at the NMJ, causing a reduction in the amount of acetylcholine released.

The periodic paralyses

Hyperkalaemic periodic paralysis	Hypokalaemic periodic paralysis
sodium-channel mutations, chromosome 17	calcium-channel mutations, chromosome 1
autosomal recessive	autosomal dominant
occurs with rest after exercise and may have periocular myotonia	occurs after meals and with rest after exercise
short attacks of weakness (about 1 hour) which may be aborted by exercise at onset	weakness for several hours

Fig. 12.7 The potassium channel periodic paralyses. Note that the presentations are often identical, and the conditions cannot often be differentiated clinically.

Lambert–Eaton myasthenic syndrome is associated in up to 60% of cases with a small cell lung carcinoma. Patients presenting this way should be fully investigated.

- Describe the key clinical features of Charcot–Marie–Tooth disease.
- What are the features of carpal tunnel syndrome. What clinical tests could you do to make the diagnosis?
- Describe the different ways in which a nerve may be traumatized.
- Give an example of a postinfectious neuropathy, and discuss its sequelae.
- What are the possible consequences of diabetic neuropathy?
- What is neurofibromatosis? How is it classified and diagnosed?
- Compare Duchenne and Becker muscular dystrophies.
- Describe the underlying abnormality in myasthenia gravis. How is it diagnosed and treated?

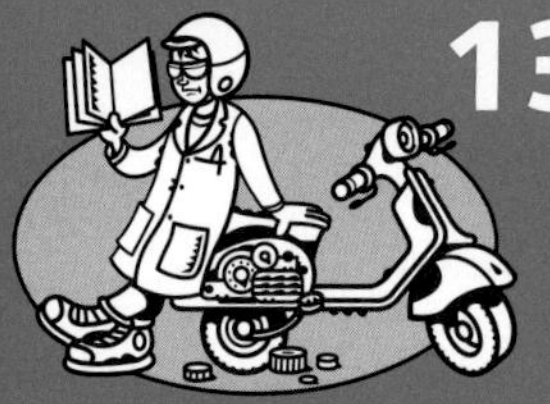

13. Higher Centres of the Central Nervous System

In this chapter, you will learn about:

- The functions of different areas of the cerebral cortex.
- Mechanisms of learning and memory.
- The limbic system and its functions.
- Cognition and cognitive impairment.
- Disorders of higher central nervous system function.
- Antiemetic drugs.
- General anaesthetics.

Localization of function and behaviour

Structural and functional asymmetry

There are structural differences between hemispheres.

The planum temporale (superior aspect of the temporal lobe lying within the lateral sulcus) is larger on the left side in the majority of people. Wernicke's area lies in the posterior part of the planum temporale, and speech is affected by damage to this area of the temporal lobe on the left, but not on the right. Along with the fact that the left hand side of the brain controls the right hand (dominant in most people), this has led to the concept of 'left hemisphere dominance'. A small, but significant number of left-handed people have right-hemisphere speech.

The localization of functional areas has been experimentally demonstrated by:

- Positron emission tomography (PET) or functional magnetic resonance imaging of normal subjects performing a range of tasks.
- Wada's test, where sodium amytal is injected into one carotid artery, which temporarily anaesthetizes one hemisphere so that tasks can be processed only by the other one. For example, injection of sodium amytal into the left carotid artery will temporarily block speech in most subjects.

Although the left and right hemispheres are connected through the corpus callosum, they carry out different functions. The evidence for this comes from:

- Patients with lesions localized to one hemisphere (e.g. patients who have aphasia following a left hemisphere stroke).
- Patients with severe grand mal epilepsy who have undergone sectioning of the corpus callosum (commissurotomy) to prevent spread of seizures.
- 'Split-brain' animal studies, in which a commissurotomy has been carried out.

In a classical experiment on commissurotomy patients, subjects were presented with a picture of an apple solely to their right visual field. A patient would report seeing an apple, as might be expected. However, if this was presented to the left visual field (and therefore to the right hemisphere), the patient reported seeing nothing. The patient had not lost his left visual field, as he was able to point to an apple, or to pick it out using tactile clues. In other words, a subject's right hemisphere could not name the object, but could identify it by nonverbal means.

Split-brain experiments may not give us the whole story, as there is some evidence that the ability of a hemisphere to carry out a task may deteriorate after commissurotomy. However, in a simplified view, lateralization can be summarized:

- The left hemisphere is involved in intellectual reasoning and language.
- The right hemisphere is more concerned with spatial construction (including depth perception and the internal 'map' of our surroundings) and emotion.

This will not be true for all patients, and the existence of commissural connections complicates this picture.

There is an element of plasticity in the location of function. In children who sustain damage to one hemisphere, the other one can take over its functions so that there is no appreciable deficit. This is not the case in adults, as shown by the effects of a stroke.

Cortical localization

Different cortical regions perform different functions. This is because of their different input and output connections.

Regions within different lobes can be split up into functional units:

- Primary sensory or motor areas, which receive information from outside the brain or project outside the brain.
- Higher-order sensory or motor areas. These areas carry out further processing on information from one modality. For example, visual areas V2–V5 segregate information into the colour, form and motion channels. The supplementary motor area has a role in planning movements by integrating inputs from the prefrontal cortex, basal ganglia and cingulate cortex.
- Association areas, where information from different modalities is brought together for processing that encompasses more than just vision, hearing, etc. (e.g. the posterior parietal cortex has a role in integrating visual information with somatic information to give an awareness of one's presence in space).

Frontal lobes

The frontal lobes have:

- An association area that plans sequences of responses, changes response patterns to fit current demands and controls emotional states.
- Higher-order motor processing areas that have motor control functions for eye movements (the frontal eye fields) and speech (Broca's area on the dominant side).

Therefore frontal cortex damage can produce:

- Inability to organize responses to solve problems.
- An error pattern of 'perseveration' in tasks where changes must be responded to. The Wisconsin card-sorting test is based on asking a subject to sort cards according to one rule (e.g. same colour), and then the examiner changes the rule (e.g. to same pattern). The subject works out the new rule by feedback from the examiner about correct or incorrect card sorting. Perseveration occurs when subjects do not change from using a previously correct rule that has become incorrect.
- Personality changes occurring along emotional dimensions. Patients typically become more impulsive, aggressive and subject to rapid changes in emotional state. This is referred to as disinhibition.
- Disordered eye movement scanning of a visual scene.
- Damage to Broca's area produces problems in speech production with hesitant, limited speech (described as 'telegrammatic').
- Disordered working memory (with distractability).

It is rare for these patients to have insight into their condition.

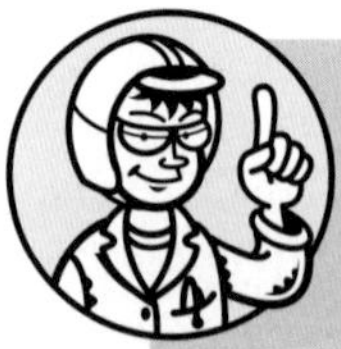

Perseveration may be an important feature in dementia. When asked their name, patients may answer correctly, but subsequent (different) questions will elicit the same answer.

Temporal lobes

The temporal lobes have:

- Association areas that are involved in learning.
- Higher-order sensory areas involved in the comprehension of language (Wernicke's area) and visual object recognition.

The consequences of temporal damage are:

- Disorders in learning verbal information in left-sided lesions.
- Disorders in learning visuospatial information in right-sided lesions.
- Problems in understanding spoken and written language but no reduction in fluency of language production (receptive aphasia). This results in meaningless or irrelevant speech.
- Object agnosia, where patients cannot recognize objects from visual information but can do so from other modalities (e.g. touch).

Parietal lobes

The parietal lobes have:

- A primary sensory area receiving somatosensory information.
- A higher-order sensory area.
- An association area where many sensory modalities and motor inputs converge to build up a picture of how the body is positioned in the environment (incorporating attentional

mechanisms) and how the environment is structured.

Damage can therefore produce:

- Lack of conscious sensation on one half of the body.
- Attentional deficits presenting as neglect (usually of the left half of space after a right-sided lesion).
- Inability to make voluntary eye movements and optic ataxia after bilateral parieto-occipital damage (Balint syndrome).
- Constructional apraxia, which is an inability to organize movement in space (seen with right-sided lesions). It is tested by attempting to copy a figure by drawing, typically interlocking pentagons in the mini mental state examination.
- Disorders of spatial awareness (also mainly seen with right-sided lesions). This manifests as a defect in route finding.
- Disorders of language (mainly with damage to the dominant parietal lobe, although there may be aspects of speech which are processed in the non-dominant hemisphere).
- Agnosia—this is the inability to perceive objects normally. People with parietal damage may have astereognosia—an inability to recognize objects by touch. For example, they could not pick out a particular coin from a selection in a pocket by touch alone, without looking at the coins.

Each hemisphere represents the contralateral half of space in the parietal cortex. However, there is an unequal amount of space represented in each hemisphere. The left hemisphere represents only the right side of space. The right hemisphere represents the left and some of the right side of space. The right side of space is therefore slightly over-represented.

This means that lesions of the left parietal cortex will not affect processing of the right side of space severely because this is also being carried out to some extent in the right parietal cortex.

Right-sided lesions will produce more severe effects on the processing of the left half of space because it is not carried out anywhere else.

Learning and memory

Learning is the acquisition of new information. Memory is the retention of learned information, and can be divided into two basic parts:

- Declarative memory for facts (semantic memory, e.g. London is the capital of England) and events (episodic memory, e.g. I had a sandwich for lunch). This is easy both to acquire and to lose.
- Procedural memory for skills/behaviour, which is hard to acquire and also hard to lose (even in profound loss of declarative memory, e.g. you never forget how to ride a bike).

Declarative memory can be split into three parts, as shown in Fig. 13.1:

- Sensory memory.
- Working memory.
- Long-term memory.

Sensory memory

Sensory memory is a store of all the sensory information that has just been processed. It is held in stores that are modality specific (e.g. visual stores, tactile stores) with a very high capacity, but that are limited in the time which information can be held (fading after 0.5 s).

There is no conscious access to sensory memory. Its function is in selective attention, filtering the inputs that will be consciously processed by working memory.

Working memory

Working memory contains the information that we are processing 'right now' and we have conscious access to it. Inputs to working memory are from sensory memory or long-term memory.

- Its span (maximum capacity) is typically less than a dozen units of information (number, word, etc.).
- It functions as a push-down stack, so that new units of information displace the oldest units from the working memory store. Units are generally thought to only be stored for a few minutes at most.
- It has a visual store and a verbal store. Words are more likely to be coded by their acoustic properties than by semantic properties (what the words mean).

Long-term memory

Long-term memory is a collection of different types of memory that are grouped together by the nature of the information stored. As a general principle of long-term memory properties, these stores show unlimited capacity, but limitations in the capacity of the retrieval mechanism.

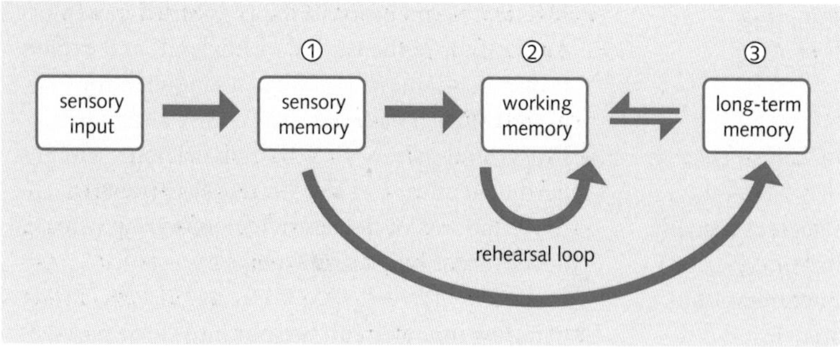

Fig. 13.1 The three-stage model of memory.

Distinctions between long-term memory and working memory

Studies of amnesia

In Wernicke–Korsakoff syndrome, the amnesia affects memory for events in adult life (sparing childhood memories) but patients have a preserved working memory span.

The serial position effect

After giving normal subjects a list of data, then asking them to recall the information freely in any order, the first and last units of information are preferentially recalled (the primacy and recency effects, respectively). After a delay before testing recall, the recency effect is lost. This suggests that working memory holds the most recently given data and that first few units of information have made it into the long-term stores.

The coding strategy for holding verbal information

Working memory uses an acoustic strategy (evidence for this comes from error patterns made by normal subjects when recalling verbal information) whereas long-term memory stores verbal information in terms of meaning (typically, we can remember the 'gist' of what people have said without recalling the actual words used).

Capacity for information

Working memory is limited in terms of the amount of information it holds and the time for which it is held. Long-term memory has an unlimited capacity for information and the information held has a much longer 'shelf life'. Over time, there is either gradual loss of storage space or, more likely, a diminished capacity to retrieve the information stored. Thus, we tend to get more forgetful as we get older.

Amnesia and localization of memory function

Amnesia is the loss of memory and/or the ability to learn, either caused by brain injury (organic amnesia) or for psychological reasons such as great stress (psychogenic amnesia).

- Retrograde amnesia is a loss of memory for things before the injury. Memories which have recently been transferred from the short-term to long-term stores may be more vulnerable to disruption.
- Anterograde amnesia is an inability to form new memories after injury.

Medial temporal lobe structures (e.g. the hippocampus and parahippocampal gyrus) have been implicated in memory function, and damage in these areas produces disruption of declarative memory, sparing procedural memory. This area receives highly processed information from association cortices and, as a possible cellular basis for memory, long-term potentiation (see below) has been recorded in cells in the hippocampus.

Memory disruption may also occur after frontal and thalamic lesions.

The limbic system

Overview of the limbic system

The limbic system is a complex system of fibre tracts and grey matter. It is located on the medial aspect of each temporal lobe, encircling (limbus = border) the upper part of the brainstem.

- It serves as the 'nervous system' for emotional feelings and behaviour.
- It has extensive connections to both lower and higher parts of the central nervous system, which give the system an ability to integrate a wide variety of stimuli.

- It has connections with the hypothalamus to provide a substrate for a variety of nervous, hormonal and visceral interactions.

The limbic system is in a position to influence both higher cognitive processes and lower homoeostatic regulatory processes. Emotion, by its very nature, seems to bridge these two types of processing, requiring dimensions of thought and physical sensations. Memory plays a role in emotion, particularly in guiding behavioural responses to the environment, but the memory functions of the limbic system are not restricted to emotionally-laden stimuli.

Although this picture of different functions may seem confusing, it highlights the areas to be aware of when dealing with patients who have suffered damage to these regions.

Structure of the limbic system

Fig. 13.2 shows the arrangement of limbic structures. We can consider the complicated connections of the limbic system as two simpler systems:

- A system primarily involved in learning and memory.
- A system involved with the processing of emotion, particularly its behavioural and endocrine aspects.

There are modulatory inputs from the reticular formation. The locus coeruleus sends a noradrenergic input and the raphe nuclei send a serotonergic input.

Hippocampal circuit

The hippocampal circuit runs from the medial temporal lobe (hippocampus and parahippocampal gyrus) to the mammillary bodies and thalamus, and is involved in learning and memory. The connections offer some guide as to how information flows in the circuit, as shown in Fig. 13.3.

There is some debate about the precise role of this circuit, particularly the hippocampus, parahippocampal gyrus and mammillary bodies, but the following points are clear:

- Damage to the medial temporal lobe involving the hippocampus and parahippocampal gyrus (e.g. after herpes simplex encephalitis) produces a profound defect in declarative memory acquisition. This leads to anterograde amnesia. Long-term memories are probably stored in the overlying cerebral cortex.
- The physiological properties of cells in the hippocampus allow them to give increased responses to certain patterns of input. This occurs via long-term potentiation, which is an increase in the efficacy of a synapse with repetitive stimulation. It is mediated by NMDA glutamate receptors, which are plentiful in the hippocampus. Repeated depolarization of the post-synaptic

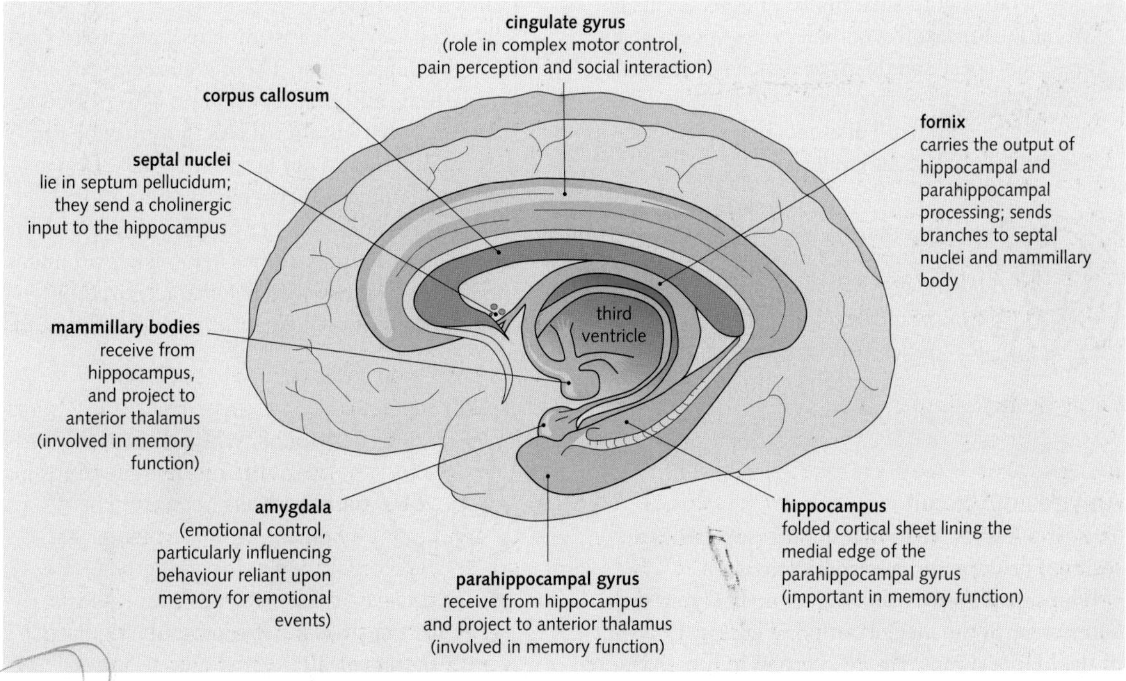

Fig. 13.2 Outline of the limbic system.

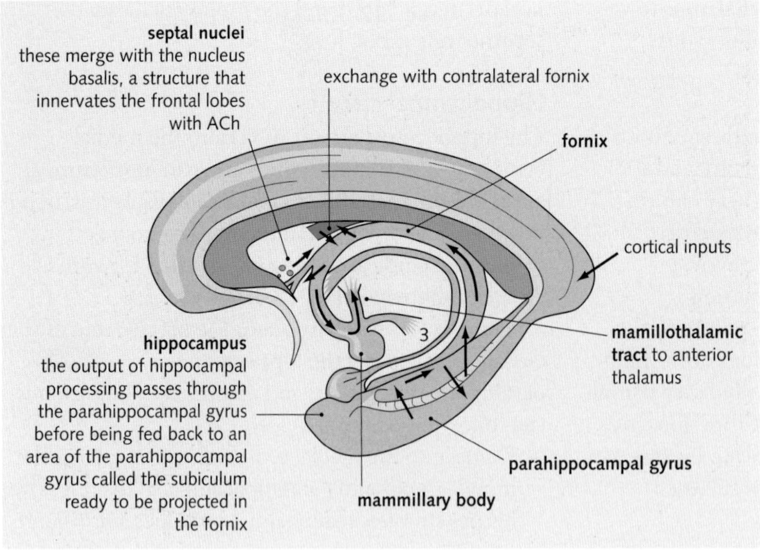
septal nuclei
these merge with the nucleus basalis, a structure that innervates the frontal lobes with ACh
exchange with contralateral fornix
fornix
cortical inputs
3
hippocampus
the output of hippocampal processing passes through the parahippocampal gyrus before being fed back to an area of the parahippocampal gyrus called the subiculum ready to be projected in the fornix
mamillothalamic tract to anterior thalamus
parahippocampal gyrus
mammillary body

Fig. 13.3 Processing in the hippocampal circuit. To trace the pathway start at the hippocampus and follow the arrows.

membrane causes an alteration in the NMDA receptor, allowing calcium to enter the cell. This causes protein kinase activation, and phosphorylation of the AMPA glutamate receptor (the receptor used under normal circumstances at glutamatergic synapses). Recent evidence suggests that this may lead to a duplication of the presynaptic terminal (by an unknown mechanism) and consequent strengthening of the synapse. The sequence of events is summarized in Fig. 13.4.

- Degeneration of the mammillary bodies occurs in Wernicke–Korsakoff syndrome, where a combination of alcohol abuse and thiamine deficiency results in a memory disorder with anterograde amnesia. There may also be poor recall of events before the onset of the disease (retrograde amnesia).

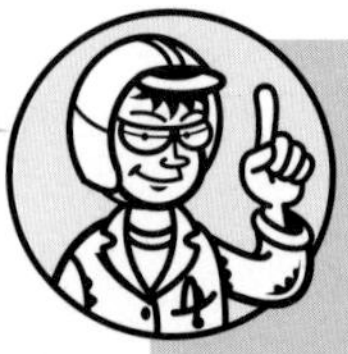

Alzheimer's disease is typified by the inability to form new memories, and is due to the deposition of neurofibrillary tangles and amyloid plaques in the parahipppocampal areas.

Amygdaloid circuit

This circuit is less clear in function, possibly as a result of its rather diffuse connections.

The amygdala is a collection of nuclei lying at the anterior tip of the medial temporal lobe just in front of the hippocampus. Fig. 13.5 shows inputs to the amygdala. Its outputs are simply connections travelling to the sources of input (reciprocal connections), but the largest output is to the hypothalamus through the stria terminalis.

There are many potential functions for the amygdala, though no 'unifying theory' has yet been proposed.

- Lesion experiments on animals examining the function of the lateral part of the amygdala suggest that this circuit is involved in governing behaviour towards stimuli associated with reward (particularly food).
- When the amygdala is stimulated, patients report strong feelings of fear. There is an accompanying sympathetic autonomic response. This has led to the theory that emotional reactions may be partly determined by activity in the amygdala. Lesions may cause impaired recognition of emotional facial expressions of other people. Ablation of the amygdala and hippocampus in monkeys produces the Klüver–Bucy syndrome, characterized by decreased emotionality, withdrawal, tendency to

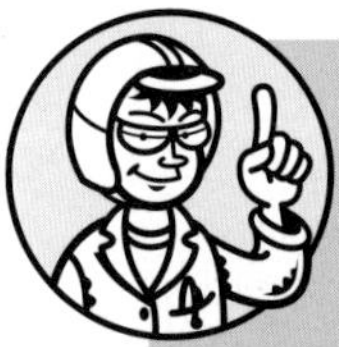

The inability of autistic children to 'read' the facial expressions of others has been used as evidence for there being damage in the amygdala. The social isolation which is characteristic of autism is more typical of cingulate damage.

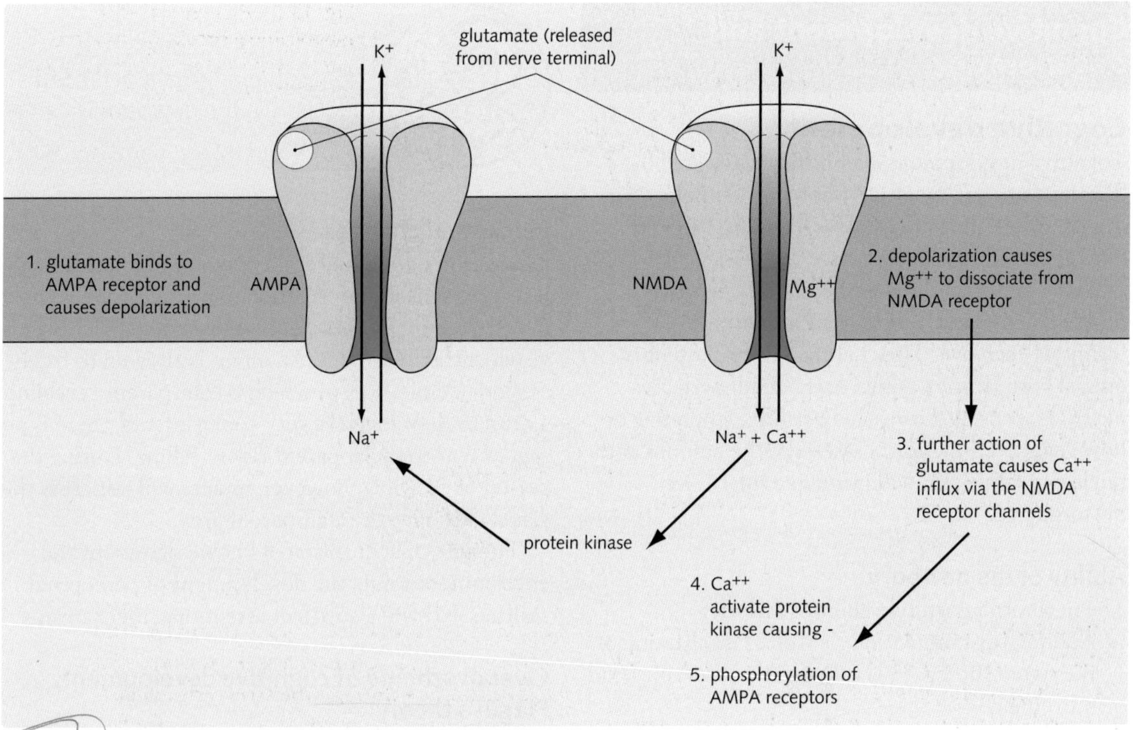

Fig. 13.4 Proposed mechanism of long-term potentiation.

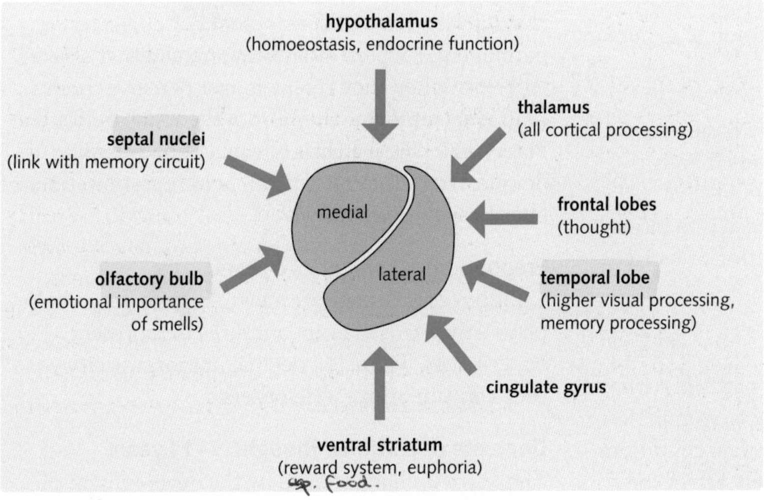

Fig. 13.5 Connections of amygdala.

put everything in their mouths and hypersexuality. Patients with temporal lobe epilepsy tend to show the opposite of these symptoms.

- The amygdala is implicated in learning, particularly the association of a stimulus and an emotional response.

The cingulate gyrus

The cingulate gyrus loops around the limbic system and lateral ventricles. It has a role in complex motor behaviours, pain perception and social interactions.

Patients with lesions in this area are typically socially isolated individuals, and may be so withdrawn as to be akinetic (not moving) and mute.

Cognitive development and degeneration

Cognitive development

Cognitive development in children is assessed by learning tests and by observation of their behaviour. There are set 'milestones' which children should have achieved by certain ages.

Many factors influence the rate of cognitive development and the level that individuals ultimately achieve. The chemical environment is crucial both *in utero* and in early childhood, as is nutritional status during this period. Depending on how cognitive function is assessed, the amount and quality of education will influence final performance.

Ability of the newborn

The newborn's cognitive abilities include:

- Auditory discrimination, as well as localization of the sound source. This is tested by observing head movements.
- Operant learning where, if certain responses are rewarded, babies will be more likely to make those responses.
- The production of smooth pursuit eye movements.
- Preferential interest in certain stimuli (e.g. human faces).

The newborn's motor capabilities are basic motor programmes (e.g. reaching movements if body weight is supported).

The social behaviour of the newborn is to interact with the primary care-giver by imitation of facial movements.

Motor changes

New motor abilities emerge in a set pattern, with the rate of appearance varying according to stimulation and encouragement of the child. Certain conditions (e.g. Down's syndrome) will adversely affect the attainment of these milestones.

Visual input is crucial to the natural development of reaching movements. Babies who are congenitally blind need special devices, such as echo locators, to develop appropriate reaching movements.

The fundamental changes in motor development as the child gets older are greater control over fine movements and greater fluidity of a series of movements.

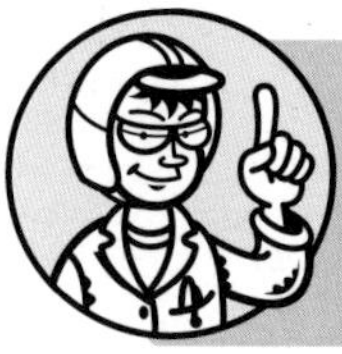

Detection of blindness (e.g. from congenital cataracts) and deafness in the newborn is essential.

Perceptual changes

Changes in perceptual ability involve learning how to interpret sensory information. One milestone is the development of depth perception shown by Gibson's visual cliff experiment. An infant is allowed to freely explore a table, part of which is transparent revealing a drop to floor level. In very young infants, there is no sign of fear to the apparent risk of falling. During the period of crawling, however, infants will not cross the visual cliff onto the transparent area.

The rate of acquisition of knowledge about the environment limits the development of perceptual abilities and will also affect attentional mechanisms.

Overall scheme of cognitive development: Piaget's theory

Sensorimotor stage: 0–2 years

Exploration of the environment occurs, and the child learns to distinguish themselves from it (the beginnings of self-awareness). This stage is also characterized by the development of object permanence, where infants understand that objects still exist when they can no longer perceive them (e.g. after removing them from the visual field). For Piaget, this was the basis of thought because it demonstrates that infants can hold representations of objects in their minds.

Preoperational stage: 2–7 years

Children at this stage are able to engage in symbolic play—using language and pictures to represent experiences. There is a decline in egocentricity—they can empathize with others.

Concrete operational thought: 7–11 years

This stage is characterized by the development of conservation, where children can appreciate that some aspects of objects remain the same, despite changes in appearance. This is displayed with the pencils test—two identical pencils are placed so that they have their bases and tips aligned. One is then moved relative to the other so that it looks longer than the other (if one ignores the fact that the bases have moved relative to each other). Children who conserve will not infer that, when the pencils have moved, one must be longer than the other. Children at this stage are capable of logical thought—seeing relationships between things and applying rules to new situations, but cannot undertake tasks involving abstract reasoning.

Formal operational thought: 11–15 years

At this stage, the ability of abstract reasoning develops.

Language acquisition

The process of language acquisition is not well understood, but current thinking (based on the theories of Chomsky and Pinker) is that there is a preprogrammed way of understanding language construction.

This inbuilt understanding of the workings of language allows rapid learning at a young age, no matter how that language is presented (i.e. learning and ease of use is the same for verbal and sign systems; deaf children learn sign language more quickly and use it in a far richer fashion than their hearing parents).

Children with delayed speech should have urgent investigation for hearing deficits, as language may be more difficult to acquire as the child gets older.

Cognitive degeneration

The ageing brain

The gross changes in the brain include reductions in total volume, weight and size of gyri, and an increase in ventricular size. This is due to atrophy (i.e. the shrinkage of cells) along with nerve cell loss. There are changes in the distribution of cell types. There is a steady decrease in the number of large neurons, accompanied by an increase in both small neurons and glial cells from the age of 20 years onwards.

Neuronal death may be due to pre-programming, sensitivity to certain factors, or accumulated mutations.

Successful ageing

A decline in mental function is not an inevitable consequence of ageing. Compensatory sprouting of dendrites by remaining neurons can help to maintain the total number of synaptic connections. This process is called reactive synaptogenesis.

Reactive synaptogenesis explains why there is an increase in the length of dendrites in hippocampal granule cells between middle and old age. The mean dendritic length begins to fall back after 80 years, suggesting that there is a limit to how long this process can continue protecting against the effects of cell loss.

Dementia

Dementia has emerged as a modern disease, owing to increases in life expectancy. Of individuals aged over 65 years, 5% are severely demented.

The most common form of dementia is the Alzheimer type, where there is a cognitive decline affecting all aspects of cognition and personality (e.g. memory, attention, orientation, etc.). The neuronal pathology is characteristic, including:

- Disturbances of the cytoskeleton, called neurofibrillary tangles, composed of paired helical filaments of a protein called t (tau), which is an abnormally phosphorylated form of a microtubule-associated protein.
- Extracellular deposits of protein rich in β-amyloid and apolipoprotein E, called senile plaques. The precursor of β-amyloid is a cell membrane protein acting as a protease inhibitor. Mutations in the gene coding for the precursor protein may be responsible for some of the familial cases of Alzheimer's disease.

There is a characteristic decrease in brain weight and cortical atrophy. There is marked loss of neurons, usually most prominent in the hippocampus, parahippocampal gyrus and the frontal, anterior temporal, and parietal cortices (mainly affecting glutamatergic pyramidal neurons).

Cell loss also occurs in the basal forebrain complex notably the basal nucleus (of Meynert), which gives rise to a diffuse acetylcholine projection to most of the neocortex, and the medial septal nuclei which give a diffuse cholinergic innervation to the hippocampus. Therapeutic strategies to increase acetylcholine release in the brain have had some limited success.

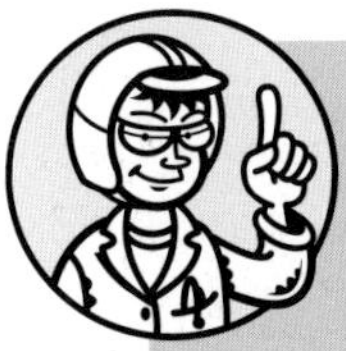

Vascular dementia (so-called 'multi-infarct dementia') is characterized by a stepwise deterioration in cognitive function.

Psychological aspects of ageing

The normal changes in cognitive function begin at between 50 and 60 years of age and comprise:

- Reduction in the ability to perform problem-solving tasks, particularly if the problems are very novel or involve switching between different types of response.

- Slowing of responses in certain cognitive tests, due to reductions in decision speed rather than motor function.
- Memory function decreases, affecting visual information more than verbal information, and recall more than recognition.
- Alterations of motor functions (particularly proprioceptive dysfunction, changes in gait and muscle weakness).

Often, there are changes in social functioning, so-called disengagement behaviour, where there is withdrawal from social contact. This may be caused by a lack of opportunity for social contact due to physical limitations on travel or financial limitations. As such, this may not represent a personality change, but may be a symptom of depression.

Mood changes after the age of 60 years typically include depression and anxiety as reactions against a perceived loss of a role in society, loss of social support and bereavement. This should not be assumed to be 'normal'.

Pharmacology of higher central nervous system function

Anxiolytics and hypnotics

Anxiety is an exaggeration of a normal state with a cognitive component (unpleasant feelings of fear and restlessness) and an autonomic component (tachycardia, gastrointestinal upset, sweating). Anxiolytics reduce the symptoms of anxiety, whereas hypnotics enable people to sleep. This distinction is not clear-cut, particularly if anxiety is the main impediment to normal sleep.

Benzodiazepines

Benzodiazepines bind to-$GABA_A$ receptors (ligand-gated Cl^- channels), increasing their affinity for GABA (γ-aminobutyric acid). This increases the inhibitory effect of GABA on the postsynaptic cell.

Benzodiazepines have four main actions:

- Anxiolysis (both the cognitive and somatic symptoms).
- Sedation and sleep.
- Anticonvulsant.
- Reduction in voluntary muscle tone.

Their clinical uses are in anxiety states, preoperative sedation, status epilepticus, acute alcohol withdrawal, and sedation during endoscopy and bronchoscopy.

Their main side effects are:

- Psychomotor impairment and drowsiness.
- Incoordination, weakness, diplopia.
- Amnesia.
- Disinhibition (leading to inappropriate behaviours, including aggression).
- Dependence.

Fig. 13.6 shows the mechanism and site of action of benzodiazepines.

Dependence is shown after 4–6 weeks and is both psychological and physical. The withdrawal syndrome (in 30% of patients) comprises rebound anxiety and insomnia, tremors and twitching. Withdrawal is more severe after taking a short-acting benzodiazepine.

In overdose, benzodiazepines alone will produce a long sleep but, particularly if alcohol is taken as well, the central nervous system depressant effects are potentiated and fatal respiratory depression can result. Treatment is with a benzodiazepine antagonist, flumazenil.

- Flumazenil antagonizes the effect of benzodiazepines (anxiolytic, anticonvulsant) and also antagonizes the effect of a class of drugs called β-carbolines (anxiogenic, proconvulsant). β-Carbolines therefore bind to the same receptor as benzodiazepines but they have opposing effects, possibly due to fluctuations in the conformational shape of the binding site and receptor function.
- As β-carbolines have the reverse effect of benzodiazepines and can have their effects blocked, they are called inverse agonists.

Fig. 13.7 outlines the differences between the benzodiazepines. Some have active metabolites with

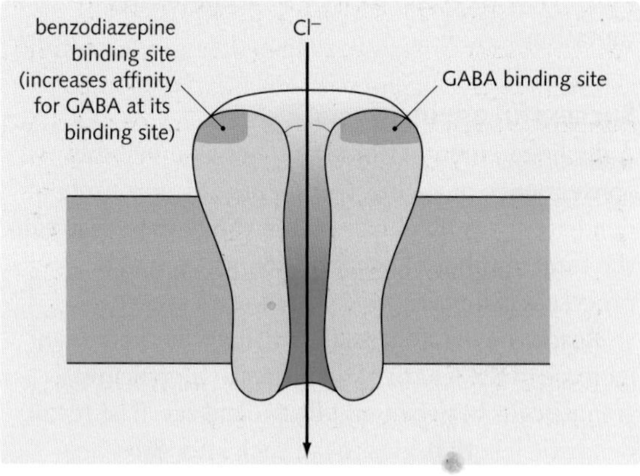

Fig. 13.6 Mechanism and site of action of benzodiazepines.

Properties of benzodiazepines			
Drug (half-life in brackets)	Metabolite (half-life in brackets)	Duration (h) of action	Clinical use
lorazepam (1–12 h)	none	12–18	anxiolysis, hypnosis, anticonvulsant
temazepam (8–12 h)	none	12–18	anxiolysis, hypnosis
diazepam (20–40 h)	nordiazepam (60 h)	24–48	anxiolysis, anticonvulsant
clonazepam (50 h)	none	24–48	anxiolysis, anticonvulsant (absense seizures)

Fig. 13.7 Properties of benzodiazepines.

a half-life longer than that of the administered parent drug. This is important if the drug is taken for a long time, particularly in the elderly, as a prolonged sedated state could result.

5-Hydroxytryptamine modulators

- There is a 5-hydroxytryptamine (5-HT) theory of anxiety that implicates altered functioning of the cortical innervation from the raphé nuclei.
- The drive to develop drugs affecting the 5-HT systems is to find an anxiolytic drug that does not cause sedation and incoordination. So far, the only one that has made it into clinical practice is busipirone (a 5-HT agonist). This may seem counter-intuitive because high levels of 5-HT in the brain were always thought to cause anxiety. It is thought that busipirone may act on presynaptic receptors to decrease the release of endogenous 5-HT. In general, it has a much better side-effect profile than the benzodiazepines (less sedation, psychomotor retardation and dependence). The side effects that it does produce are markedly different: dizziness, nervousness, excitement. The main factor limiting its prescription is cost.

Drugs used in affective disorders

Affective disorders involve a disturbance of mood and can be thought of as pathological extremes along a normal continuum of mood change. They are classified according to which extremes they encompass and the type of symptoms that patients report.

- Unipolar affective disorders present either with mania (euphoria, increased motor activity, flight of ideas and grandiose delusions) or depression (misery, malaise and despair).
- Bipolar affective disorder involves swings between episodes of depression and mania.

Attempts have been made to classify types of depression, focusing on two clear groups of symptoms:

- 'Reactive' depression, where there is a clear psychological cause, involving less-severe symptoms and less likelihood of biological disturbance. This might happen, for example, in response to a bereavement.
- 'Endogenous' depression, where there is no clear cause. More severe symptoms (e.g. suicidal thoughts) are seen and there is a greater likelihood of biological disturbance (e.g. sleep disturbance, anorexia, weight loss or gain). Depressions with some of these features tend to respond better to drug therapy.

Monoamine theory of depression

For many years, it was thought that depression was due to reduced activity of monoamines (dopamine, noradrenaline). These observations explain why:

- Monoamine oxidase inhibitors can improve mood by reducing the catabolism of monoamines.
- Tricyclic antidepressants can improve mood by blocking the uptake of noradrenaline from the synaptic cleft.
- Reserpine produces a depression-like syndrome in animal models by causing a depletion of amines.
- Methyldopa produces depression by inhibiting noradrenaline synthesis.

The monoaminergic theory cannot explain why:

- Amphetamine, cocaine and L-dopa, which all affect monoamine systems, do not elevate the mood of depressed patients.
- Atypical antidepressants (e.g. iprindole) work without manipulating monoaminergic systems.
- There is a 'therapeutic' delay of 2 weeks between the full neurochemical effects of antidepressants and the start of their therapeutic effect.

It is unlikely that monoamine mechanisms alone are responsible for the symptoms of depression.

Tricyclic antidepressants (TCAs)

This class of drugs acts by reducing the uptake of noradrenaline and 5-HT from the synaptic cleft. Examples are imipramine and amitriptyline and they have a similar efficacy.

The side-effect profile includes:

- Muscarinic blocking effects—dry mouth, blurred vision, constipation.
- α-Adrenergic blocking effects—postural hypotension.
- Noradrenaline uptake block in the heart, causing arrhythmia (greater with amitriptyline).
- Central effects—sedation (greater with amitriptyline), convulsions, mania.
- Weight gain.
- Interactions with alcohol and antihypertensive drugs.

In overdose, patients present with confusion, mania and dysrhythmia.

The main use of TCAs is in depression with 'endogenous' features, and amitriptyline helps in disturbed sleep but is to be avoided if patients are apathetic or seriously suicidal. They also help in phobic disorders, obsessive–compulsive disorder and panic disorder.

Monoamine oxidase inhibitors (MAOIs)

MAO has two main forms, MAO_A and MAO_B, which differ in terms of substrate preference. Inhibition of the A form correlates best with antidepressant efficacy. These drugs reduce the activity of MAO, mainly affecting 5-HT and noradrenaline nerve terminals. Examples are phenelzine (irreversible inhibitor) and moclobemide (selective for MAO_A).

The side-effect profile includes:

- Interactions with indirectly acting amines, either tyramine in food (cheese, wine) or over-the-counter cold cures containing ephedrine or phenylephrine. Inhibition of MAO in the liver means that indirectly acting amines, which would normally be metabolized, can gain access to the systemic circulation. This causes noradrenaline release, resulting in large blood pressure increases and possibly death from a cerebrovascular accident.
- Central nervous system stimulation: excitement, tremor.
- Sympathetic blockade: hypotension.
- Muscarinic blockade: dry mouth, blurred vision, constipation.
- Phenelzine can be hepatotoxic.

In overdose, patients present with convulsions.

MAOIs, particularly moclobemide, are mainly used in severe depression.

Selective serotonin reuptake inhibitors (SSRIs)

SSRIs are as effective as TCAs, suggesting that 5-HT mechanisms, rather than noradrenaline mechanisms, are partly responsible for depression. Examples are fluvoxamine and fluoxetine.

Their side-effect profile is much better than that of TCAs and MAOIs, as there are no amine interactions, anticholinergic actions, adrenergic blockade or toxic effects in overdose; however, it includes:

- Nausea and headache.
- Insomnia.
- Rare serotonin syndrome of hyperthermia and cardiovascular collapse when used in conjunction with MAOIs.

SSRIs are now the most widely prescribed antidepressants.

Lithium

Given as lithium carbonate, it acts as a mood stabilizer with antimanic and antidepressant activity. It is restricted to treatment of bipolar disorder. Its mechanism of action is unclear but probably involves modulation of second-messenger pathways of cAMP and inositol triphosphate (IP_3).

It has a very narrow therapeutic window and plasma lithium levels need to be monitored because of its severe side effects:

- Central nervous system: tremor, weakness, headache.
- Nausea and vomiting.
- Nephrogenic diabetes insipidus.
- Hypothyroidism.
- Oedema and weight gain.

In overdose, patients present with vomiting, diarrhoea, tremor, ataxia and coma.

Atypical antidepressants

Examples are mianserin and iprindole. They have no common action and, for iprindole, no effect on amine mechanisms.

Overview

An overview of the pharmacological actions of antidepressant drugs is given in Fig. 13.8.

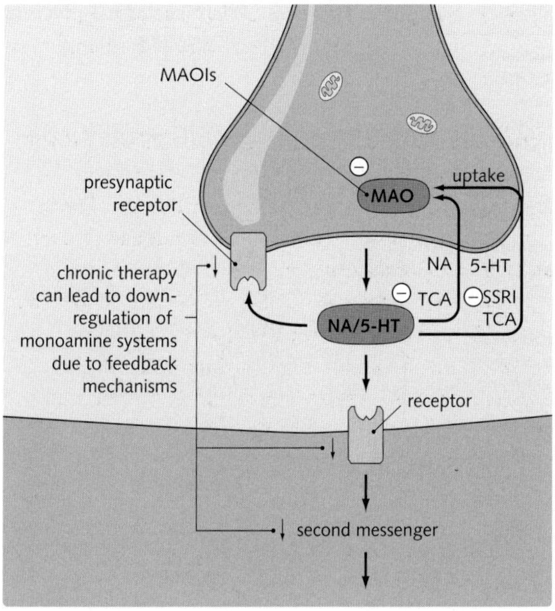

Fig. 13.8 Mechanism of action of antidepressants.

Antipsychotics (neuroleptics)

Antipsychotic drugs are used in the treatment of schizophrenia, which can be thought of as a collection of disordered thoughts, perceptions and behaviours. Some symptoms tend to occur together, and different types of schizophrenia can be described according to this grouping:

- Positive symptoms (delusions, hallucinations, impaired reasoning).
- Negative symptoms (social withdrawal, lack of drive, behavioural disorders).

The presentation and pattern of illness is very variable. In general, the positive symptoms tend to occur acutely and then a chronic course develops, involving more of the negative symptoms.

Of the population, 1% have schizophrenia (a finding found across many cultures); in 75% of cases, the onset is between 17 and 25 years and 64% of patients are male.

Theories of the cause of schizophrenia

A theory of the cause of schizophrenia must allow for genetic factors (monozygotic twins will both have schizophrenia in 50% of cases, dizygotic twins only in 17%) and environmental factors (stressful events often precede onset and influence the course of the illness).

The dopamine theory—increased dopamine transmission:

- Evidence for this is that the clinical dose of an antipsychotic is proportional to its ability to block the D_2 receptor. PET ligand scans show that there are increased D_2 receptors in the nucleus accumbens. Psychiatric side effects are seen in drugs that increase dopaminergic transmission (L-dopa, amphetamine, bromocriptine).
- Evidence against this is that the level of dopamine metabolites in the cerebrospinal fluid of patients is normal or low. This suggests that dopamine is not the only factor causing symptoms.

The developmental theory—disordered development:

- Evidence for this is that schizophrenic patients show reduced temporal lobe size compared with controls. Those born in winter months are more likely to develop schizophrenia, possibly because of viral infection of the mother before birth.
- Evidence against is that not all studies agree on their findings and the theory does not explain the efficacy of neuroleptic drugs.

Neuroleptic side effects: dopamine pathways

There are three main dopamine pathways in the brain:

- Mesolimbic dopamine, running from the midbrain to the nucleus accumbens and amygdala, affecting thought and motivation.
- Nigrostriatal dopamine, running from the midbrain to the caudate nuclei, affecting motor control.
- Tubero-infundibular, running from the hypothalamus to the pituitary gland, regulating prolactin secretion.

The side-effect profile of neuroleptics is explained by:

- Disruption of the dopamine pathways.
- Blockade of muscarinic receptors.
- Blockade of α-receptors.

A summary of the profile is shown in Fig. 13.9.

Phenothiazines

This class of compounds is split up into three groups by the side chain on the general formula producing different side-effect patterns:

- Aliphatic side chains (e.g. in chlorpromazine) produce strong sedation, moderate autonomic side effects and moderate extrapyramidal motor disturbance.
- Piperadine side chains (e.g. in thioridazine) produce moderate sedation, more autonomic

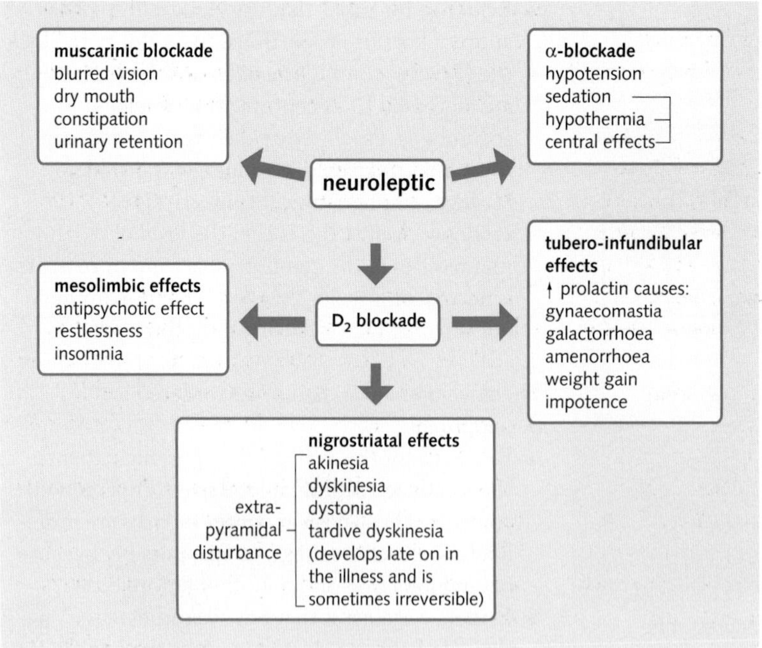

Fig. 13.9 Pharmacological effects of neuroleptic medication.

effects and mild extrapyramidal motor disturbance.
- Piperazine side chains (e.g. in fluphenazine) produce low sedation, mild autonomic effects and strong extrapyramidal motor disturbance.

Thioxanthines and butyrophenones

These two groups of compounds have a similar profile to the piperazine group of phenothiazines, with low sedation, mild autonomic effects and strong motor disturbance.

- Flupenthixol is a thioxanthine.
- Haloperidol is a butyrophenone.

Atypical neuroleptics

Drugs that have antipsychotic action but produce less intense motor side effects are termed 'atypical'.

Clozapine has 5-HT, α-adrenergic and histamine blocking effects. It has minimal central antidopaminergic activity, and therefore produces few extrapyramidal side effects. The main risk with its use is agranulocytosis, and patients need close monitoring. It is particularly useful in those who are refractory to classical antipsychotics, or who experience extreme side effects.

Other drugs which are gaining popularity due to their favourable side-effect profile include:

- Risperidone.
- Olanzepine.
- Quetiapine.
- Amisulpride.

Overall neuroleptic side-effect profile

As well as the autonomic, endocrine, behavioural and motor effects explained by clear disturbances of transmitter function, there are other effects:

- Toxic response. Agranulocytosis due to toxic bone marrow depression, particularly with clozapine. Cholestatic jaundice occurs in 2–4% of cases. Skin rashes occur in 5% of patients.
- Ocular problems. Deposits in the cornea and lens occur with chlorpromazine and thioridazine.
- Malignant neuroleptic syndrome. An idiopathic response with fever, extrapyramidal motor disturbance, muscle rigidity and coma.

Brainstem-acting drugs and general anaesthetics

Nausea and vomiting

The vomiting response consists of:

- Reverse peristalsis, where the contents of the duodenum and jejunum are propelled back into the stomach.

- Closure of the glottis.
- Relaxation of the lower oesophageal sphincter.
- Contraction of the muscles of the abdominal wall.

These events, together with the sensation of nausea, are coordinated by an area in the medulla. This is known as the vomiting centre, which sends outputs to the dorsal motor nucleus of cranial nerve X and to the spinal motor neurons innervating the abdominal musculature. The types of stimuli that produce a vomiting response are explained by the inputs to the vomiting centre.

The chemoreceptor trigger zone in the area postrema in the medulla senses information about circulating compounds as it is not protected by the blood–brain barrier. Its neural circuits have many receptors (e.g. D_2, 5-HT_3, opioid) that allow pharmacological intervention to reduce information flow about chemical triggers. Drugs inducing nausea include L-dopa, opioids, anticancer agents (e.g. cisplatin), digitalis and anaesthetics.

The vestibular system sends balance information to the vomiting centre. In motion sickness (pallor, sweating, nausea, and vomiting), there is a conflict between the visual and vestibular systems. This can be treated behaviourally or with drugs that reduce vestibular input. Vestibular disease presents with vertigo (false sense of rotary movement), particularly in:

- Labyrinthitis (seen acutely in viral infection, with symptoms of vertigo, nausea and vomiting).
- Ménière's disease (vertigo, nausea, vomiting, tinnitus, and deafness) produced by increased endolymphatic pressure.

The solitary nucleus sends viscerosensory information about chemicals in the gut collected by cranial nerve X. The enteroendocrine system in the gut wall responds to gut contents and by 5-HT mechanisms can affect the firing of cranial nerve X afferent neurons.

The spinal cord sends information about trauma: nausea can accompany physical injury.

The limbic cortex sends information from the special senses: certain odours and sights can cause nausea.

Fig. 13.10 summarizes the connections of the medullary vomiting centre and the sites of drug action.

Antiemetics

Fig. 13.11 shows the action, uses, and side effects of some antiemetic drugs.

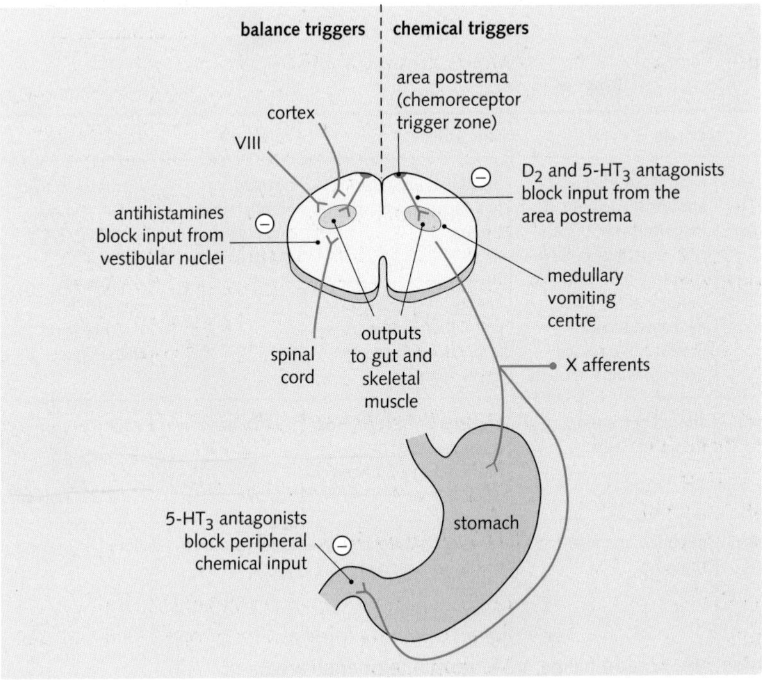

Fig. 13.10 Sites of action of antiemetics.

Drugs acting on brainstem monoaminergic systems

The brainstem monoaminergic systems project into the thalamus and cortex with a rather diffuse innervation. This is because these systems have a general modulatory function. Drugs acting on these systems are usually self-administered as drugs of abuse because of their effects on monoaminergic systems that modulate processing of thought and emotion (Fig. 13.12).

General anaesthesia

All general anaesthetic agents produce:

- Loss of consciousness, of reflex responses to noxious stimuli, of spatial orientation, of volitional

Antiemetic drugs				
Class	**Drug**	**Site of action**	**Uses**	**Side effects**
antimuscarinic	**hyoscine**	vomiting centre, antagonizing vestibular input	motion sickness	drowsiness, dry mouth, blurred vision, impaired short-term memory
antihistamine	**cinnarizine and cyclizine**	vomiting centre, antagonizing vestibular input	motion sickness, vestibular disease	less than antimuscarinics
histamine analogue	**betahistine**	reduces endolymphatic pressure in the membranous labyrinths	Meniere's disease	
D_2 antagonists	**metoclopramide and domperidone**	chemoreceptor trigger zone reducing sensitivity to chemical triggers in the blood	reduces drug-induced nausea and vomiting; combination with paracetamol to treat migraine	drowsiness, fatigue, motor restlessness
$5\text{-}HT_3$ antagonist	**ondansetron and granisetron**	chemoreceptor trigger zone and peripherally in the gut reducing transmission from 5-HTergic enteroendocrine cells in response to chemical triggers in the gut	reduces drug-induced nausea and vomiting. Addition of dexamethasone (steroid) increases efficacy in chemotherapy patients requiring high doses	headache, gastrointestinal upset

Fig. 13.11 Antiemetic drugs.

Drugs of abuse						
Class	**Drug**	**Action**	**Effects**	**Side effects**	**Tolerance**	**Dependence**
psychomotor stimulants	amphetamine	causes release of NA and DA from terminals	central DA effects: euphoria, excitement, locomotor stimulation with repetitive behaviour (stereotypies), anorexia; peripheral NA effects: increased blood pressure, decreased gastrointestinal motility	insomnia, irritability, headache, psychosis, tremor	develops as amphetamine depletes terminals of transmitter	increases activity in DA reward system (VTA to nucleus acumbens), producing psychological dependence
	cocaine	blocks NA and DA uptake (uptake 1)		cardiac dysrhythmias, convulsions, respiratory and vasomotor depression		
hallucinogens	lysergic acid diethylamide (LSD)	$5\text{-}HT_2$ partial agonist	altered perception, thoughts, feelings	persistent effects lasting several weeks, flashbacks to previous 'trips'	quickly develops	none
	MDMA (Ecstasy)	amphetamine-like and LSD-like	euphoria and altered thoughts	idiosyncratic responses—coma, convulsions, hyperpyrexia, rhabdomyolysis	cross tolerance with LSD	none

Fig. 13.12 Drugs of abuse (DA, dopamine; NA, noradrenaline; VTA, ventral tegmental area).

control, and of memory, and reductions in respiratory rate and blood pressure.
- Death at high doses, caused by respiratory depression and cardiovascular depression by actions on the medulla; in addition, cardiac depression may be brought about by direct effects on the myocardium.

Anaesthesia used to be characterized by an initial excitatory phase (modern anaesthetics act very quickly so that this phase is no longer prolonged or troublesome) followed by a dose-dependent increase in anaesthetic depth. This was seen with agents such as ether. Single anaesthetic agents are rarely used in modern practice, as their complementary effects allow lower doses to be employed. This leads to fewer side effects. Often a combination of intravenous and inhalational agents is used to exploit their different kinetic properties.

The principles of surgical anaesthesia are to produce:
- Loss of consciousness.
- Analgesia.
- Muscle relaxation.

There is no obvious pharmacological structure–activity relationship for anaesthetic agents; their mechanisms of action are complex, either by affecting the reticular formation (most anaesthetics) or by a direct depression of cortical activity (e.g. propofol).

The potency of any anaesthetic is directly related to its hydrophobic nature, generally measured as its lipid solubility as the oil : gas (for gases and vapours) and oil : water (for aqueous agents) partition coefficient. One possible mechanism of action is that anaesthetics interact with a hydrophobic region (either lipid, protein or lipoprotein) of the neuronal membrane, causing membrane expansion and consequent malfunction. Evidence for this is that anaesthesia in mammals may be reversed by high ambient pressure (in excess of 100 atm; 10.1 MPa).

Induction and recovery

Induction and recovery describe how quickly anaesthesia occurs after administration, and how quickly the body recovers from anaesthesia. The speed of induction with, and recovery from, an anaesthetic depends upon the physical properties of the anaesthetic and how quickly it can equilibrate between the lungs, blood and central nervous system for inhalants and gaseous agents, or from blood and central nervous system for aqueous agents.

Intravenous agents (e.g. propofol) are often used for the induction of anaesthesia as they can produce unconsciousness in approximately 20 seconds. This is

Anaesthetic drugs

Route	Drug	Potency (oil:gas)	Induction/recovery	Notes and side effects
inhaled	N_2O	low (1.4)	fast	Only analgesic by itself. Used 60% O_2/40% N_2O as carrier for other agents
	halothane	high (220)	medium	Depresses myocardium, baroreceptor reflex, sympathetic system producing hypotension. 20% metabolized and may cause hepatic damage
	enflurane	medium (98)	medium	Depresses myocardium producing hypotension. 2% metabolized so no hepatic damage. May cause seizures
	isoflurane	medium (91)	medium	Causes vasodilatation producing hypotension. Only 0.2% metabolized. Less epileptogenic than enflurane but may cause myocardial ischaemia
injected	thiopentone	high	fast	Depresses myocardium and respiratory centre. No analgesic effect. Duration of unconsciousness 5–10 minutes due to liver, kidneys etc., and then to muscle. Eventual redistribution to body fat so almost total
	propofol		fast ~ 20 s	Cardiovascular and respiratory depression. Rapidly metabolized and suitable for total intravenous anaesthesia

Fig. 13.13 Anaesthetic drugs.

generally preferable for patients as many find facemasks can make them feel claustrophobic.

Inhalational anaesthetics (e.g. isoflurane) are more commonly used for the maintenance of anaesthesia. This is because they give a more rapid control of the level of consciousness.

After equilibration, 95% of the administered anaesthetic is in the body fat. Fat has a low blood flow and so it takes a long time for anaesthetics to enter and leave the body fat. A very fat-soluble anaesthetic can build up gradually in adipose tissue, and then be released back into the circulation over a long period of time.

The most common general anaesthetics are compared in Fig. 13.13.

- Give some examples of functional asymmetry in the cortex.
- What consequences would damage to the left parietal lobe have, if that were the dominant hemisphere?
- Explain the difference between declarative and procedural memory.
- How might long-term memory be laid down, and where in the brain is this localized? What stages are proposed in memory formation?
- What effect does damage to the limbic system have? Relate this to its functions.
- Describe the stages of development identified in Piaget's theory.
- What changes take place in the brain as we age? Compare these with the changes seen in dementia.
- Relate the mode of action of benzodiazepines to their clinical effect.
- If a child had taken an accidental overdose of benzodiazepines, what clinical features might you expect, and how would you treat it?
- What is the monoamine theory of depression? Explain the possible flaws in this theory.
- What are the problems with lithium therapy? How do you monitor for these?
- What is the dopamine theory of schizophrenia? What other theories are there for the development of this condition?
- Name the classes and side effects of commonly used neuroleptics.

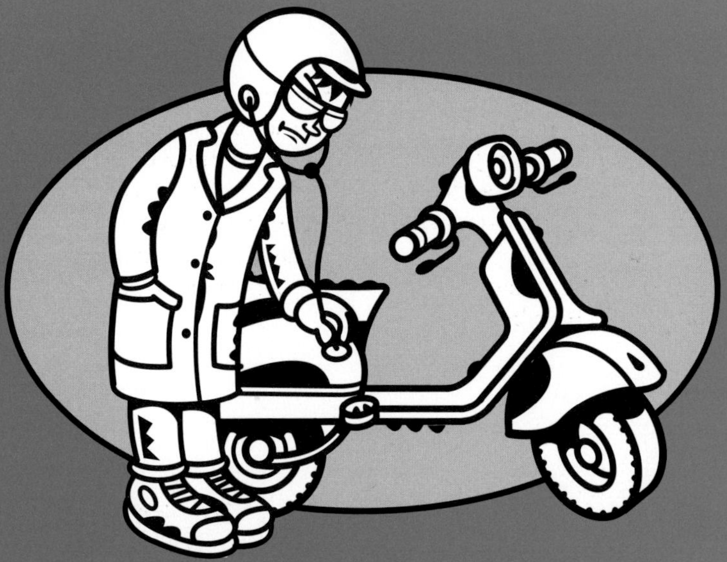

CLINICAL ASSESSMENT

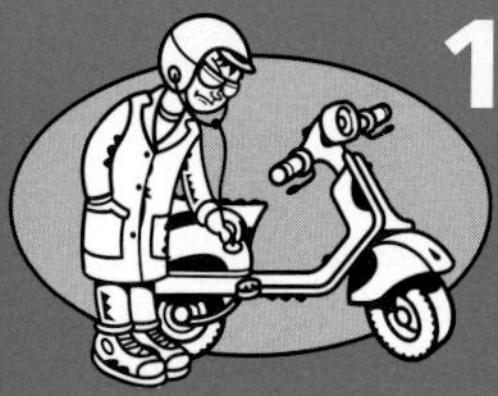

14. Common Presentation of Neurological Disease

In this chapter, you will learn about:

- Common causes and diagnostic algorithms for common neurological complaints.
- Differential diagnoses are given for:
  - Headache.
  - Central nervous system infection.
  - Dementia.
  - Numbness and tingling.
  - Dizziness.
  - Gait disturbances.
  - Weakness.
  - Coma.
  - Sudden onset of hemiparesis.
  - Seizures.

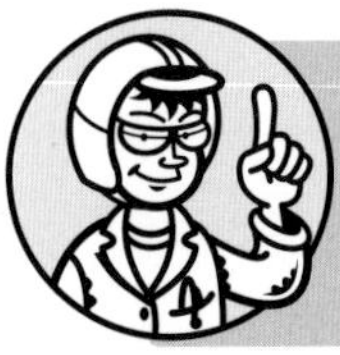

The most common causes of each complaint are indicated by asterisks. You should consider these first.

Common presenting complaints

Headache

Differential diagnosis (Fig. 14.1)

- Migraine*.
- Tension/stress headache*.
- Chronic daily headache*.
- Cluster headache.
- Hypertension.
- Increased intracranial pressure (ICP) (space-occupying lesion, SOL; cerebral vein thrombosis).
- Infection (meningitis, abscess, postherpetic neuralgia).
- Trauma (head injury, subdural haematoma).
- Vascular (intracerebral haemorrhage, subarachnoid haemorrhage).
- Drug/toxin-related (vasodilators, caffeine withdrawal, carbon monoxide exposure).

Central nervous system infections

Differential diagnosis (Fig. 14.2)

This is not strictly a 'presenting complaint' but is an important cause of a group of presenting features, as shown in Fig. 14.2.

The list of organisms that may cause central nervous system infection is huge. The most important are listed in Chapter 11.

Dementia

Differential diagnosis (Fig. 14.3)

Again, not in itself a 'presenting complaint' of the patient, but an important clinical presentation with many underlying causes.

The surgical sieve, as outlined below, will enable you to remember all the causes of this, but it is more sensible to relate them in an approximate order of likelihood (i.e. think of the asterisked causes first).

Congenital

- Huntington's disease.
- Presenile dementia.
- Adrenoleucodystrophy.
- Canavan's disease.

Acquired

Remember these using the mnemonic 'INVITED MD'.

- Infective: human immunodeficiency virus, syphilis, Creutzfeldt–Jakob disease, postencephalitis/postmeningitis, progressive multifocal leucoencephalopathy, Whipple's disease.
- Neoplastic: intracranial tumour (benign/malignant, primary/secondary), paraneoplastic.
- Vascular: multi-infarct dementia*.
- Inflammatory: multiple sclerosis.
- Trauma/idiopathic: head injury*, subdural haematoma, normal pressure hydrocephalus, depression*.
- Endocrine: hypo*/hyperthyroidism.
- Degenerative: Alzheimer's disease*, Pick's disease, Parkinson's disease*, Lewy body disease.
- Metabolic: B_{12} deficiency*, see congenital causes, organ failure, anoxia.
- Drugs/toxins: sedatives, chronic alcoholism.

Numbness and tingling

Differential diagnosis (Fig. 14.4)

- Generalized peripheral neuropathy (see Chapter 15). The most common causes are:
  - Diabetes*: by far the commonest.
  - Vitamin B_{12} and B_1 deficiency.

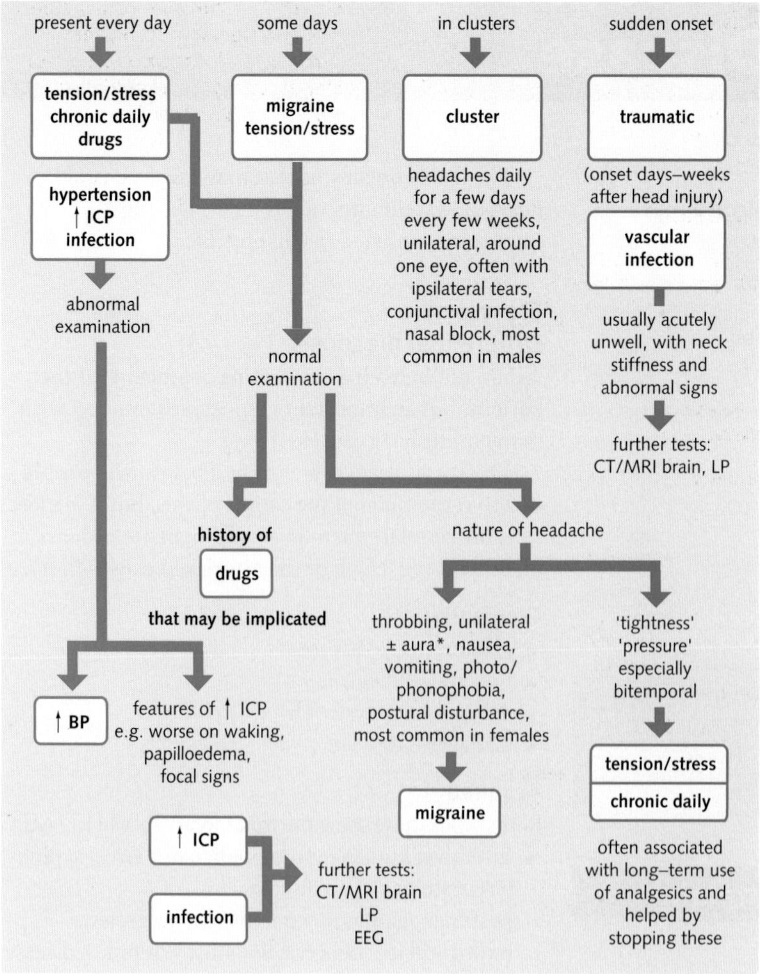

Fig. 14.1 Headache algorithm. *Migrainous auras are transient focal cerebral or brainstem symptoms that accompany the headache (e.g. visual — especially scintillating scotomata; flickering lights in homonomous field) (EEG, electroencephalogram; ICP, intracranial pressure; LP, lumbar puncture).

  - Alcohol.
  - Carcinomatous.
  - Drug-induced.
- Isolated mononeuropathy:
  - Trauma/compression.
  - Mononeuritis multiplex.
- Vascular:
  - Ischaemia (transient ischaemic attack, peripheral vascular disease).
- Other central nervous system causes:
  - Multiple sclerosis.
- Anxiety* (particularly fingers and toes).
- Idiopathic*.

Dizziness

A very common complaint in neurological practice. Patients may use the term dizziness to describe a wide variety of sensations, including vertigo (a subjective sensation of movement, usually spinning), syncope (faintness and light-headedness caused by decrease in cerebral blood flow), fitting, confusion, nausea, headache, numbness or tiredness. Be aware of this and check what the patient is describing.

Most commonly, dizziness describes episodes of either vertigo or syncope. A 'funny turn' in neurological practice is usually either one of these or is epileptic in nature.

Differential diagnosis (Fig. 14.5)

Vertigo

- Peripheral (inner ear):
  - Benign paroxysmal positional vertigo*.
  - Benign recurrent vertigo.
  - Vestibular neuronitis (also described as peripheral vestibulopathy, or viral labyrinthitis)*.
  - Ménière's disease*.
  - Infection*.

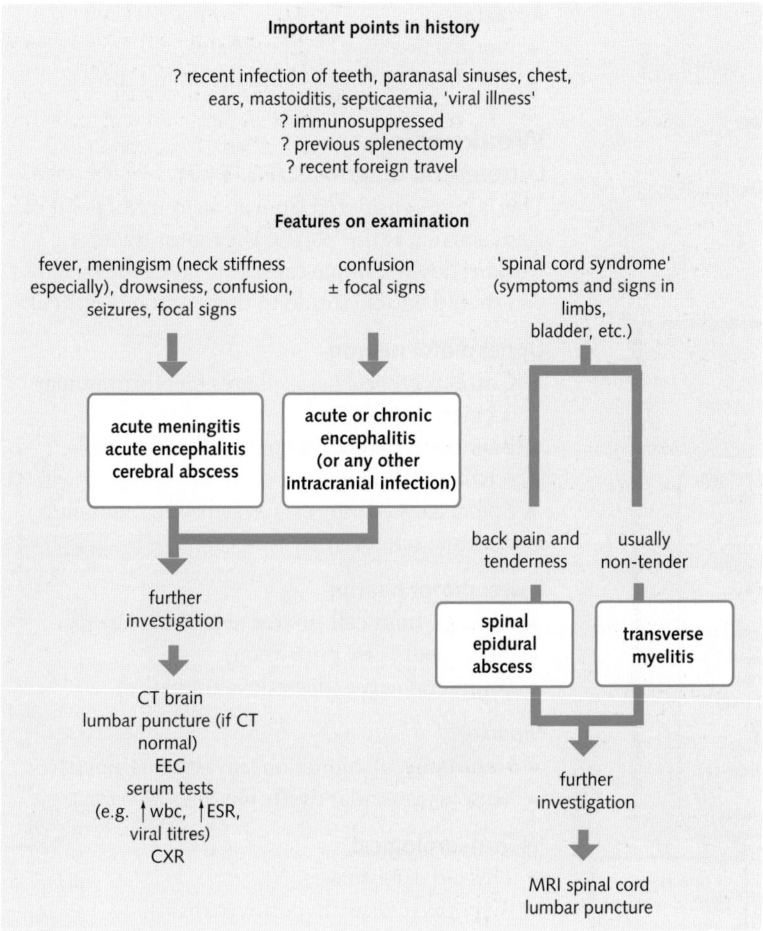

Fig. 14.2 Central nervous system infection algorithm (CXR, chest X-ray; EEG, electroencephalogram; ESR, erythrocyte sedimentation rate; wbc, white blood cells).

    - Head injury.
    - Drugs (e.g. aminoglycosides).
- Central (in the brainstem or cranial nerve VIII):
    - Multiple sclerosis*.
    - Brainstem ischaemia.
    - Basilar migraine.
    - Cerebellopontine angle (CPA) tumours.

Syncope

- Simple faint (vasovagal attack)*.
- Hypotension, especially postural*. (drugs, dehydration, pregnancy, cardiac).
- Transient ischaemic attack* (carotid disease, cardioembolism)*.
- Cardiac arrhythmia*.
- Syncope induced by micturition, cough, straining, cold foods (ice-cream syncope).

Epilepsy (see Chapter 11)

Gait disturbances

Differential diagnosis (Fig. 14.6)

Weakness

- Upper motor neuron.
- Hemiparesis (stroke*, cerebral tumour, multiple sclerosis), paraparesis (multiple sclerosis*, spinal cord infarction, tumour, cord compression, midline meningioma).
- Lower motor neuron (footdrop*, spinal claudication, root disease).

Ataxia

- Cerebellar disease.
- Proprioceptive loss (peripheral neuropathy).

Extrapyramidal disease

- Parkinson's disease*.
- Other extrapyramidal disorders.

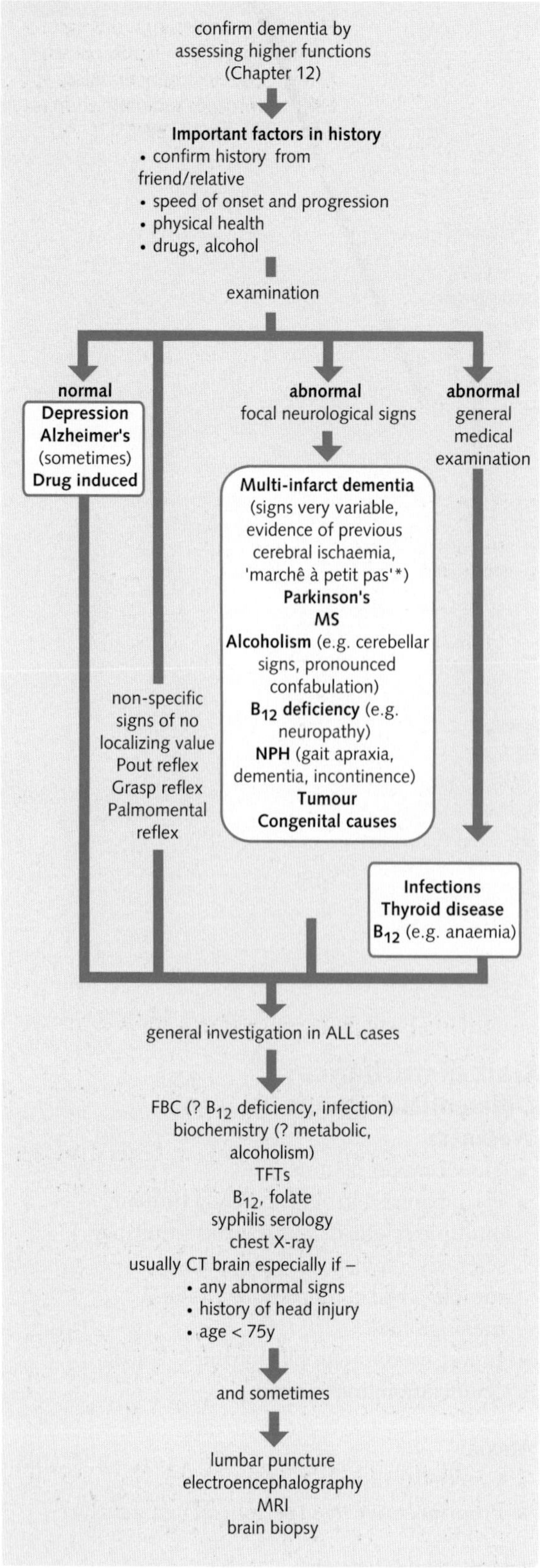

Fig. 14.3 Dementia algorithm. *Describes small-stepped gait typical of (but not specific to) multi-infarct disease (TFTs, thyroid function tests).

Apraxia

- Normal pressure hydrocephalus.
- Marche à la petit pas of multi-infarct disease.

Weakness

Differential diagnosis (Fig. 14.7)

This is best considered from an anatomical point of view, starting at the 'top' of the motor tracts and working down. Simple causes are given for each, but you should be able to add to these without difficulty.

Upper motor neuron

- Cortex/cerebral hemispheres (cerebrovascular accident, tumour).
- Brainstem/cerebellar connections (multiple sclerosis, tumour).
- Spinal cord (compression, ischaemia, tumour, multiple sclerosis).

Lower motor neuron

- Anterior horn cell (motor neuron disease).
- Nerve root (disc protrusion).
- Peripheral nerve (diabetic neuropathy).

Muscle

- Neuromuscular junction (myasthenia gravis).
- Muscle (muscular dystrophy, polymyositis).

'Non-neurological'

- Thyroid disorders (hypothyroidism/hyperthyroidism).
- Malnutrition/dehydration.
- Cachexia (underlying carcinoma).
- Electrolyte disturbances (hyponatraemia, hypernatraemia, hypokalaemia, hyperkalaemia).
- Pain/stiffness caused by joint disease (arthritis).

Coma

Differential diagnosis (Fig. 14.8)

Intracranial

- Infection* (meningitis, encephalitis, abscess, malaria; see Chapter 11).
- Tumour.
- Cerebrovascular accident* (haemorrhage more commonly than infarction, subarachnoid haemorrhage).
- Anoxic brain injury (following cardiac arrest, head injury, anaesthetic accident, respiratory failure).
- Head injury*.

Metabolic

- Hypoglycaemia*.
- Diabetic coma* [ketoacidosis, hyperosmolar non-ketotic coma (HONK)].

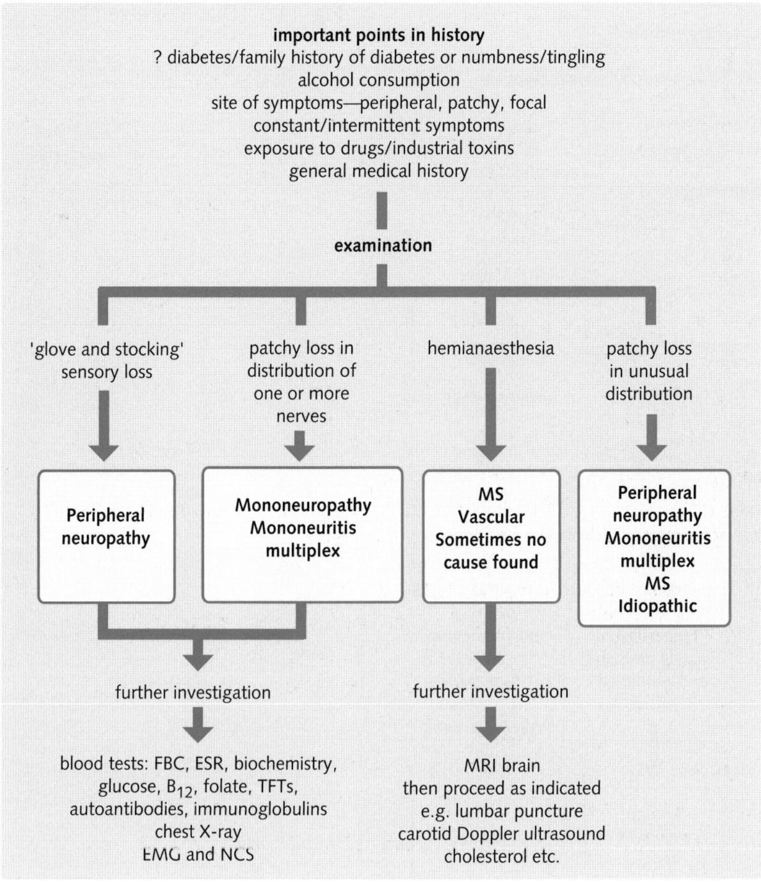

Fig. 14.4 Numbness and tingling algorithm (EMG, electromyogram; ESR, erythrocyte sedimentation rate; FBC, full blood count; NCS, nerve conduction studies; TFTs, thyroid function tests).

- Liver failure.
- Renal failure.
- Addison's disease, Cushing's disease.
- Hypopituitarism.
- Hyperammonaemia (liver failure, amino acid disorders, sodium valproate).

Toxic

- Drug-induced* (including drugs of abuse; heroin, Ecstasy, benzodiazepines and overdose* of most medications).
- Alcohol (excess, Wernicke's encephalopathy).
- Carbon monoxide.
- Hypothermia.

Conditions that may mimic coma

- Akinetic mutism (persistent vegetative state).
- Locked-in syndrome.
- Non-convulsive status epilepticus.
- Catatonia.

Sudden onset of hemiparesis

Differential diagnosis

Stroke is most likely and may be caused by any of the following:

- Atherothrombotic carotid disease* (predisposing factors — family history, smoking, hypertension, diabetes).
- Cardioembolic disease* (atrial fibrillation, cardiac valve disease).
- Cardiac arrhythmia*.
- Hyperviscosity syndrome (multiple myeloma, Waldenström's macroglobulinaemia, leukaemia).
- Hypotensive episode (watershed infarcts).

However, the differential diagnosis of a patient presenting with sudden collapse with or without focal neurological signs also includes:

- Epilepsy (see also Chapter 11).
- Syncope (see above).
- Most of the causes of coma, especially:

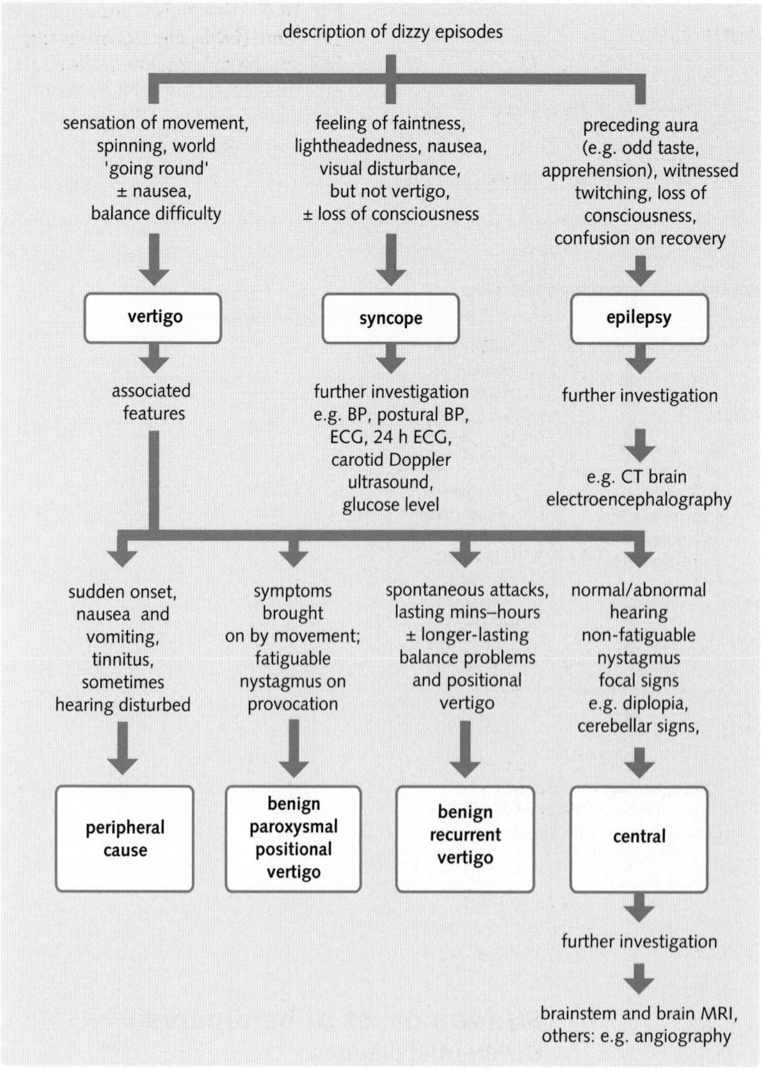

Fig. 14.5 Dizziness algorithm.

- Hypoglycaemia.
- Cerebral tumour.
- Subarachnoid haemorrhage.

Seizures (see Chapter 11)

Differential diagnosis (Fig. 14.9)

- Primary generalized epilepsy*.
- Secondary generalized epilepsy.
- Partial (focal) seizures*:
  - Simple (no impairment of consciousness).
  - Complex (with impairment of consciousness).
- Seizures due to focal structural (tumour, stroke*, infection, trauma) or metabolic (hypoglycaemia*; liver failure; drugs*, including overdose; toxins, especially alcohol and alcohol withdrawal*) causes.

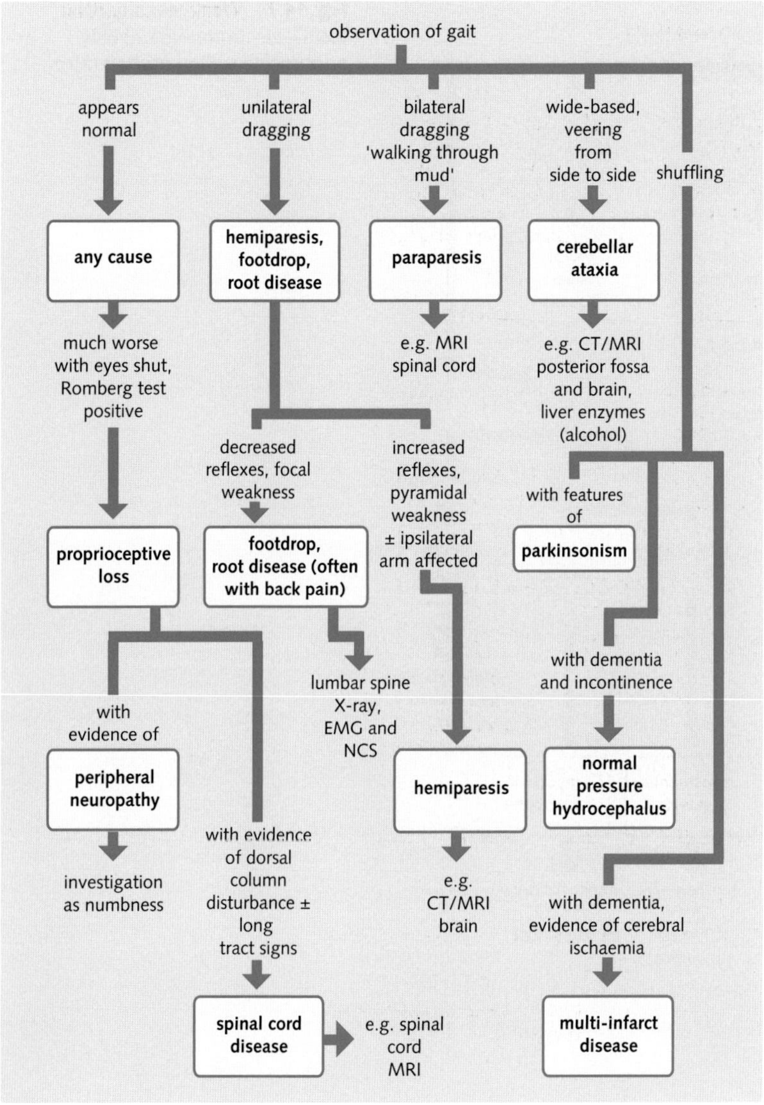

Fig. 14.6 Gait disturbance algorithm (EMG, electromyogram; NCS, nerve conduction studies).

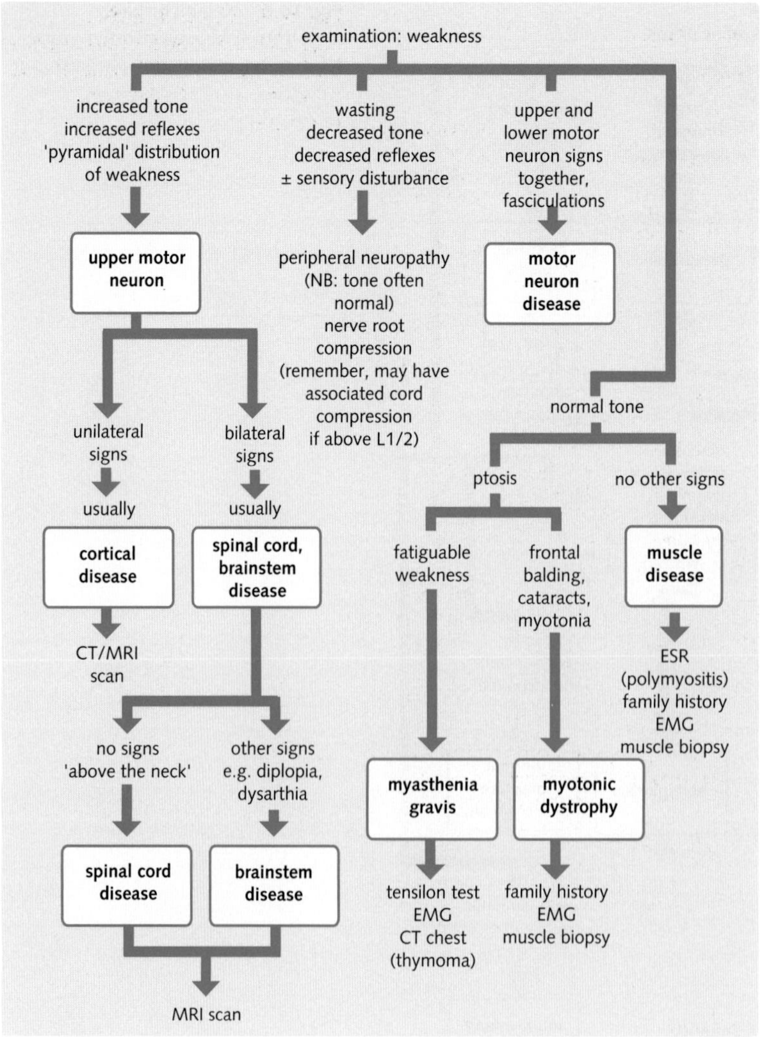

Fig. 14.7 Weakness algorithm (EMG, electromyogram; ESR, erythrocyte sedimentation rate).

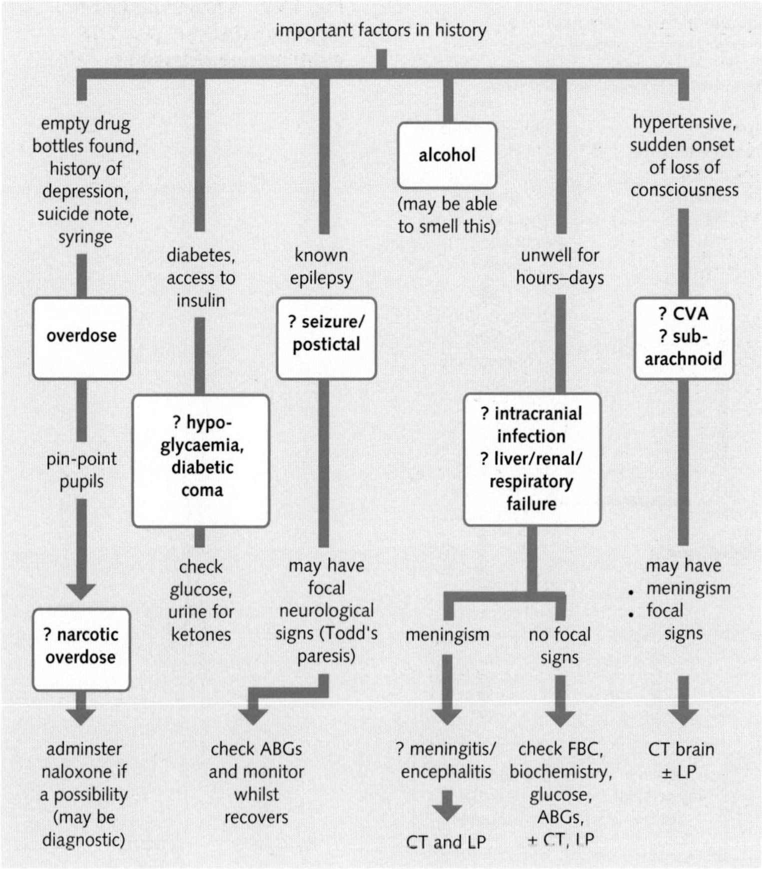

Fig. 14.8 Coma diagnostic algorithm (ABG, arterial blood gases; CVA, cerebrovascular accident; FBC, full blood count; LP, lumbar puncture).

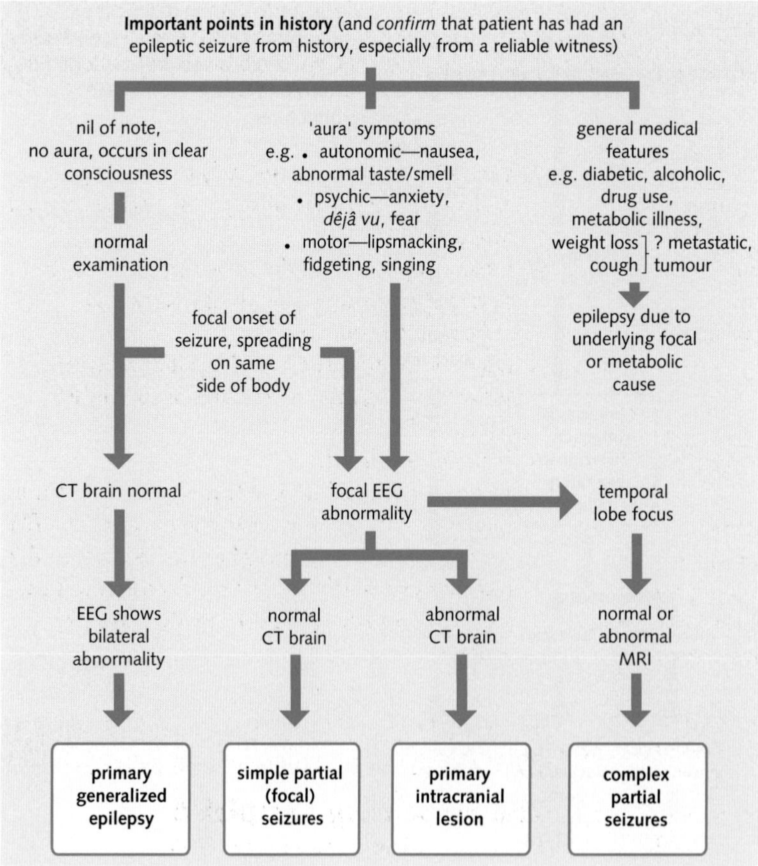

Fig. 14.9 Seizures diagnostic algorithm (EEG, electroencephalogram).

- Outline the important features of the history of a 65-year-old man presenting with confusion.
- How would you approach the management of a 30-year-old woman who complains of a 1-year history of frontal headache?
- A 50-year-old man has been having dizzy spells for a month. What would you do?
- Outline your management of a 20-year-old man who presents to an Accident and Emergency Department unconscious.
- How would you distinguish the different types of seizure from history and examination?

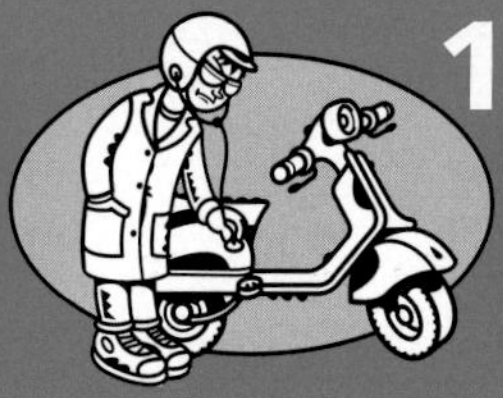

15. The Neurological Assessment

In this chapter, you will learn about:

- The observation of a neurological patient.
- Communication skills particularly relevant to patients with neurological problems.
- Examination of the nervous system.
- The examination and assessment of an unconscious patient.

Beginning the interview

Taking a history is the most important part of assessment of the patient with neurological symptoms. Many diagnoses are based on clinical findings alone; the investigations in neurology tend to be expensive and complex, so avoiding them is a bonus.

Observation of the patients as they walk into the examination room or as you approach the bed is vital.

- Do they appear unwell?
- Do they use walking aids (sticks, crutches, frame, wheelchair, callipers)?
- Do they appear to be independent, or clearly need help from others?
- Are there any obvious morphological abnormalities (e.g. weakness on one side, drooping of the face, wasting of the muscles)?

As with all clerkings, begin your interview by:

- Introducing yourself.
- Explaining who you are.
- Asking if you may talk to and examine them.
- Asking their age and occupation.
- Asking whether they are right- or left-handed—if you do not ask this at the beginning, you will forget about it until your consultant asks you!

In hospital, general observation of the patient's environment is always important.

- Notice the sputum pot and diabetic urine-tests.
- Cards and flowers from friends and relatives may indicate a supportive home network.

Immediately, you will observe important points regarding their neurological status.

- Do they respond appropriately (indicating probable preservation of important higher mental functioning)?
- Do they appear to be depressed (which may be part of their neurological condition or may indicate a reaction to it)?
- Do they appear to be elated (again, a feature of some neurological illnesses such as multiple sclerosis)?
- Is their speech normal?
- You may notice additional features such as tremor, agitation, twitches and abnormal movements. Do not worry about what may be causing these at this stage, as things will become much clearer as you progress through a systematic history-taking process.

The structure of the history

The presenting complaint

From the patient's point of view. Ask:

- 'What is the main problem?'
- 'What was it that caused you to go to your doctor/come to the hospital?'

When presenting the history to others, use the patient's own words (e.g. 'this woman complains of seeing double' rather than 'this woman has horizontal diplopia').

The history of the presenting complaint:

- When was it first noted by the patient?
- Has it worsened, improved or stayed the same since?
- What is its nature (e.g. headache may be sharp, dull, an ache, a throb, etc.)?
- Is there anything that makes it better (e.g. medicines, sleep, exercise) or worse (e.g. time of day, posture, exercise)?
- Have any other symptoms developed since this first complaint was noticed (e.g. main complaint may be weakness of the hand, but a numb patch may have developed more recently)?
- Have any tests already been performed, and if so where and by whom?

- Has the patient ever had other neurological symptoms in the past (these may be related, e.g. an episode of transient visual loss 5 years previously in a young woman now complaining of difficulty in walking)?
- It is often worth running through a checklist of neurological symptoms.

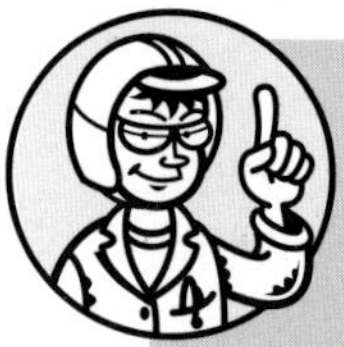

Neurological symptoms
Remember these by working from the 'head down':
- Headache.
- Memory problems.
- Speech difficulty.
- Dizzy turns.
- Swallowing.
- Weakness.
- Numbness.
- Bladder or bowel disturbance.
- Walking difficulty.

Review of systems

Do not underestimate the importance of going through these categories (if only briefly). Co-existent disease may have a huge impact on disability, and may be linked to the presenting complaint (e.g. weight loss and back pain may be indicative of a tumour, which may be related to new-onset neurological symptoms). Things to ask about include:

- Gastrointestinal: appetite, weight loss/gain, swallowing, bowel function (change?).
- Cardiovascular: chest pain, breathlessness, claudication.
- Respiratory: cough, breathlessness.
- Genitourinary: bladder function, impotence, sexual function.
- Musculoskeletal: joint pain, stiffness.

Past medical history

- Any serious illnesses in the past or now? It is useful to write an abbreviated list of important negatives in your clerking, to show that these have been checked. The mnemonic 'MJTHREADS' is commonly used as a reminder: myocardial infarction, jaundice, tuberculosis, hypertension, rheumatic fever, epilepsy, asthma, diabetes, stroke.

Drug history

- Is the patient taking any medicines now, or have any been taken for some time in the past?
- Are there any known drug allergies?

Family history

- Are there any 'family illnesses'? Are parents, siblings, and children alive and well, and if not, what did they die from and at what age? Draw a family tree (Fig. 15.1) if appropriate.

Social history

- Home circumstances: own home, stairs, social-service help, family support, responsibilities for children/disabled relatives, etc.
- Smoking (ever).
- Alcohol (ever heavy consumption).
- Diet (are they likely to have a vitamin deficiency? Ask about supplementation).
- Heterosexual or homosexual (use your judgement as to whether this is an appropriate question—in a 90-year-old lady with dementia, it is likely to cause eyebrows to be raised!)

Summary

When presenting the history, run through the categories described above, always starting with the same pattern (e.g. 'Miss Randolph is a 40-year-old right-handed administrator who complains of numbness in the feet').

- Describe the history of the presenting complaint, past medical history and review of systems. You

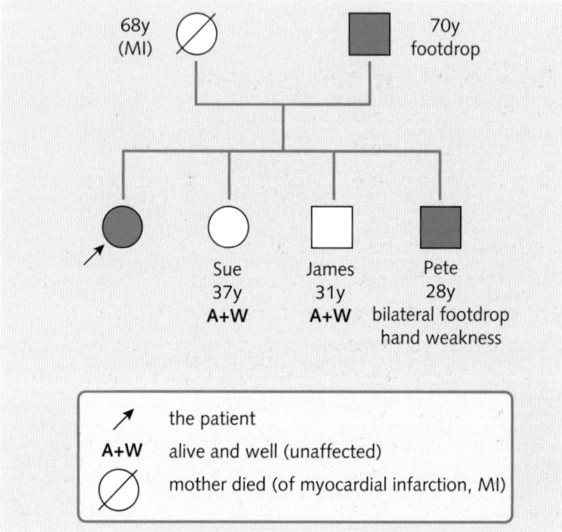

Fig. 15.1 The Lane family tree: an example of autosomal dominant inheritance. In this case, hereditary motor and sensory neuropathy (HSMN).

do not have to mention specifically all negative points, but it is worth pointing out those that are important (e.g. 'she has no history of diabetes').

- Say whether the patient is taking any medication.
- Describe the family history, if relevant; if not, explain that 'there is no relevant family history'.
- Describe important social points (e.g. 'she drinks only moderate alcohol and has never smoked').

You will then move on to your examination findings.

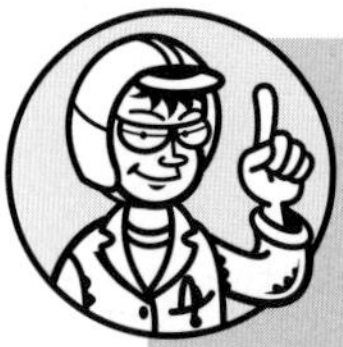

When presenting the history, aways start with the same sequence:

- Name.
- Age.
- Handedness.
- Occupation.
- Complaint (in the patient's words).

Communication skills

Patients with neurological problems often present particular problems with communication. This can make them daunting to approach, as we feel embarrassed about our fumblings. Remember that these people have to deal with discrimination and ignorance all the time, and the most important thing you can do is to respect them.

Approaching the patient

Always make sure that you look respectable (it is better to temporarily abandon your white coat if it is dirty or blood stained until you get a clean one). Introduce yourself to the patient and ask their permission for you to talk to them. Always speak to the patient first, rather than any relatives who may be around, even if they appear to be unconscious or incapable of responding. Surprisingly, relatives prefer this too! Many older people like to shake their doctor's hand, but do be aware of cultural differences (see later). Ensure that the patient is comfortable, but that you are too! You don't want to be distracted by cramp halfway through the history. Ask the patient's permission to perch on the end of the bed, or sit on a chair. Preferably you should be at eye level with them, or slightly lower. Eye contact is important in building trust with a patient, which you will need when embarking on the examination. It is worth making sure you are in a comfortable position to write.

Beginning the conversation

If possible, leave your note taking until later—perhaps just jotting down important dates of operations, etc., that you might otherwise forget. Start by checking the patient's name, age, occupation and handedness. This is a good opportunity to build a relationship with them—show interest in their occupation, or where they live. Patients often have fascinating stories to tell, if only people have the time to listen to them!

Begin your history taking with open questions such as 'tell me what led you to come to hospital' or 'tell me what has been happening with your health lately'. Be wary of asking 'what brought you into hospital', it is hard to chuckle at the 25th patient who says 'an ambulance, doc!'.

Problems in neurological patients

Be sensitive to any disability that the patient has. If they are deaf, make sure you enunciate your words very clearly, and raise your voice if appropriate. Remember that neurological conditions often leave cognitive functions unaffected, so do not speak to any adult patient as if they were a child. Give patients plenty of time, and try not to interrupt—if a patient finds speaking difficult and slow, they probably find it much more frustrating than you do!

Culture and gender

As with all patients, if you are of a different gender, be aware that you may embarrass them by asking them to remove all their clothes. If you need to expose the genital area (or the breasts in females), make it as quick and painless as possible. Cover any part of the patient you are not examining at that moment with a blanket. It is advisable to ask someone of the same sex as the patient to chaperone you in any intimate examination.

Different cultures approach the gender issue very differently. For example, Muslim women may not feel comfortable shaking the hand of a male doctor. Ask for a chaperone if you are in any doubt about how appropriate it is for you to be alone with the patient. This is for your own protection too!

Most patients will not mind you making mistakes with their culture's customs, as long as you apologize and try to learn for next time. It goes without saying that all cultures should command the same degree of respect from their doctor. However, do not be afraid of patients from a different culture from your own—they will be able to teach you more than the patients who are most similar to you!

The neurological examination

Speech

This will probably be one of the first things you assess, albeit unconsciously, during the history.

Speech production is organized at three levels: phonation, articulation and language production.

Phonation

Phonation is the production of sounds as the air passes through the vocal cords. A disorder of this process is called dysphonia.

Assessment

In dysphonia, the speech volume is reduced and the voice sounds rather husky. Dysphonia is usually due to lesions of the recurrent laryngeal nerves, or to respiratory muscle weakness (e.g. Guillain–Barré syndrome).

Articulation

Articulation is the manipulation of sound as it passes through the upper airways by the palate, the tongue and the lips to produce phonemes. A disorder of this process is called **dysarthria**.

Assessment

To assess articulation, ask the patient to repeat 'British Constitution', 'baby hippopotamus', and 'West Register Street'. If the speech articulation is abnormal, this could be caused by:

- Cerebellar dysarthria: speech is slurred (sounds like they are intoxicated), with 'staccato' or scanning quality.
- Extrapyramidal dysarthria: speech is soft and monotonous.
- Pseudobulbar dysarthria: speech is high pitched with a 'strangulated' quality and sounds like 'Donald Duck' speech.
- Bulbar dysarthria: speech has a nasal quality that may worsen as the patient continues to speak (suggesting myasthenia gravis).

Language production

Language production is the organization of phonemes into words and sentences, and is controlled by the speech centres in the dominant hemisphere. A disorder of this process is called **dysphasia**.

Assessment

To assess language production:

- Establish the patient's handedness. Dysphasia is a feature of dominant hemisphere dysfunction.
- Listen to the patient's spontaneous speech, assessing its fluency and contents.
- Assess the patient's comprehension by observing his or her response to simple commands: 'open your mouth, look up to the ceiling'.
- Assess the patient's ability to name objects. Use your wrist-watch (face, hands, strap, buckle).
- Assess the patient's ability to repeat sentences: 'no ifs, ands, or buts'.
- If any of these features is abnormal, the patient may be dysphasic (but they must be distinguished from a patient who is depressed and has psychomotor retardation, or severe dysarthria).

Cerebrovascular disease and brain tumours are the commonest causes of dysphasia. Dysphasia is classified according to speech fluency and content, comprehension and anatomical location of the lesions (Figs 15.2 and 15.3).

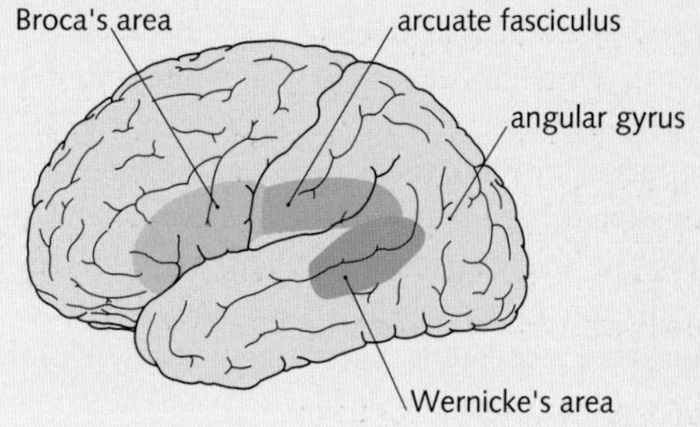

Fig. 15.2 Broca's and Wernicke's areas and their connecting arcuate fasciculus.

Classification of dysphasia					
Type	**Lesion**	**Speech fluency**	**Speech content**	**Comprehension of speech**	**Associations**
Expressive	Broca's area	Non-fluent	Normal	Normal	Telegrammatic speech, dysarturia
Receptive	Wernicke's area	Fluent	Impaired	Impaired	Neologisms, excessive speech
Conductive	Arcuate fasiculus	Fluent	Normal	Normal	Impaired function in repetitive tasks
Global	Parietal lobe/dominant hemisphere	Non-fluent	Impaired	Impaired	Contralateral visual/sensory inattention, defects in written language, variable extent of other disabilities according to size of lesion

Fig. 15.3 Classification of dysphasia.

Mental state and higher functions

Consciousness

Consciousness is the state of being aware of self and the environment. It has two components:

- The level of arousal.
- The content of consciousness.

The level of arousal

A number of ill-defined terms are used to describe the different levels of arousal:

- Full awakefulness and responsiveness—normal arousal status.
- Obtundation—patient is drowsy and not fully responsive.
- Stupor—patient appears to be asleep, with little or no spontaneous activity; however, he or she is rousable when stimulated.
- Coma—patient is unresponsive and unrousable.

This aspect of consciousness is conventionally assessed using the Glasgow Coma Scale.

The content of consciousness

The content of consciousness is dependent on the patient's level of cognitive functioning. The content of consciousness can be assessed only when a reasonable degree of arousal is present. This aspect of consciousness is conventionally assessed using the mini-mental state examination (see below).

Appearance and behaviour

Assessment of the patient's mental state begins as soon as you meet him or her. The physical appearance can be helpful. Demented patients may look bewildered but unconcerned, or apathetic and withdrawn. Look for evidence of self-neglect, which is often concealed by relatives. Observe the patient's response to your questions during the history-taking, assessing his or her comprehension and whether he or she retains insight into his or her problem.

Affect

Ask the patient if he or she has been feeling anxious, depressed or irritable, and decide if his or her mood is appropriate. Euphoric and manic patients look inappropriately cheerful and energetic, and tend to ignore or play down their problems and disabilities. Patients with emotional lability have sudden unprovoked outbursts of laughing or crying, which can be very distressing to them.

In cognitive impairment, patients' emotional reactions vary according to the severity of their illness:

- At the early stages, anxiety and depression might result from preserved insight into the increasing intellectual difficulties.
- In advanced stages, a flattening of the affect becomes apparent, and may lead to the patient being apparently totally unresponsive.

Attention and orientation

Attention

Ensure that the patient's comprehension is normal. Formal assessment of attention is carried out using serial reversals:

- 'Can you spell 'world' backwards for me, please'.
- 'Can you name the months of the year backwards, starting with December'.
- 'Can you count backwards from 20'.

Orientation

Assess the patient's orientation in time, place, and person. To test the parient's orientation in time, ask:

- 'What day of the week is it today?'
- 'What month are we in?'
- 'What time of day is it?'—this is a very sensitive marker for dementia.

To test the patient's orientation in place, ask:

- 'Can you tell me where are you now?'
- 'What city are we in?'

To test the patient's orientation in person, ask:

- 'Who is this person?' (point to a family member, a nurse or a doctor).

Memory

Immediate memory (recall)

Establish that the patient's comprehension and attention are normal. Immediate recall is tested with digit span: 'can you repeat these numbers after me, please'. Start with two or three figures, avoiding recognizable sequences. A normal individual can repeat a five- to seven-digit sequence.

Recent memory

Ask the patient about recent political, social or sporting events, taking into account his or her premorbid intelligence and socio-economic status.

Ask the patient to memorize a short address (try '23 West Register Street'). Ask him or her to repeat the address after you to ensure that it has been registered. Distract the patient for the next 10 minutes (by continuing your assessment of his or her mental status), then ask him or her to repeat the address. Most normal individuals will be able to recall all the data in 10 minutes.

Visual memory can be tested by displaying a drawing for 5 seconds and asking the patient to redraw the design 10 seconds later (Fig. 15.4). Patients with visuospatial disorders will have difficulty with the task, even if their visual memory is intact.

Remote memory

Ask the patient about childhood, schooling, work history or marriage. The accuracy of his or her answers should be verified by a relative. If no relative is available, ask a question about a time period relevant to the patient. In elderly people, this might be 'in what year did World War One start?' or, in younger patients 'in what year did England win the football world cup?'. These questions should again be adjusted for premorbid intelligence and socio-economic status.

Immediate and recent memory is usually affected early in dementia. However, remote memory is relatively spared in patients with minor degrees of brain damage, but is always affected in those with advanced dementia.

Calculation

This should be tested in the light of the patient's education. Give the patient simple addition or subtraction sums. Serial sevens or threes (subtracting sevens or threes serially from 100) is a useful test.

Dyscalculia is a prominent feature of Gerstmann's syndrome (dyscalculia, right–left disorientation and finger agnosia), caused by dominant parietal lobe lesions.

Abstract thinking

This is tested by asking the patient to interpret common proverbs:

- 'A bird in the hand is worth two in the bush'.
- 'People in glass houses should not throw stones'.

Abstract thinking can also be tested by assessing the patient's ability to identify the similarities between pairs of objects: 'cow and dog, air and water'.

Constructional ability and neglect

Constructional ability and neglect are tested by asking the patient to construct simple designs

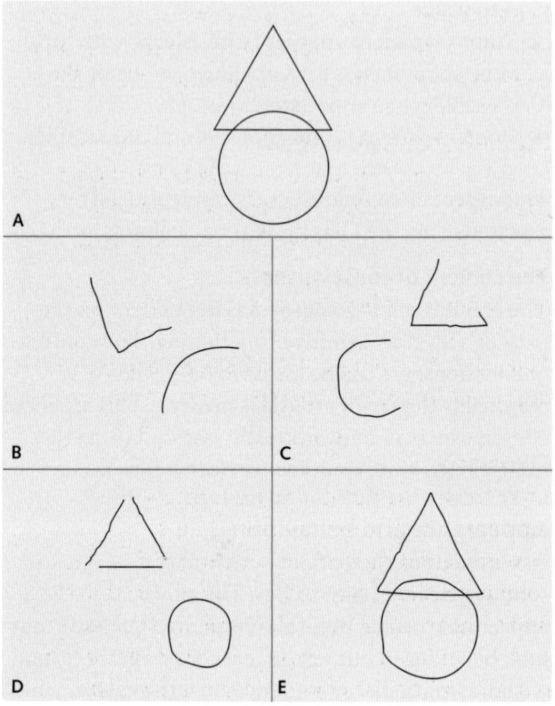

Fig. 15.4 Visual memory test showing (A) the standard design and (B–E) reproductions scored from 0–3.

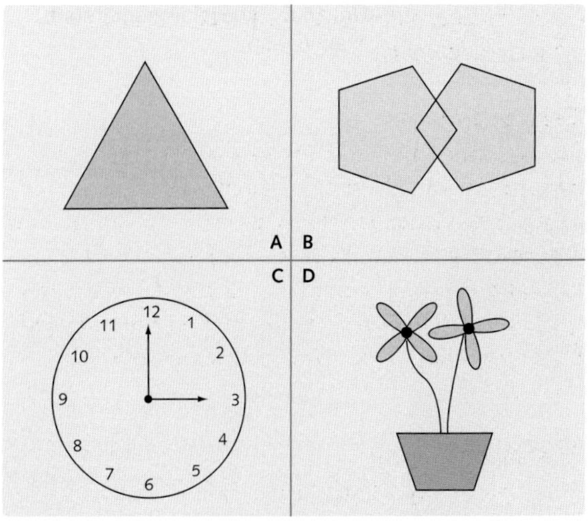

Fig. 15.5 Constructional tests: drawings of increasing complexity to be reproduced by the patient.

(triangle, square) using match-sticks, and to draw or copy designs of increasing complexity (Fig. 15.5):

- 'Please draw a clock, put the hours on it, and set the time at 3 o'clock'.

Patients with non-dominant parietal lesions have poor constructional ability (which is often associated with neglect to the contralateral side of the body, including the visual fields), which is often reflected in the patients' drawings (they copy only the right side of the design, or they draw and put the numbers on the one side, usually the right side, of the clock).

Right–left disorientation

Establish that the patient's comprehension is normal. Right–left disorientation is assessed by giving the patient simple commands of increasing complexity:

- 'Show me your right hand'.
- 'Put your left hand on your right ear'.

Right–left disorientation is seen in patients with dominant parietal lobe lesions.

Dyspraxia

Dyspraxia is the inability to perform a skilled movement in the absence of weakness, incoordination, sensory loss or abnormal comprehension. Dyspraxia can be confined to the limbs, the trunk or the buccofacial musculature.

Dyspraxia is tested by asking the patient to carry out particular tasks of increasing complexity:

- 'Stick out your tongue'.
- 'Pretend to whistle'.
- 'Show me how to use a toothbrush'.
- 'Show me how to take the cap off a toothpaste tube and squeeze the toothpaste onto a brush'.

There are some special forms of dyspraxia:

- Dressing dyspraxia.
- Constructional dyspraxia.
- Gait dyspraxia.

Agnosia

Agnosia is the inability to recognize a sensory input in the absence of primary sensory pathway dysfunction. It can affect a certain sensory modality in a global fashion (visual agnosia, auditory agnosia), or can affect a specific class of stimuli (colour agnosia).

Agnosia is tested by showing the patient a few objects and asking him or her to name each one. Allow the patient to manipulate the objects, which might improve recognition (by allowing him or her to use a different sensory input). Assess other sensory modalities:

- Auditory agnosia (inability to recognize sounds).
- Tactile agnosia (inability to recognize objects placed in the hand: astereognosis).
- Finger agnosia (inability to name fingers).
- Topographic agnosia (inability to comprehend three-dimensional sense).

Mini-mental state examination

It is often difficult to perform an extensive testing of higher cortical functions in every patient. Screening tests have been devised to allow rapid assessment. The mini-mental state examination (Fig. 15.6) is one of many such tests. This is a helpful screening test, but has its limitations.

- The maximum score is 30.
- Scores 28–30 do not support the diagnosis of dementia.
- Scores 25–27 are borderline.
- Scores < 25 are suggestive of dementia (if acute confusional state and depression are unlikely).

Cortical and subcortical dementia

Learn to differentiate between the features of cortical and subcortical dementia (Fig. 15.7). Patients with cortical dementia retain the ability to answer questions at a relatively normal speed. However, their answers are irrelevant and 'hopeless'.

- Q: How many arms do you have?
- A: Oh, not many!

Mini-mental state examination

Orientation
1. What is the year, season, date, month, day? (one point for each correct answer)
2. Where are we? Country, county, town, hospital, floor? (one point for each answer)

Registration
3. Name three objects, taking 1 second to say each. Then ask the patient all three once you have said them. One point for each correct answer. Repeat the questions until the patient learns all three

Attention and calculation
4. Serial sevens. One point for each correct answer. Stop after five answers. Alternative: spell 'world' backwards

Recall
5. Ask for names of three objects asked in question 3. One point for each correct answer

Language
6. Point to a pencil and a watch. Ask the patient to name them for you. One point for each correct answer
7. Ask the patient to repeat 'No ifs, ands, or buts'. One point
8. Ask the patient to follow a three-stage command: 'Take the paper in your right hand; fold the paper in half; put the paper on the floor.' Three points
9. Ask the patient to read and obey the following: CLOSE YOUR EYES. (Write this in large letters). One point
10. Ask the patient to write a sentence of his or her own choice. (The sentence must contain a subject and an object and make some sense.) Ignore spelling errors when scoring. One point
11. Ask the patient to copy two intersecting pentagons with equal sides (Fig 12.4B). Give one point if all the sides and angles are preserved, and if the intersecting sides from a quadrangle

Maximum score = 30 points

Fig. 15.6 The mini-mental state examination.

Features of cortical and subcortical dementia

	Example	Cognition	Insight	Memory	Response time	Personality	Mood
cortical dementia	Alzheimer's disease, Pick's disease	severely disturbed	absent	difficulty learning new information	normal	unconcerned	may be depressed
subcortical dementia	Parkinson's disease, Huntington's chorea	impaired problem solving	partially retained	difficulty retrieving learned information	slow	apathetic	often depressed

Fig. 15.7 Features of cortical and subcortical dementia.

Patients with subcortical dementia have difficulty in retrieving memories and their response time is therefore long. They are not totally 'hopeless' and often find the right answer with some help.

- Q: Who is the monarch on the throne in England now?
- A: Erm . . . I don't know.
- Q: Is it George, Victoria or Elizabeth?
- A: Queen Elizabeth.

Clinical syndromes associated with specific focal hemispheric dysfunction

Frontal lobe

Conditions associated with frontal lobe dysfunction are:

- Altered personality, altered mood, loss of interest, loss of initiative.
- Expressive dysphasia (dominant hemisphere) and dyspraxia.

- Hemiparesis and primitive reflexes.
- Sphincter incontinence (bifrontal lesions).

Parietal lobe

Conditions associated with parietal lobe dysfunction on the dominant side are:

- Dysphasia, dyslexia, dysgraphia.
- Dyscalculia.
- Right–left disorientation.
- Finger agnosia.

Conditions associated with dysfunction of the non-dominant side are:

- Neglect to the contralateral side of the body.
- Constructional and dressing dyspraxia.
- Topographic agnosia.

Conditions associated with dysfunction of the non-dominant or dominant side are:

- Hemisensory disturbance or inattention.
- Lower quadrant homonymous field defect.

Temporal lobe

Conditions associated with temporal lobe dysfunction are:

- Amnesic syndromes.
- Dysphasia (dominant lobe).
- Upper quadrant homonymous field defect.

Occipital lobe

Conditions associated with occipital lobe dysfunction are:

- Visual field defects.
- Distortion of vision.
- Impaired visual recognition (visual agnosia).

Gait

In normal gait, the erect moving body is supported by one leg at a time while the other swings forward in preparation for the next support move. Only one foot will be on the floor at any time, although both the heel of the anterior foot and the toes of the posterior foot will be on the ground momentarily when the body weight is transferred from one leg to the other. Normal gait requires input from the motor, sensory, cerebellar and vestibular systems.

Assessment

The gait of a patient is assessed as follows:

- Ask the patient to walk up and down the examination room in his or her usual fashion, with his or her arms loose by his or her side.
- Observe the patient's posture, the pattern of his or her arm and leg movements and the control of his or her trunk.
- If gait appears normal, ask the patient to heel–toe walk ('I would like you to walk heel to toe as if

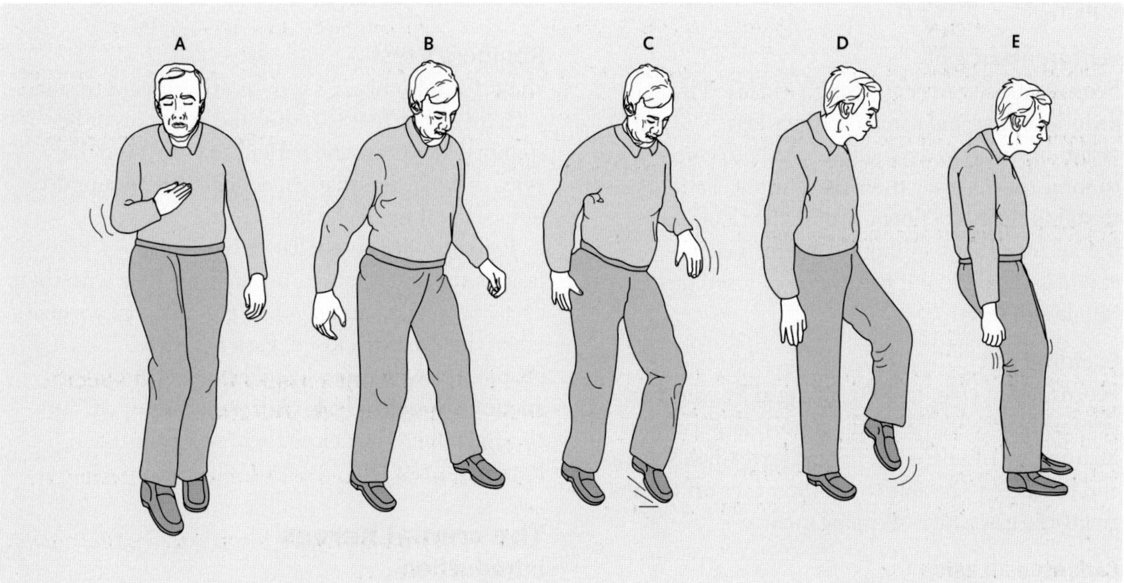

Fig. 15.8 Gait disorders. (A) Hemiplegic, (B) cerebellar ataxia, (C) sensory ataxia, (D) unilateral footdrop and (E) parkinsonian.

you are walking on a tightrope'). Walk alongside the patient to support him or her if he or she appears unsteady.
- If gait appears abnormal, classify it into one of the following patterns:

Hemiplegic gait
Hemiplegic gait (Fig. 15.8A) is caused by unilateral upper motor neuron leg weakness. The ipsilateral arm is held flexed and adducted while the ipsilateral leg is extended (pyramidal pattern of weakness). To move the affected leg, patients tilt their pelvis to be able to swing the affected leg forward in a 'circumduction' manner.

Spastic gait
Spastic gait is caused by bilateral upper motor neuron leg weakness. Both legs are spastic and patients walk in small steps with their toes pressing firmly on the floor as if they are walking in mud. The legs are held in adduction with the knees touching each other, giving the gait a 'scissored' quality.

Cerebellar ataxic gait
Cerebellar ataxic gait (Fig. 15.8B) is caused by cerebellar (and occasionally vestibular) lesions. Patients walk on a wide base and appear unsteady, with erratic body movements. They stagger to the affected side in unilateral lesions (backwards if the lesion is in the cerebellar vermis). The condition may be embarrassing for the patient as people assume that they are drunk. Mild cases can be detected only by asking patients to walk on a narrow base (heel–toe walking).

Sensory ataxic gait
Sensory ataxic gait (Fig. 15.8C) is caused by proprioceptive and somatosensory loss. The gait is rather unsteady but patients are able to compensate to some extent using their visual input. Patients tend to stamp their feet down against the floor, owing to the loss of all sensory input. Patients become very ataxic in the dark or if the eyes are closed (see Romberg's test).

Footdrop gait
Footdrop gait (Fig. 15.8D) is caused by common peroneal nerve lesion (if unilateral), or peripheral neuropathy (if bilateral). Patients over-flex the hip and the knee to be able to lift their toes off the floor, giving the gait a high-stepping quality.

Parkinsonian gait
Parkinsonian gait (Fig. 15.8E) is slow and shuffling with small stride length, flexed posture and reduced arm swinging. Patients often have problems in starting to walk and in turning while walking, which is achieved by using an exaggerated number of steps. This gait should be differentiated from the less common *marche à petit pas* seen in bilateral frontal lobe lesions, in which gait is shuffling but the arms and the trunk are not affected.

Waddling gait
Waddling gait is caused by proximal myopathy. Patients have exaggerated lumbar lordosis. They bend their pelvis forward and walk with a waddle, tilting from one side to the other.

Antalgic gait
Antalgic gait is caused by painful musculoskeletal conditions. Patients walk with a 'limp' in an attempt to minimize the use of the painful leg.

Apraxic gait
Apraxic gait is caused by parietal lobe lesions. Patients have no difficulty in manipulating their limbs when sitting or lying, but when attempting to walk they experience great difficulty in organizing their gait and placing their feet in the right positions. Gait appears to have an odd and bizarre character. Patients are liable to 'freeze' to the ground, unable to initiate movements.

Hysterical gait
Hysterical gait is erratic and unpredictable. Patients stagger widely with exaggerated arm movements. Falls and injuries are unusual but their presence does not exclude this diagnosis.

Romberg's test
To perform Romberg's test, ask the patient to stand with his or her feet together and assess his or her stability. Next, ask the patient to close his or her eyes, making sure that you will be able to support him or her if he or she falls.

Patients with cerebellar or vestibular lesions are usually ataxic on a narrow base with their eyes open. Their ataxia might get marginally worse when the eyes are closed. Patients with propioceptive sensory loss might be slightly ataxic on a narrow base with their eyes open, but they fall when they close their eyes (positive Romberg's test).

The cranial nerves
Introduction
Examination of the cranial nerves plays an important part in the central nervous system assessment. They

provide a number of neurological signs that aid localization, particularly in unconscious patients.

Olfactory nerve (I)

To test the olfactory nerves, first ask patients about any recent change in their sense of smell (anosmia, parosmia, olfactory hallucination) (Fig. 15.9). Then, test their ability to smell coffee, cinnamon and tobacco, by examining each nostril in turn. Avoid using very irritating odours (e.g. ammonia or camphor), which could stimulate the trigeminal nerve endings, even in anosmic patients.

Unilateral loss of smell is usually asymptomatic. Bilateral loss of smell is usually associated with an altered sense of taste (loss of the ability to appreciate aromas).

Remember to examine the olfactory nerve in all patients presenting with personality changes, disinhibition or dementia (frontal lobe tumours) and, in all cases of head injury.

Causes of olfactory symptoms

Anosmia (loss of smell)
- congenital
- nasal sinuses infections/tumours
- head injury/cranial surgery
- frontal lobe tumours
- subfrontal meningiomas

Parosmia (persistent unpleasant smell)
- nasal infections/tumours
- head injury
- depression

Olfactory hallucination
- temporal lobe epileptic seizures

Paroxysmal, unpleasant smell (burning rubber, smell of gas)
- psychosis

Fig. 15.9 Causes of olfactory symptoms.

The eye (II and III)

Visual acuity (VA)

Visual acuity is tested using a Snellen chart in a well-lit room. Seat or stand the patient 6 m from the chart. Small, hand-held Snellen charts can be read at a distance of 2 m.

Near visual acuity is tested using reading charts, but this does not necessarily correlate well with distance acuity.

Correct the patient's refractive errors with glasses or a pinhole. Ask the patient to cover each eye in turn with his or her palm, and find which line of print he or she can read comfortably. Visual acuity is expressed as the ratio of the distance between the patient and the chart to the number of the smallest visible line on the chart (normally 6/6) (Fig. 15.10).

If the patient is unable to read characters of line 60 (visual acuity less than 6/60), assess his or her ability to count your fingers at 1 m (VA: CF), see your hand movements (VA: HM), or perceive a torch light (VA: LP). If unable to perceive light (VA: NLP), then the patient is medically blind.

Colour vision

Colour vision is tested using Ishahara plates in a daylight-lit room. Test each eye separately. If 13/15 plates or more are read correctly, colour vision can be regarded as normal. This test is designed principally to detect congenital colour vision defects, but is sensitive in detecting mild degrees of optic nerve dysfunction.

Visual fields

Sit about 1 m from the patient with your eyes at the same horizontal level. Start by testing for visual inattention. Ask the patient to look into your eyes

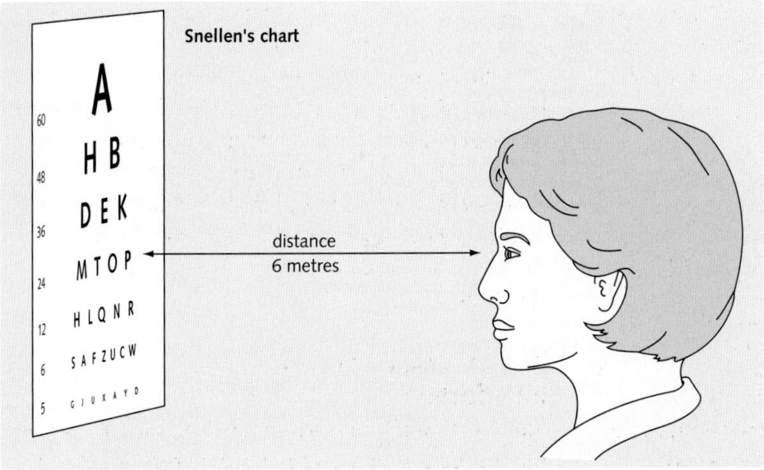

Fig. 15.10 Visual acuity. The patient is able to read line number 24, but not number 12. Visual acuity is 6/24.

and hold your hands outstretched halfway between you and the patient. Stimulate the patient's visual fields by moving each hand separately and then both hands together, and ask the patient to indicate which of your hands has moved each time.

In patients with parietal lobe lesions, a visual stimulus presented in isolation to the contralateral field is perceived, but it is missed when a comparable stimulus is presented simultaneously to the ipsilateral field (neglect).

Visual fields are examined by confrontation, during which you compare your own visual fields with the patient's (provided that yours are normal). The patient's visual field will match yours only if your head positions are exactly comparable and if your hand is exactly halfway between you and the patient; this is seldom the case.

Visual fields in poorly cooperative patients are assessed by using visual threat (sudden, unexpected hand movement into the patient's visual field).

Peripheral fields Examine each eye in turn. To test the patient's right visual field, ask him or her to cover his or her left eye with his or her left palm and to look into your left eye throughout the examination.

Cover your own right eye with your right hand, and test the patient's peripheral field by bringing the moving fingers of your left hand into the upper and then the lower quadrants of the patient's temporal fields. Ask the patient to inform you as soon as he or she sees your fingers.

Now cover your own right eye with your left hand and examine the patient's nasal fields with your right hand using the same method.

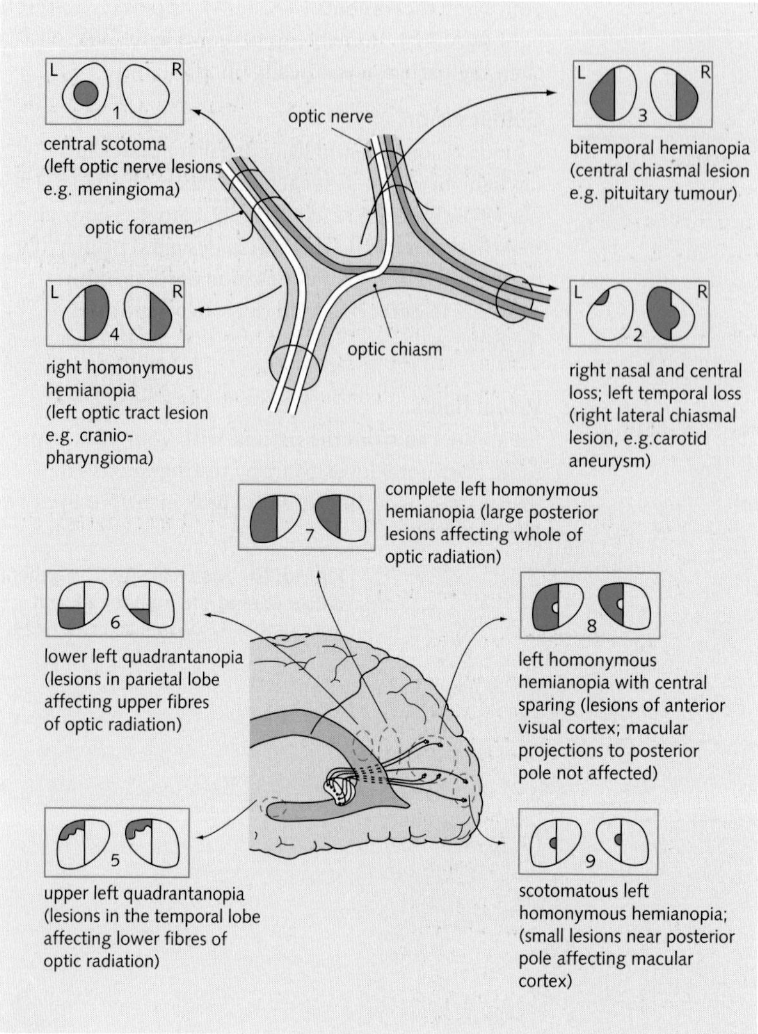

Fig. 15.11 Visual field defects (courtesy of Dr Ross, St Thomas's Hospital, London).

Blind spot The blind spot is tested using a 10 mm red hat pin. Ask the patient to cover his or her left eye and focus on looking at your nose. Move the pin from the central into the temporal field along the horizontal meridian, having explained to him or her that the pin will disappear briefly and then reappear again, and that he or she should indicate when this happens. Once you have found the patient's blind spot, you can map its shape and compare its size with yours.

Central field The central field is tested by moving a red hat pin along the central visual field (fixation area) in the horizontal meridian. Ask the patient to indicate if the pin disappears (absolute central scotoma) or if the colour appears diminished (relative scotoma). A central scotoma extends temporally from the fixation area into the blind spot.

Visual field defects Bedside testing of visual fields can detect only large scotomas. Different patterns of visual field defects can be recognized clinically (Fig. 15.11).

Eyelids and pupils

Inspection Note the position of the eyelids. If there is a ptosis, decide whether it is partial or complete; assess its fatiguability by asking the patient to sustain upward gaze for at least 1 minute. Next, assess the size and shape of the pupils. They should be circular and symmetrical (Fig. 15.12).

Light response Light responses should be assessed using a bright torch light. Ask the patient to fixate on a distant target and shine the light in each eye in turn from the lateral side. Observe the direct (ipsilateral) and the consensual (contralateral) responses.

Assess the presence of an afferent pupillary defect by swinging the light from one eye to the other, dwelling 3 seconds on each. As you swing the light from, say, the right eye to the left, the pupil of the latter (which has just started to dilate because of loss of its consensual reaction) should immediately constrict. A delayed constriction indicates loss of sensitivity of the afferent pathways (optic nerve damage).

Accommodation Hold your finger 50–60 cm from the patient and ask him or her to fixate on it. Bring your finger towards the patient's eyes. Observe the normal reaction of bilateral pupillary constriction and convergence (adduction).

Fundoscopy

This is often the most feared part of the neurological examination. The key to picking up signs is simply a matter of practice—try to look at the fundi of every patient you clerk.

Ask the patient to fixate on a distant target, avoiding bright lights. Using an ophthalmoscope, examine the patient's right eye using your right eye, and the patient's left eye using your left eye. Warn the patient that you will have to get close to them to do this, and try to keep breathing!

Adjust the ophthalmoscope lens until the retinal vessels are in focus and trace them back to the optic disc. Assess the optic disc shape, colour and clarity of its margins. The temporal disc margins are normally slightly paler than the nasal margins. The physiological cupping varies in size but does not extend to the disc margins.

unilateral		reaction to light	associated signs
third nerve palsy		negative	ptosis (partial or complete) external ophthalmoplegia
Horner's syndrome		poor reaction to shade	ptosis (always partial) anhydrosis endophthalmus
Holmes–Adie syndrome		slow reaction	constriction to pilocarpine (0.1%) lower limb areflexia
bilateral			
Argyll Robertson	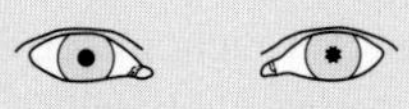	negative	depigmented iris normal accommodation neurosyphilis
midbrain compression	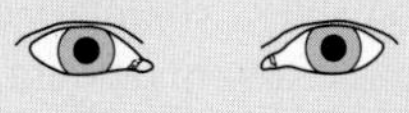	negative	coma lateralizing signs
pontine stroke		negative	coma hyperventilation hyperpyrexia

Fig. 15.12 Pupillary abnormalities.

Fig. 15.13 Common fundoscopic abnormalities.

Common fundoscopic abnormalities		
Structure	**Abnormality**	**Pathology**
optic disc	papilloedema	raised intracranial pressure, venous obstruction (e.g. cavernous sinus thrombosis, orbital tumour), high CSF protein (e.g. Guillain–Barré syndrome, spinal cord tumours), malignant hypertension, hypercapnia
	optic atrophy	optic neuritis (e.g. multiple sclerosis, Devic's disease), optic nerve/chiasmal compression (e.g. meningioma, optic nerve gliomas, pituitary tumours, Paget's disease of the skull, arachnoiditis), toxic/metabolic (e.g. methyl alcohol, B_{12} deficiency), long-standing raised intracranial pressure), infections (e.g. neurosyphilis), hereditary (e.g. Leber's optic atrophy)
retinal arteries	silver-wiring, increased tortuosity, arteriovenous nipping	hypertension
	gross narrowing with retinal pallor and reddened fovea	central retinal artery occlusion
	cholesterol or platelet emboli	cerebrovascular disease
retinal veins	venous engorgement	papilloedema (see above), central retinal vein occlusion
retina	haemorrhages	superficial flamed-shaped (hypertension) and deep dot-shaped (diabetes) subhyaloid between the retina and the vitreous (subarachnoid haemorrhage)
	exudates	soft cotton-wool and hard exudates (diabetes)
	pigmentation	retinitis pigmentosa (e.g. hereditary, Refsum's disease, Kearns–Sayre syndrome), choroidoretinitis (e.g. toxoplasmosis, sarcoidosis, syphilis), post-laser treatment (diabetes)

Next, assess the retinal vessels. The arteries are narrower than the veins and brighter in colour. The vessels should not be obscured as they cross the disc margins. Look for retinal vein pulsation, which is present in about 80% of normal individuals and is an index of normal intracranial pressure. This is seen best at the disc margins where the veins cross over the arteries. Note the width of the blood vessels and look for arteriovenous nipping at the crossover points.

Assess the rest of the retina, noting any evidence of discoloration, haemorrhages or white patches of exudate. Ask the patient to look at the light of the ophthalmoscope, which brings the macula into view. Classify fundoscopic abnormalities into those affecting the optic disc, retinal vessels or the retina (Fig. 15.13).

Patients with acute optic neuritis might have fundoscopic abnormalities similar to papilloedema. However, in optic neuritis, eye movements can be painful and visual acuity is substantially reduced.

Eye movements (III, IV, and VI)

Inspect the eyes and note the position of the eyelids and the presence of any strabismus (squint). Strabismus is concomitant (usually asymptomatic) if it remains constant throughout the range of eye movements, and incomitant (paralytic) if it varies.

If the patient is capable of voluntary eye movements, the pursuit and saccadic systems should be tested to assess whether eye movements are conjugate, and to detect the presence of diplopia and nystagmus.

Isolated painful third nerve palsy is suggestive of a posterior communicating artery aneurysm.

Pupil-sparing third nerve palsy is suggestive of vascular aetiology, particularly diabetes.

Monocular diplopia is suggestive of either refractive defects (cornea or lens) or hysteria.

Very complicated and variable diplopia is suggestive of myasthenia gravis. Look for orbicularis oculi weakness in these cases.

Pursuit eye movements

Steady the patient's head with one hand and hold the index finger of your other hand 40–50 cm in front of his or her eyes. Ask the patient to follow your slowly moving finger throughout the range of binocular vision in both the horizontal and the vertical planes in a letter 'H' pattern.

Assess the smoothness, speed and magnitude of the movements. Look for nystagmus, and ask the patient to report any diplopia. In the presence of diplopia, identify the direction of the maximum separation of images and the two muscles responsible for moving the eyes in this direction (Fig. 15.14). Identify the source of the outer image, which comes from the defective eye, by covering each eye in turn. This will allow you to name the muscle(s) and the nerve(s) involved.

Saccadic eye movements

Ask the patient to keep his or her head still, and to look left, right, up and down as quickly as possible. Assess the velocity and the accuracy of the movements. Look for slow or absent adduction (internuclear ophthalmoplegia) (Fig. 15.15).

If pursuit or saccadic eye movements are absent, oculocephalic reflex (doll's eye movements) will differentiate between supranuclear and nuclear ocular paralysis. Ask the patient to fixate on your eyes while you rotate his or her head in the horizontal and the vertical planes. In supranuclear lesions the reflex is intact, allowing the patient's eyes to remain fixated on yours.

Ocular nerve paresis

Clinical signs of ocular nerve paresis are shown in Fig. 15.16. Causes of ocular paresis are shown in Fig. 15.17.

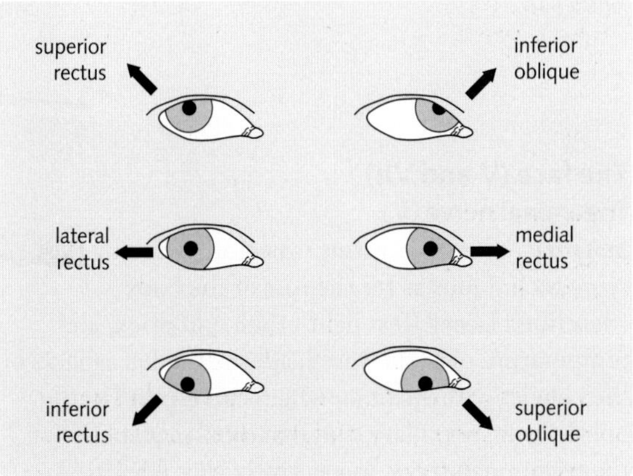

Fig. 15.14 Muscles responsible for eye movements in particular directions.

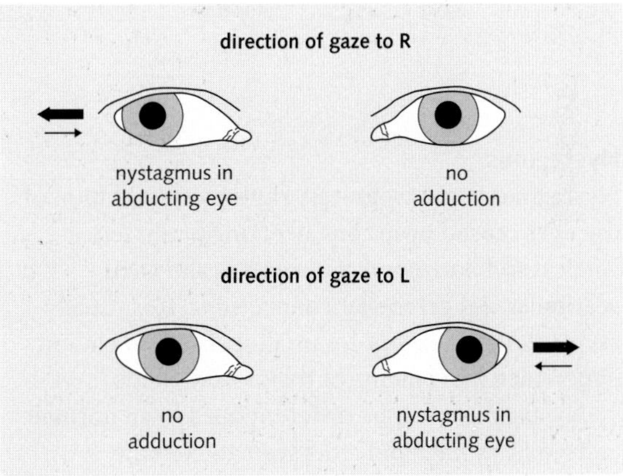

Fig. 15.15 Bilateral internuclear ophthalmoplegia.

Clinical signs of ocular nerve paresis

Nerve	Signs
III	ptosis, eye is deviated laterally and slightly downwards (divergent strabismus), pupil may be dilated and unresponsive (pupil staring in diabetes and vascular causes)
IV	impaired depression (and intortion) of the fully adducted eye, head might be tilted to the opposite side to avoid diplopia when reading or looking down
VI	impaired abduction (convergent strabismus)

Fig. 15.16 Clinical signs of ocular nerve paresis.

Fig. 15.17 Causes of ocular paresis.

Causes of ocular paresis		
Type		**Pathology**
supranuclear gaze paresis	horizontal	frontal lobe lesions: eyes deviated to the side of the lesion. Common massive stroke, head injury. Paralysis and voluntary conjugate gaze, with preserved brainstem reflexes (e.g. to coloric stimulation). brainstem pretecral lesions: eyes deviated to opposite side
	vertical	brainstem pretectal region: Parinaud's syndrome (vertical gaze paralysis, pupillary dilation, absent accommodation reflex) extrapyramidal diseases (e.g. Parkinson's disease, progressive supranuclear palsy): impaired vertical gaze (initially upward)
nuclear and nerve (III, IV, VI) palsies	brainstem	vascular lesions, tumours, demyelination, Wernicke's encephalitis
	peripheral	raised intracranial pressure (VI as a false localizing sign, III caused by tentorial herniation) vascular lesions (e.g. atheroma, diabetes, temporal arteritis, syphilis) aneurysms (posterior communicating artery: III, cavernous sinus: III, IV, VI) meningeal inflammation and malignant infiltration skull base tumours (nasopharyngeal carcinoma, chordoma) cranial polyneuropathy (Guillain–Barré syndrome, sarcoidosis) orbital tumours and granulomas, sinus disease
muscle disease		myasthenia gravis, thyroid eye disease, mitochondrial cytopathy

Nystagmus

Nystagmus is an involuntary rhythmic oscillation of the eyes caused by lesions affecting brainstem vertical and horizontal gaze centres and their vestibular and cerebellar connections. It is usually asymptomatic, except for oscillopsia when patients experience movements of their visual fields.

Nystagmus must be differentiated from normal end-point nystagmoid jerks seen at extreme deviation of gaze, and from the voluntary rapid oscillation of eyes. Both are brief and unsustained.

Testing Note the presence of nystagmus in the primary position of gaze (when looking forward), and while examining eye movements, and decide whether it is pendular or jerky, and whether the movements are horizontal, vertical, rotatory or of mixed nature.

Record its amplitude (fine, medium, coarse), persistence and the direction of gaze in which it occurs (the direction of nystagmus is, by convention, the direction of the fast component). Causes of nystagmus are shown in Fig. 15.18.

The face (V and VII)

Trigeminal nerve (V)

Sensory Sensory testing is performed using the same techniques as for the rest of the body (described later). Test light touch, pin prick, and temperature over the forehead, the medial aspects of the cheeks, and the chin, which correspond to the ophthalmic, maxillary, and mandibular branches of the trigeminal nerve, respectively (Fig. 15.19). A partial loss can be detected by comparing the response to the same stimulus on the other sites on the face.

Corneal response is elicited by lightly touching the cornea (not the conjunctiva) with a wisp of cotton wool. Synchronous blinking of both eyes occurs. An afferent defect (Vth cranial nerve lesion) results in depression or absence of the direct and consensual reflex. An efferent defect (VIIth cranial nerve lesion) results in an impairment or absence of the reflex on the side of the facial weakness. The clinical pattern of sensory loss depends on the anatomical site of the lesion (Fig. 15.20).

Causes of nystagmus		
Type	**Description**	**Pathology**
pendular	oscillations of equal velocity	long-standing impaired macular vision (since early childhood), miner's nystagmus
jerky	fast phase towards the side of the lesion	unilateral cerebellar lesions
	fast phase to the opposite side of the lesion	unilateral vestibular lesions
	direction of nystagmus varies with the direction of gaze	brainstem pathology
	upbeat nystagmus	lesions at or around the superior colliculi
	downbeat nystagmus	lesions at or around the foramen magnum
rotatory	specific to one head position, and fatigues with repeated testing	unilateral labyrinthine pathology
rotatory or mixed	all other types	brainstem pathology

Fig. 15.18 Causes of nystagmus.

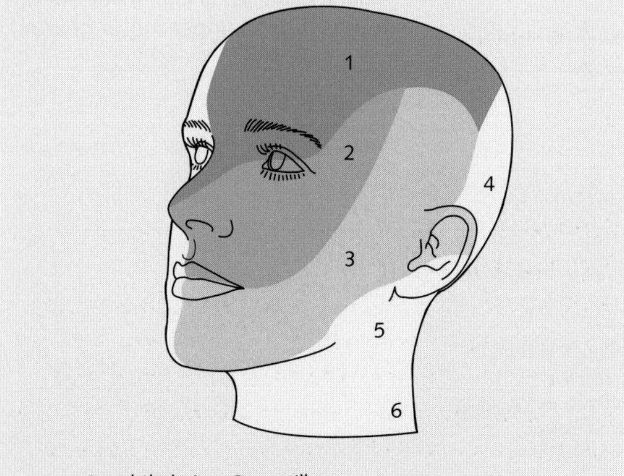

Fig. 15.19 Trigeminal sensory innervation to the face.

Motor Inspect for wasting of the temporalis muscles, which produces hollowing above the zygoma. Ask the patient to clench his or her teeth together and palpate the masseters, noting any wasting. The pterygoid muscles are assessed by resisting the patient's attempts to open his or her mouth. In unilateral trigeminal lesions, the lower jaw deviates to the paralytic side as the mouth is opened.

Jaw jerk Jaw jerk is a brainstem stretch reflex. Ask the patient to open his or her mouth slightly. Rest your index finger on the apex of the jaw and tap it with the patella hammer. The response, mouth opening, is due to a contraction of the pterygoid muscles. An absent reflex is not significant, but the reflex could be brisk in pseudobulbar palsy (see later).

Facial nerve (VII)

Motor response Inspect the patient's face, looking for asymmetry of the nasolabial folds and the position of the two angles of the mouth. Assess the movements of the upper part of the face by asking the patient to elevate his or her eyebrows, close his or her eyes tightly and resist your attempt to open them. Movements of the lower side of the face are assessed by asking the patient to blow out his or her cheeks with air, purse his or her lips tightly together and resist your attempt to open them, show his or her teeth, or whistle. Finally, ask the patient to smile, and observe any facial asymmetry.

If you detect any weakness or asymmetry, decide if the weakness is confined to the lower part of the face (upper motor neuron lesion) or both the upper and the lower parts of the face (lower motor neuron lesion) (Figs 15.21 and 15.22).

Do not miss bilateral facial weakness. In this case, the face appears to sag, with lack of facial expression.

Clinical syndromes of the trigeminal nerve		
Site of lesion	**Signs**	**Pathology**
dorsal pons	altered light touch, with preserved pain and temperature.	vascular, tumour
high central medulla	'onion-skin' circumoral analgesia which advances outwards	syringobulbia
low central medulla or high intrinsic cervical lesion above C2	'onion-skin' analgesia which starts at the peripheral parts of the face and advances towards the nose and the mouth	syringomyelia
lateral medulla	ipsilateral loss of pain and temperature	lateral medullary syndrome
upper cervical cord, foramen magnum	generalized sensory loss which starts first in ophthalmic division and advances downwards	cervical spondylosis, meningiomas
sensory root or ganglia	generalized sensory loss of all modalities	acoustic neuroma, meningioma, angioma
peripheral branch	selective sensory loss of all modalities	orbital tumours, neuromas

Fig. 15.20 Clinical syndromes of the trigeminal nerve.

Clinical syndromes of facial weakness		
Site of lesion	**Signs**	**Common pathology**
supranuclear	contralateral (or ipsilateral) UMN weakness	vascular, tumour
brainstem	ipsilateral LMN weakness	vascular, tumours, syrinx, demyelination
cerebellopontine angle	Ipsilateral LMN weakness	acoustic neuromas, meningiomas, angioma
basal meninges	often bilateral LMN weakness	sarcoidosis, malignant meningitis
petrous bone	ipsilateral LMN weakness	middle ear infections, Bell's palsy, geniculate herpetic zoster
face	ipsilateral LMN weakness	parotid tumours, trauma
muscle disease	usually bilateral LMN weakness	myasthenia gravis, myotonic dystrophy, muscular dystrophy
others	usually bilateral LMN weakness	Guillain–Barré syndrome

Fig. 15.21 Clinical syndromes of facial weakness (LMN, lower motor neuron; UMN, upper motor neuron).

Look for Bell's phenomenon (eyeball rotates upwards and outwards on attempting to close the eye). The lack of this sign may indicate that the patient is not attempting to close his or her eye, raising the suspicion of a psychological reason for their symptoms.

Taste Formal assessment of taste is rarely of practical benefit. Taste is examined by applying a solution of salt, sweet (sugar), or sour (vinegar) to the anterior two-thirds of the tongue and comparing the response on the two sides. The mouth should be rinsed with water between testing. Cranial nerve VIII lesions proximal to the middle ear will cause loss of taste.

Hyperacusis Hyperacusis (undue sensitivity to noise) is suggestive of a lesion proximal to the middle ear, affecting the nerve to the stapedius.

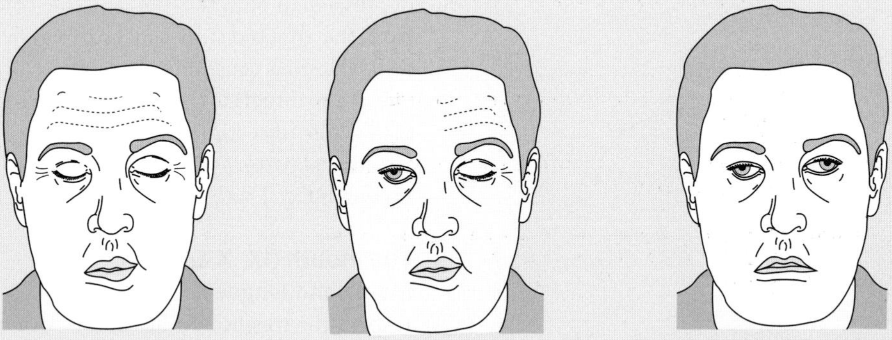

Fig. 15.22 Facial weakness. The patient is asked to close his or her eyes and purse his or her lips. Note the defective eye closure and Bell's phenomenon in B and C (LMN, lower motor neuron; UMN, upper motor neuron).

Auditory nerve (VIII)

Hearing

Clinical bedside assessment of hearing is not sensitive, and can detect only gross hearing loss. Audiometry is usually required for detailed assessment. Assess each ear separately while masking the hearing in the other ear by occluding the external meatus with your index finger. Test the patient's hearing sensitivity by whispering numbers into his or her ear and asking him or her to repeat them.

If hearing is impaired, examine the external auditory meatus and the tympanic membrane with an auroscope to exclude infections or wax. Determine if the hearing loss is conductive (middle ear pathology) or perceptive (inner ear pathology) by performing Rinné and Weber's tests.

Rinné test Place a vibrating 512 Hz tuning fork on the mastoid process (bone conduction) and then hold it close to the ear (air conduction). Ask the patient to determine which sound is loudest. Normally, air conduction is louder than bone conduction (positive Rinné). In sensorineural deafness, this will be the same; whereas in conductive deafness, bone conduction will be louder.

Weber's test Place a vibrating 512 Hz tuning fork at the midline over the vertex and ask the patient to determine whether the sound is perceived equally loudly in both ears (normal status), or in one ear more than the other. Sound is heard louder in the affected ear in conductive deafness, and in the unaffected ear in perceptive deafness.

Vestibular functions

Sensory information from the vestibular system is important in the control of posture and eye movements. The vestibular functions are assessed by examining these two areas:

- Posture: patients with vestibular lesions complain of vertigo and are mildly ataxic but usually able to compensate, using their visual input. However, patients with acute vestibular lesions can be markedly ataxic, with a tendency to fall towards the affected side.
- Nystagmus: unilateral vestibular dysfunction causes jerky/rotatory nystagmus with the fast phase towards the unaffected side (see nystagmus).

Hallpike's manoeuvre Hallpike's manoeuvre should be performed in all patients with positional vertigo (vertigo precipitated by a particular head position).

Sit the patient at the side of a couch facing away from the edge. Pull the patient quickly backwards and to one side so that the head hangs about 30–45° below the horizontal plane rotated to one side (Fig. 15.23). Ask the patient to keep his or her eyes open and to report any vertigo, and look for nystagmus. Sit the patient up and observe any nystagmus. Repeat the manoeuvre to the other side.

If positive, repeat the manoeuvre to the same side and determine if the pathology is central or peripheral (not always easy) (Fig. 15.24).

Caloric testing This test is not routinely done in all neurological examinations.

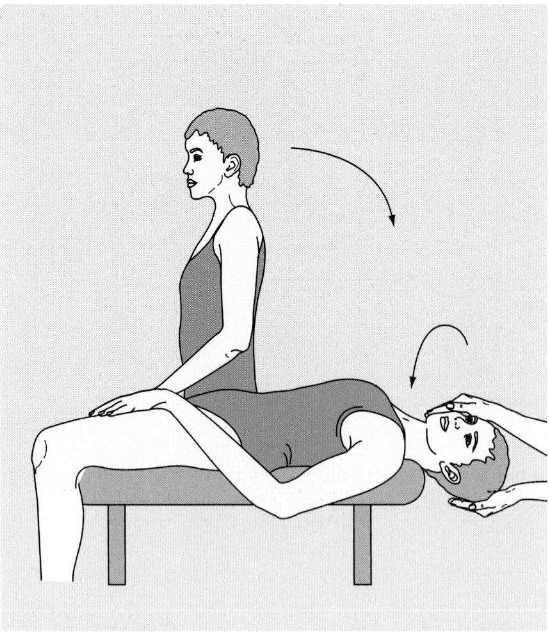

Fig. 15.23 Technique for exhibiting positional nystagmus (Hallpike's manoeuvre).

Features of peripheral and central positional nystagmus		
	Peripheral	Central
site of pathology	semicircular canals	brainstem
vertigo	always present	may be absent
nystagmus	rotatory	horizontal/rotatory
onset	delayed by 3–10 seconds	immediate
repeated testing	response fatigues	usually does not fatigue

Fig. 15.24 Features of peripheral and central positional nystagmus.

Establish that the patient's tympanic membranes are intact. With the patient lying supine with the head elevated at 30°, flush 250 mL of cold water (30°C) into the external auditory meatus. After a delay of 20 seconds, this produces a tonic deviation of the eyes to the same side with compensatory nystagmus to the opposite side lasting for more than 1 minute. Unconscious patients with intact vestibular function will have the tonic deviation only.

The test is repeated 5 minutes later with hot water (44°C), which induces tonic deviation of the eyes to the opposite side and compensatory nystagmus to the side of the irrigated ear.

Labyrinthine or vestibular nerve lesions cause depression of both the 'hot' and the 'cold' responses from the affected side (canal paresis), whereas central lesions cause an enhancement of nystagmus in one of the directions, whether triggered by hot or cold water (directional preponderance).

Clinical patterns of cranial nerve VIII lesions are shown in Fig. 15.25.

The mouth (IX, X and XII)

Mouth and tongue

Inspect the tongue as it lies in the floor of the mouth for evidence of wasting (unilateral or bilateral), fasciculations (shimmering movements at the surface of the tongue) or other involuntary movements (Huntington's chorea, orofacial dyskinesia). Ask the patient to protrude his or her tongue, and then move it rapidly from side to side.

Abnormalities can be caused by unilateral or bilateral upper motor neuron or lower motor neuron lesions (Fig. 15.26).

Pharynx and gag reflex

With the patient's mouth wide open, inspect the soft palate, the uvula, and the posterior pharyngeal wall at rest and during phonation (by asking the patient to say 'aah').

If you suspect a positive finding, press the end of an orange stick into the posterior pharyngeal wall, first on one side then the other. Assess the afferent pathway of the gag reflex (IXth cranial nerve) by asking the patient if the sensation is comparable on the two sides, and the efferent pathway (Xth cranial nerve) by inspecting the normal response of a symmetrical rise of the soft palate in the midline. This is a very unpleasant sensation for the patient, and should be carried out with care.

The upper motor neuron innervation of the palatal and pharyngeal muscles is bilateral, and unilateral lesions cause no significant dysfunction. In unilateral lower motor neuron lesions, the palate lies slightly lower on the affected side and deviates to the intact side during phonation or while testing the gag reflex.

Minor and inconsistent deviations of the uvula should be ignored.

The larynx

Formal assessment of the vocal cords is usually performed by indirect laryngoscopy, which is not part of the clinical examination. Bedside evaluation is confined to the assessment of phonation and cough.

Clinical patterns of VIIIth nerve lesions

Site of lesion	Clinical features	Pathology
peripheral	auditory and/or vestibular symptomatology	cranial trauma barotrauma infections occlusion of the internal auditory artery Ménière's disease toxins and drugs
central	auditory or vestibular symptomatology, often with other cranial nerve involvement (V, VII) and long tract signs	cerebrovascular disease multiple sclerosis cerebellopontine angle tumours brainstem tumours syringobulbia

Fig. 15.25 Clinical patterns of VIIIth cranial nerve lesions.

Clinical patterns of tongue weakness

lower motor neuron lesions	unilateral	focal atrophy, fasciculations, and deviation to the ipsilateral (paralysed) side
	bilateral	see bulbar palsy (Fig. 12.28)
upper motor neuron lesions	unilateral	deviation to the paralysed side
	bilateral	see pseudobulbar palsy (Fig. 12.28)

Fig. 15.26 Clinical patterns of tongue weakness.

Unilateral lesions of the recurrent laryngeal nerve cause partial upper airway obstruction with stridor, hoarseness of voice, and 'bovine' cough. Bilateral lesions cause severe stridor and aphonia.

The accessory nerve (XI)

The function of the trapezius muscles is assessed by asking the patient to shrug their shoulders, first without, and then against, resistance. The bulk and the strength of the sternocleidomastoid muscle is assessed by asking the patient to rotate their head to the contralateral side against the resistance of your hand.

Bulbar and pseudobulbar palsies (IX, X, XII)

These syndromes describe bilateral weakness of the bulbar muscles of either an upper or a lower motor neuron type (Fig. 15.27).

Clinical features and causes of pseudobulbar and bulbar palsies

	Clinical features	Cause	Pathology
pseudobulbar palsy	dysarthria (spastic), choking attacks, emotional lability; the tongue is stiff, spastic, slow but not wasted; jaw jerk and gag reflexes are brisk	bilateral upper motor neuron lesions of IX, X and XII (supranuclear)	bilateral cerebrovascular disease, motor neuron disease, multiple sclerosis, supranuclear palsy, Creutzfeldt–Jakob disease
bulbar palsy	dysarthria (nasal), dysphagia and nasal regurgitation; the tongue appears, wasted, flaccid, and fasciculating, and the gag reflex is absent	bilateral lower motor neuron lesions	• nuclear: medullary infarction, tumour, syrinx, encephalitis • peripheral nerve: cranial polyneuropathy (e.g. Guillain–Barré syndrome, sarcoidosis, diphtheria), neoplasms (e.g. meningeal infiltration, metastasis), skull base lesions (e.g. metastasis,chordoma, glomus tumour), skull base anomaly (e.g. Chiari malformation) • disorders of neuromuscular transmission: myasthenia gravis • primary muscle disease: polymyositis, muscular dystrophy

Fig. 15.27 Clinical features and causes of pseudobulbar and bulbar palsies.

Multiple cranial nerve palsies

Patchy loss of function

These palsies are usually caused by:

- Malignant meningitis (due to carcinoma, lymphoma or leukaemia).
- Granulomatous meningitis (due to sarcoidosis, tuberculosis or syphilis).
- Bone disease (due to metastasis or Paget's disease).

Diffuse loss of function

These palsies are usually caused by:

- Guillain–Barré syndrome.
- Motor neuron disease.
- Myasthenia gravis.
- Polymyositis.

The Motor System

General notes

In most cases, the cardinal sign of motor impairment is weakness. Remember that other findings (signs) will vary with the sites of pathology (Fig. 15.28).

Acute upper motor neuron lesions cause decreased tone (flaccid paralysis) and absent reflexes, although the Babinski response (see below) will be extensor.

Begin, wherever possible by an inspection of the patient's gait, as outlined earlier. In addition, while the patient is standing:

- Can the patient stand on his or her toes and heels without support?
- Can the patient hop? Most patients with significant leg weakness cannot hop.

Following this, ask the patient to lie on the bed, and make sure his or her arms and legs are exposed.

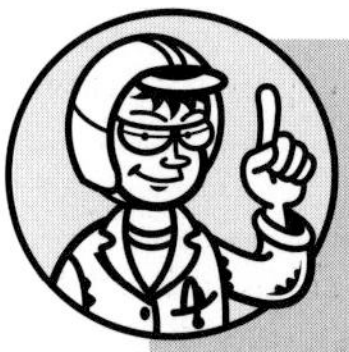

An examination of the motor system should include the following four features.

- Tone.
- Power.
- Coordination.
- Reflexes.

Inspection

When inspecting the patient, look for:

- Wasting—a reduction of muscle bulk in certain muscles compared with others. Wasted muscles are usually weak, and wasting is characteristic of lower motor neuron (i.e. anterior horn cell, nerve root and nerve) dysfunction.
- Scars—indicating previous injury or surgery, which may have damaged a nerve.
- Fasciculations—seen as rippling or twitching of a muscle at rest, a feature of lower motor neuron problems (especially, but not exclusively, motor neuron disease).
- Involuntary movements such as tremor may be obvious.

Tone

'Tone' means how floppy (decreased tone) or stiff (increased tone) a limb feels. Some patients with increased tone in the legs may complain that their legs 'jump', especially in bed.

Some patients have difficulty relaxing during an examination, which can artificially increase stiffness in their limbs. You must therefore do your utmost to put them at ease.

Variation in examination findings with site of pathology

Site of lesion	Wasting	Tone	Power	Reflexes
upper motor neuron	none	increased	decreased	increased
lower motor neuron	wasted	decreased	decreased	decreased
neuromuscular junction	rarely	usually normal, decreased	decreased (fatiguable)	usually normal
muscle	sometimes	normal	decreased	decreased

Fig. 15.28 Variation in examination findings with site of pathology. Not every patient will have every feature and occasionally patients may diverge from these features, but this remains a useful guide.

Arms

To examine tone, relax the patient and ask him or her to make him- or herself 'go floppy'.
Take his or her arm and slowly flex and extend the elbow, then hold his or her hand, with the elbow flexed, and pronate/supinate the forearm. Try to make your movements as unpredictable as possible, as cooperative patients may unconsciously try to 'help' you move their arms. If tone is increased, you may feel a 'supinator catch'—an interruption of the smooth movement on supination. Other signs in the arm include cogwheel rigidity, typically seen in Parkinson's disease.

Legs

There are several ways to examine tone in the legs:

- Rock each leg from side to side on the bed, holding it at the knee. Normally, the foot lags behind the leg. If tone is increased, the foot and leg move stiffly, as one unit. If tone is decreased, the foot flops from side to side.
- Flex and extend the knee, supporting both the upper leg and the foot.
- Place your hand under the patient's knee and quickly lift the knee about 15 cm; normally the foot will stay on the bed; if tone is increased, it may jump up with the lower leg.

Clonus describes the rhythmic contractions evoked by a sudden passive stretch of a muscle, elicited most easily at the ankle. A few beats may be normal in anxious patients, but 'sustained clonus' is characteristic of an upper motor neuron lesion.

Increased tone occurs in two main forms:

- Spasticity (derived from the Greek word spastikos, to tug or draw) is associated with upper motor neuron lesions, characterized by resistance to the first few degrees of movement, then a sudden lessening of resistance with a 'give way' (so-called clasp-knife) effect.
- Rigidity is characteristic of extrapyramidal disorders such as Parkinson's disease, distinguished clinically from spasticity by constant resistance to passive movement at a joint (lead-pipe rigidity). If tremor is superimposed on rigidity, the resistance is jerky or of 'cog-wheel' type.

Power

Power needs to be tested in each of the main muscle groups. Power in each muscle is given a grade defined by the Medical Research Council scale (Fig. 15.29), which can initially seem complicated, but is very useful for assessing changes.

The MRC scale	
Grade	**Response**
0	no movement
1	flicker of muscle when patient tries to move
2	moves, but not against gravity
3	moves against gravity but not against resistance
4	moves against resistance but not to full strength
5	full strength (you cannot overcome the movement with your equivalent muscle group)

Fig. 15.29 The Medical Research Council (MRC) scale for muscle weakness.

The scheme in Figs 15.30 and 15.31 allows testing of the main muscle groups of the arms. The scheme in Figs 15.32 and 15.33 allows testing of the main muscle groups of the legs.

Reflexes

Tendon reflexes are most easily determined by briskly stretching the tendon with a tendon hammer, held near the end and briskly tapped either onto the tendon directly or onto a finger placed over the tendon (biceps and supinator) (Fig. 15.34A). You should examine the tendon reflexes in the leg, as shown in Fig. 15.34B. These may be

- Increased.
- Decreased.
- Absent.

If absent, this should be confirmed by reinforcement (Fig. 15.34C shows this for the legs). There are two methods:

- Asking the patient to clench their teeth tightly just before you tap the reflex.
- Asking the patient to grip their hands and pull sideways (hard!) just before you tap the reflex.

The latter is obviously not appropriate when testing arm reflexes.

Tendon reflexes are conventionally notated as shown in Fig. 15.35. Abdominal reflexes can be tested as shown in Fig. 15.34D. The plantar response is elicited by scratching of the sole (Fig. 15.34E).

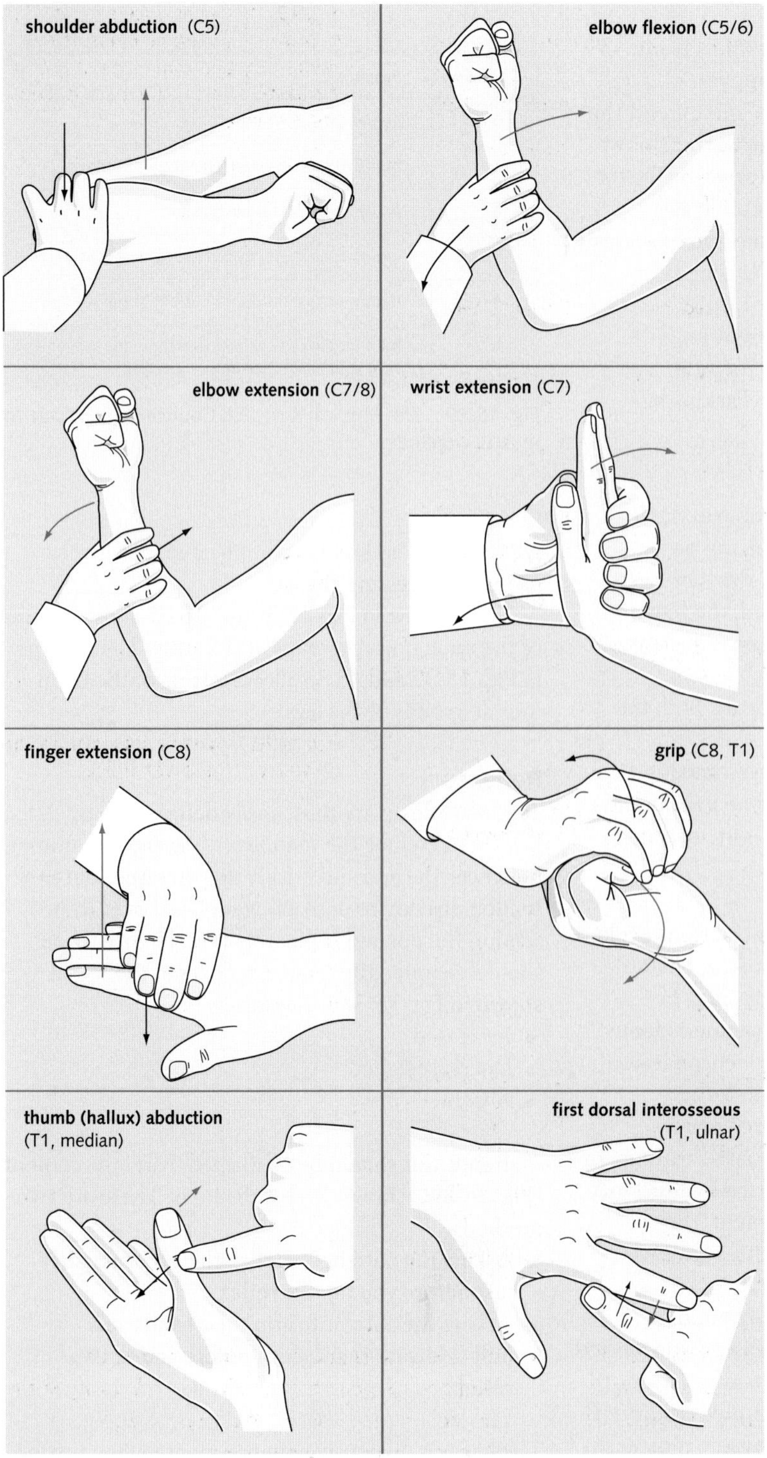

Fig. 15.30 Testing muscle groups of the upper limb. The blue arrow indicates the direction of movement of the patient, and the black arrow the direction of movement of the examiner. Each muscle group should be given a grade as defined by the MRC scale (see Fig. 15.29).

Coordination

Whether a patient can perform smooth and accurate movements is dependent partly on power in the muscles, lack of which may cause clumsiness, but more importantly on the cerebellar system. Assess:

- Gait—a wide-based, sometimes lurching gait is seen in cerebellar disease. Unsteadiness is made more obvious if the patient is asked to walk 'heel to toe'.
- Arms—the finger–nose test: ask the patient to touch your finger, held about 50 cm in front of the patient,

Scheme for examination of power in the upper limbs

Movement	Instruction	Muscle/myotome
shoulder abduction	bend your elbow and hold your arms up and out to the side. Don't let me push them down	deltoid/C5
elbow flexion	bend your elbow and don't let me straighten it	biceps/C5, C6
elbow extension	now straighten your elbow and don't let me bend it	triceps/C7, C8
wrist extension	cock your hands up like this and don't let me stop you	wrist extensors/C7
finger extension	straighten your fingers out and don't let me push them down	finger extensors/C8
grip	grip my fingers	finger flexors/C8, T1
thumb abduction	[with palms flat] Point your thumb to the ceiling and don't let me push it down	abductor pollicis brevis/C8, T1, median nerve
index finger abduction	spread your fingers wide and don't let me push them together	abductors (dorsal interossei)/T1, ulnar nerve

Fig. 15.31 Scheme for examination of power in the upper limbs. It is useful to get into the habit of giving the same instruction to each patient you examine.

Scheme for examination of power in the lower limbs

Movement	Instruction	Muscle/myotome
hip flexion	lift your leg straight off the bed, keep it up	iliopsoas/L1, L2
hip extension	straighten your knee and don't let me bend your leg	quadriceps/L3, L4
hip adduction	keep your knees together and don't let me pull them apart	hip adductors/L2, L3
knee flexion	bend your knee and keep it bent	hamstrings/L5, S1
ankle dorsiflexion	pull your foot up towards your nose, don't let me push it down	tibialis anterior and long extensors/L4, L5
plantiflexion (towards the floor)	point your foot down to the bed, keep it there	gastrocnemius/S1
knee extension	press your legs flat against the bed and don't let me pull them up	gluteal muscles/L5, S1

Fig. 15.32 Scheme for examination of power in the lower limbs.

with his or her index finger and then to touch his or her nose, then move back and forth. You may have to move the patient's finger for him or her on the first attempt. Cerebellar lesions may cause 'overshooting' of the target, missing your finger (past-pointing) or tremor (intention tremor). Dysdiadochokinesis describes the impairment of rapid alternating movements seen in such patients, and is tested by asking them to slap their palm whilst alternately pronating and supinating their other arm.

- Legs—the heel–shin test: ask the patient to place one heel on the other knee, and slowly slide the heel down the lower leg, then up again. Intention tremor may be seen.

Note that the presence of inaccuracy is the most important sign. These movements must be tested on each side in turn.

Abnormality of these movements in a patient with a cerebellar problem is described as ataxia, and

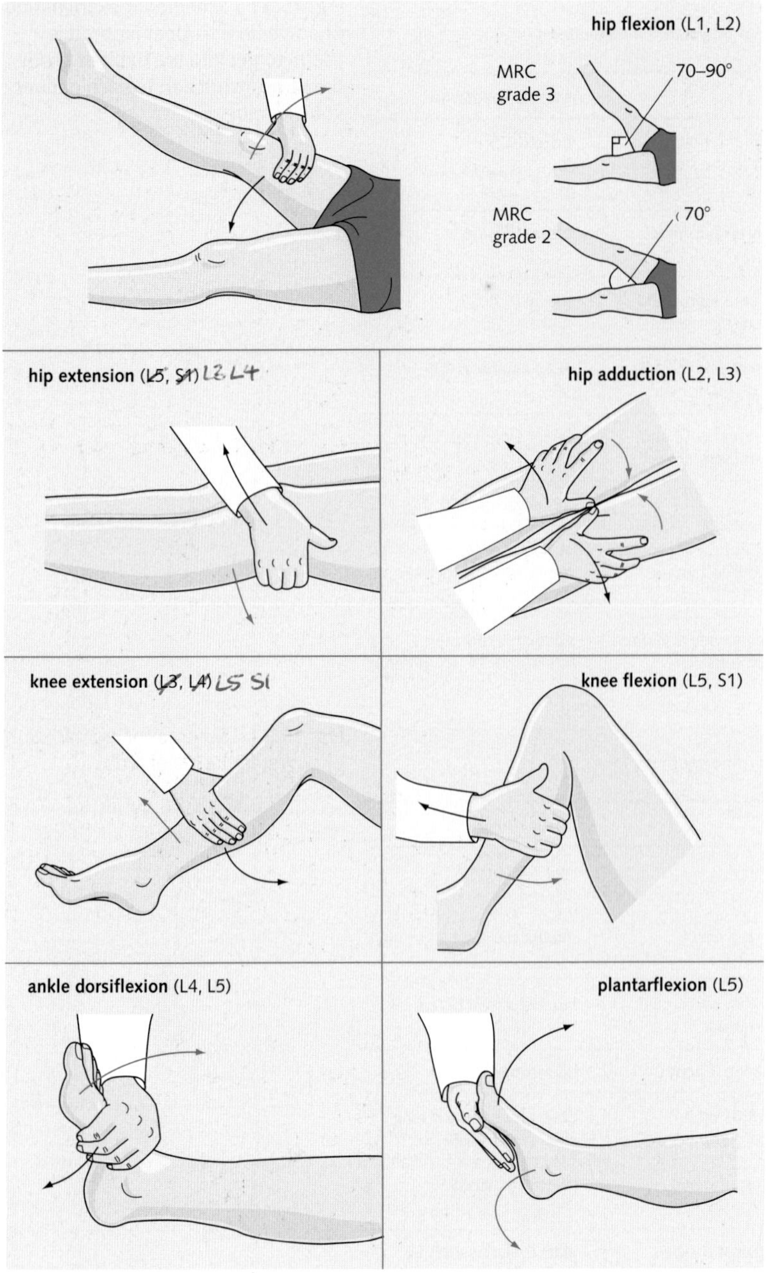

Fig. 15.33 Testing muscle groups of the lower limb. The blue arrow indicates the direction of movement of the patient, and the black arrow the direction of movement of the examiner. Each muscle group should be given a grade as defined by the MRC scale (see Fig. 15.29).

may be associated with other signs of cerebellar disease:

- Nystagmus.
- Dysarthria.

Fine movements

Early stages of an upper motor neuron or extrapyramidal disorder may be picked up by noting impairment of fine finger movements: ask the patient to pretend to play a piano, and to touch the thumb with each finger of the same hand in turn.

Abnormal movements (dyskinesias)

Abnormal movements include:

- Decreased movement (e.g. the bradykinesia of Parkinson's disease).
- Increased movement.

The main types of increased movement you will encounter are shown in Fig. 15.36, and may involve

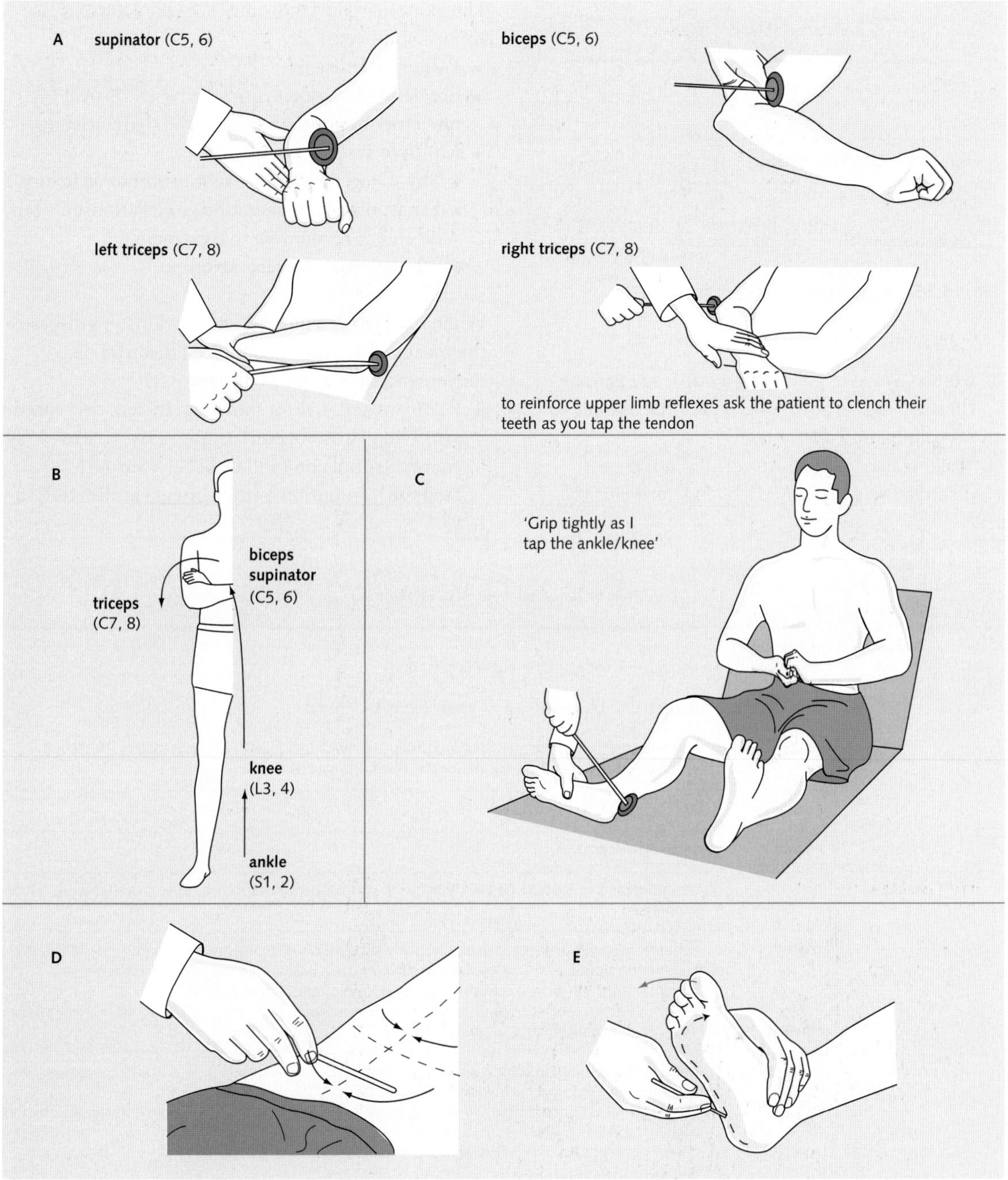

Fig. 15.34 Eliciting reflexes. (A) Upper limb tendon reflexes. (B) A simple way to remember root values of reflexes. (C) Testing ankle jerk with reinforcement. (D) Abdominal reflexes: test in four quadrants shown. (E) The normal response is a downgoing hallux. In an upper motor neuron lesion, the hallux dorsiflexes and the other toes fan out (the Babinski response).

the limbs (more usually the arms) and face. All are involuntary.

The most important aspect of examination of dyskinesias is inspection, and most of the features described in Fig. 15.36 can be elicited by this alone. In addition:

- Tremor at rest—ask the patient to sit with his or her hands overhanging his or her lap, close his or her eyes and count backwards from 100 to 'bring out' resting tremor.
- Tremor with different actions—the patient will complain if anything in particular makes his or her

Annotation of tendon reflexes	
normal	+
brisk	++
very brisk, with associated clonus	+++
absent	0
present with reinforcement only (decreased)	±

Fig. 15.35 Annotation of tendon reflexes.

tremor worse (e.g. holding a cup), so examine those actions in particular. The same applies to myoclonus and dystonias.
- Walking may exaggerate certain movement disorders (e.g. dystonias), so examine this too.

The akinetic rigid syndromes are characterized by abnormal movement:
- Parkinson's disease.
- Steele–Richardson syndrome (with vertical eye movement disturbance and mild dementia).
- Multiple system atrophy:
  - Shy–Drager syndrome (with autonomic failure).
  - Striatonigral degeneration (like Parkinson's but often not responsive to treatment).
  - Olivopontocerebellar atrophy.

When examining a patient with Parkinson's disease, the most commonly encountered disorder of movement, look in particular for:
- Festinant gait—slow, shuffling, flexed, decreased arm swing, unstable on turning, may 'freeze'. May show retropulsion (will walk backwards if stopped). Initiation of movements is affected, so

Types of abnormal movement (dyskinesia)		
Tremor	**action** physiological	 normal, low amplitude, in outstretched hands
	drug induced	exaggeration of normal (e.g. sympathomimetics, lithium)
	essential	coarser, especially when assuming a posture (e.g. holding a glass); usually autosomal dominant; especially in upper limbs; may involve the head (titubation)
	resting	ask the patient to sit with his hands in his lap, most common in Parkinson's disease
	intention	cerebellar, as above
Jerks	**tic**	abrupt, repetitive, stereotyped jerk-like movements; especially facial; no cause is often found; can be suppressed
	chorea	fleeting, irregular, semi-purposeful, disorderly movements affecting any body part; caused by (e.g.) Huntington's disease, stroke involving the subthalamic nucleus (causing ipsilateral chorea, or hemiballismus), drugs (e.g. neuroleptics), or systemic lupus erythematosus
	athetosis	slow, writhing movements, often with chorea
	myoclonus focal segmental generalized	brief, shock-like muscle contractions of 1 body part (e.g. palatal myoclonus) caused by focal disease of the spinal cord or brainstem and involving body segments supplied by this region (e.g. arm) a large number of causes including liver and renal failure, Creutzfeldt–Jakob disease, anoxia, and myoclonic epilepsy May also be *at rest*, with *action* (e.g. postanoxia), or *stimulus sensitive* (e.g. postencephalitis)
Dystonia	**focal** **segmental** **axial** **hemidystonia** **generalized**	sustained muscle contraction causing unusual postures, may be painful involving one body part (e.g. writers' cramp, torticollis) affecting adjacent body segments involving neck and back on one side of the body (e.g. cerebral palsy) all limbs and axial muscles involved (e.g. metabolic disorders—Wilson's disease, Parkinson's disease) drug-induced dystonia may be acute (e.g. metaclopramide, neuroleptics), or chronic (e.g. L-dopa, phenytoin)

Fig. 15.36 Types of abnormal movement (dyskinesia).

watch the patient rise from a chair, or start to walk from a stationary position.

- Bradykinesia (slow movements) (especially obvious on fine finger movements).
- Rigidity—carefully examine tone for cog-wheeling.
- Tremor—'pill-rolling', at rest.
- Facial akinesia—characteristic facies with poverty of movement and lack of expression. May have a 'positive glabellar tap': with the hand above the patient, repeatedly tap between the eyes. A normal person will stop blinking after a few taps, but a patient with Parkinson's disease will continue to blink. In practice, this is not particularly useful, but is a favourite with examiners. Increased salivation or drooling may also be evident.
- Handwriting—small and cramped. Keep a sample of this in your examination notes.

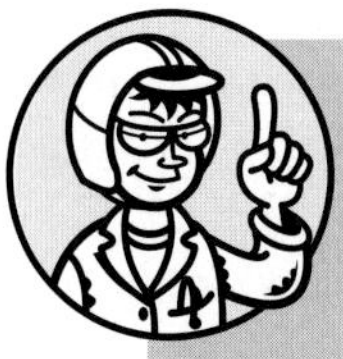

Causes of mixed upper and lower motor neuron signs:

- Motor neuron disease.
- Single spinal cord and adjacent root lesion (e.g. cervical spondylosis).
- AIDS.
- Syphilis.
- Chronic upper motor neuron weakness causing 'disuse atrophy'.

Sensation

General notes

Patients use various terms to describe sensory disturbance, including numbness, weakness, tingling/pins and needles (paraesthesiae), odd unpleasant touch (dysaesthesia) and painful touch (hyperaesthesia).

Tell the patient that you are going to test whether he or she can feel certain sensations.

Sensory testing

Do not spend hours doing this, you will exhaust the patient and yourself. Be sensible, and tailor your examination to the patient's complaint.

Remember, sensation from one side of the body travels in sensory tracts to the contralateral cerebral hemisphere.

If the patient complains of loss of sensation, start sensory testing in the abnormal area, and move out from there.

The dermatomes of the upper and lower limbs are shown in Fig. 15.37.

Pin prick

Use a sensory testing/needlework pin, not a needle. Test the pin on the sternum first—'can you feel this as sharp?'. With the patient's eyes open, start at the tips of the fingers/toes and work your way proximally. If the patient does not complain of sensory disturbance, it is not necessary to traverse the entire body with the pin. Remember, this is testing pain sensation. Ask the patient 'is it sharp or blunt?'.

Light touch

Test with cotton wool and with the patient's eyes closed. Start at fingers/toes and work proximally. Ask the patient to 'say yes when you feel me touching you'.

Joint position sense

Move the distal interphalangeal joint of the index finger/toe up or down, holding the sides of the digit. With the patient's eyes closed, ask them 'is your toe/finger moving up . . . or down?'. It is useful to demonstrate what you mean by 'up' and 'down' before testing, as patients often do not understand.

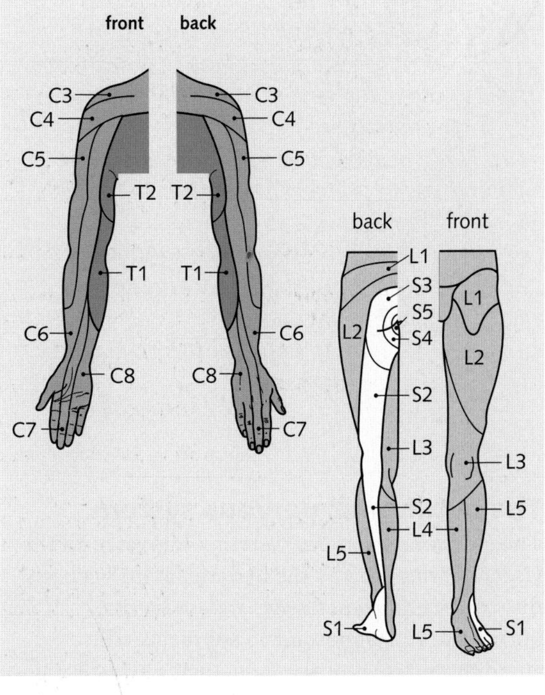

Fig. 15.37 The dermatomes of the upper and lower limbs.

Vibration sense

Use a 128 Hz tuning fork. Set it vibrating, and place it on the patient's sternum. Ask the patient 'can you feel this vibrating?'. Place the tuning fork on the distal interphalangeal joint of the finger or big toe (hallux). Ask 'can you feel it now?'.

Sensation is often lost early in neuropathies.

Two-point discrimination

Test two-point discrimination with specific compasses and with the patient's eyes closed. While testing on the pulp of the index finger (normal 3 mm) and hallux (5 mm), ask 'do you feel one point or two?'.

Temperature

With the patient's eyes closed, touch the skin with the flat forks of a tuning fork, not vibrating. Ask, 'does this feel hot or cold?'.

Lhermitte's symptom

Lhermitte's symptom is a sudden, electric-shock-like sensation travelling down the neck and back when the neck flexes, caused by a lesion in the spinal cord, most typically multiple sclerosis.

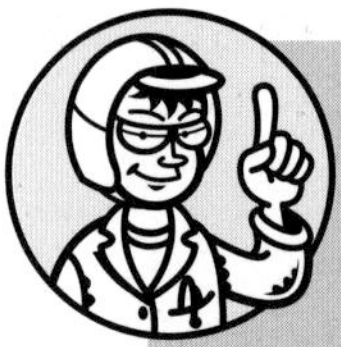

There are five sensations to test.

If the patient complains of sensory disturbance, start testing that area first. If there is no complaint, start distally and move proximally.

Test each sensation in turn in the arms, then each sensation in turn in the legs.

Pain sensation is not agony sensation and therefore do not use a blood-taking needle!

Vibration sense is often lost in neuropathies.

The autonomic nervous system

The autonomic nervous system, innervates all the viscera, influenced by the hypothalamus via both direct descending pathways and endocrine hormones. It is important to appreciate the anatomy and roles of the individual sympathetic and parasympathetic systems, especially in relation to the effects of drugs on each. However, clinically, 'autonomic failure' usually involves both systems simultaneously, most commonly presenting with a combination of symptoms, as shown in Fig. 15.38.

Thorough examination of this system is not necessary in every neurological patient, unless the patient complains of symptoms of autonomic failure or the diagnosis is suspected. The following tests may then be performed at the bedside (more specialized tests may be performed by an autonomic function laboratory).

Examination of the cardiovascular system

Measure the blood pressure after the patient has been lying down for a few minutes. Then stand the patient up, wait for a minute and take the blood pressure again. The systemic blood pressure normally rises a little. A fall of > 20 mmHg is abnormal (postural hypotension).

The pulse can be monitored by a continuous electrocardiogram recording (measurement of the R–R interval is a useful way of measuring such pulse changes) in response to posture, with deep respiration (sinus arrhythmia may be lost) and with the Valsalva manoeuvre.

The Valsalva manoeuvre

Ask the patient to take a deep breath in, then to blow out through a 20 mL syringe (they will not be able to push the plunger out). Normally, a tachycardia occurs during the forced expiration, followed by a reflex bradycardia on release. The blood pressure drops initially, then is maintained throughout the

Signs and symptoms of autonomic failure

Affected system or site	Signs and symptoms
cardiovascular system	postural hypotension (or, uncommonly, hypertension); impaired response of pulse to respiration, posture or Valsalva manouvre; resting tachycardia
genitourinary system	impotence, ejaculatory failure, changes in bladder function (including incontinence)
gastrointestinal tract	constipation or diarrhoea
secretory systems	inability to sweat; dry mouth and eyes
pupils	Horner's syndrome; dilation or constriction; sluggish or absent light response

Fig. 15.38 Signs and symptoms of autonomic failure.

expiration, before overshooting on release. This response is lost in autonomic failure.

Examination of other systems

The examination of other effects of autonomic failure is more specialized, but includes:

- The pupils (Fig. 15.39).
- Effects of stress (such as grip, arousal, mental activity) on pulse and blood pressure.
- Pharmacological tests of cardiovascular function.
- Sweating responses with heat and pharmacological agents.
- Skin responses to pharmacological agents.
- Urodynamic tests and sphincter electromyography.

Examination of the unconscious patient

Causes of unconsciousness in adults

See differential diagnosis of coma in Chapter 14.

Assessment of the patient

As with any medical emergency, resuscitation is the priority.

A. Check the airway—in danger either because protective reflexes (e.g. coughing) are suppressed or the respiratory centre is compromised. Clear debris and insert an oropharyngeal/ nasopharyngeal airway or endotracheal tube if necessary.
B. Breathing—early stages of respiratory centre depression cause 'periodic' (Cheyne–Stokes) breathing, with alternate hyperventilation and apnoea. Later, the patient may hyperventilate. Breathing then becomes irregular, then gasping, prior to respiratory arrest. Give oxygen and count the respiratory rate. Abnormality indicates that artificial ventilation may be necessary.
C. Circulation—pulse and blood pressure. Raised intracranial pressure causes raised blood pressure and a slow pulse, and progression of this indicates increasing pressure. Drug overdoses may cause arrhythmias. Hypotension may need to be corrected. Attach an electrocardiogram monitor.
D. Disability—assess the patient's general and neurological status (a rapid but careful examination of each system is mandatory). Obtain a history from a relative or friend (this is often the most helpful part of the assessment and can save a great deal of time). Look for drug bottles, prescriptions or a Medic-Alert bracelet.
E. Environment and Exposure—the patient must be examined from head to toe, but do not forget that hypothermia is an important cause of neurological disability.
G. Do not ever forget glucose!—hypoglycaemia is a common and easily treatable cause of unconsciousness (usually caused by insulin overdose); check blood glucose immediately in every unconscious patient, and treat with intravenous dextrose if low. If high, check the urine for ketones and treat as a diabetic ketoacidosis.

The Glasgow Coma Scale (Fig. 15.40) is a widely used, standard, consistent and fairly sensitive

Examination of the pupils

Test	Normal response	Autonomic failure
instillation of 1:1000 adrenaline	no effect	dilation if have sympathetic post-ganglionic denervation
instillation of 2.5% methacholine	no effect	constriction if have parasympathetic denervation

Fig. 15.39 Examination of the pupils in the presence of autonomic dysfunction.

Glasgow coma scale

Eyes (E)		
	opening spontaneously (with blinking)	4
	open to command or speech	3
	open in response to pain (applied to limbs or sternum)	2
	not opening	1
Motor function (M)		
	obeys commands	6
	localizes to pain	5
	withdraws from pain	4
	flexor response to pain (decorticate)	3
	extensor response to pain (decerebrate)	2
	no response to pain	1
Vocalization (V)		
	appropriate speech	5
	confused speech	4
	inappropriate words	3
	groans only	2
	no speech	1

Fig. 15.40 The Glasgow Coma Scale. Coma score is E + M + V. The maximum (fully conscious) score is therefore 15 and the range 3–15.

measure of the level of unconsciousness, which enables:

- Small changes in the patient's unconscious level to be noted quickly.
- Medical staff to communicate rapidly with each other regarding the patient's condition.

You should also consider:

- Narcotics (e.g. pin-point pupils, needletracks, slow respiratory rate); give naloxone.
- Is the patient fitting? If so, give intravenous lorazepam or diazepam.
- Head injury (if found, assume also has cervical spine injury until proved otherwise).
- Neck stiffness (e.g. meningitis, subarachnoid haemorrhage). If there is any suspicion of meningitis, do not delay treatment whilst a computed tomography of the brain and lumbar puncture is performed; take blood for culture and treat immediately with an intravenous antibiotic—one example is ceftriaxone but protocols may differ from hospital to hospital.

Particular points to note in the neurological assessment are:

- Pupils, eye movements (Fig. 15.41) and fundi. Papilloedema is a late stage of raised intracranial pressure, and this diagnosis cannot be excluded if the fundi are normal. Retinal haemorrhages may be seen with subarachnoid haemorrhage.
- Tone, power (is there any movement, spontaneously or in response to command or pain?) and reflexes can localize the cause. Brainstem lesions usually cause bilateral (symmetrical or asymmetrical) signs, sometimes just reflex changes. Supratentorial lesions usually cause asymmetrical signs (e.g. hemiparesis).

Investigations

Undertake urgent investigations (e.g. blood glucose, urea and electrolytes, liver function tests, full blood count, arterial blood gases, urine and blood drug screens, thyroid function tests, blood cultures).

Chest X-ray, skull X-ray, computed tomography brain scan, lumbar puncture and electroencephalogram may also be necessary.

Other management

The patient is likely to need urethral catheterization (also enables fluid balance to be monitored). Other aspects of longer-term care include:

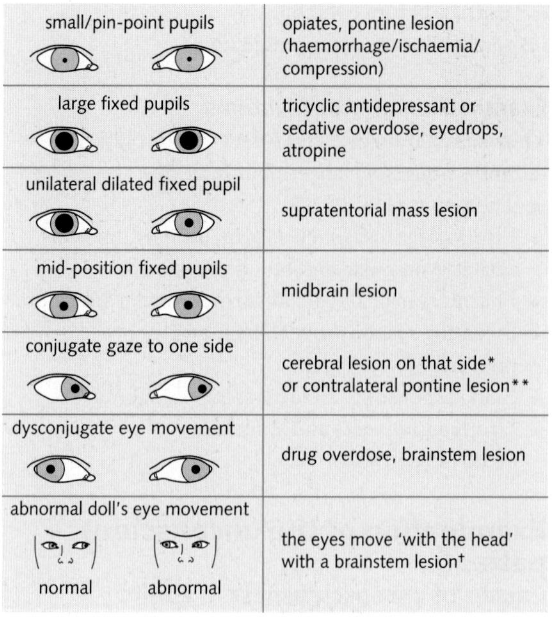
small/pin-point pupils
opiates, pontine lesion (haemorrhage/ischaemia/ compression)
large fixed pupils
tricyclic antidepressant or sedative overdose, eyedrops, atropine
unilateral dilated fixed pupil
supratentorial mass lesion
mid-position fixed pupils
midbrain lesion
conjugate gaze to one side
cerebral lesion on that side* or contralateral pontine lesion**
dysconjugate eye movement
drug overdose, brainstem lesion
abnormal doll's eye movement
normal
abnormal
the eyes move 'with the head' with a brainstem lesion†

Fig. 15.41 Pupils and eye movements in the unconscious patient. *'looking towards the lesion'; **'looking away from the lesion'; †normally, if the head is held and turned quickly from side to side, the eyes swivel in the opposite direction to the head.

- Continued monitoring of A, B, C and Glasgow coma scale.
- Turning to prevent pressure sores.
- Eye, mouth, bladder and bowel care.
- Passive limb movements to prevent contractures.

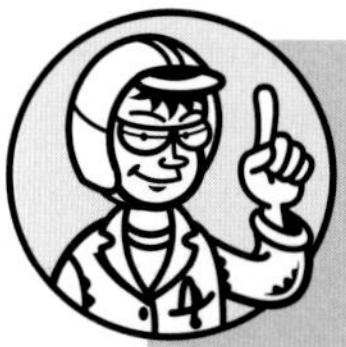

An unconscious patient is a medical emergency and, as such, resuscitation takes priority (A,B,C).

Because hypoglycaemia is easily treatable, a finger-prick glucose test should be performed immediately.

The Glasgow Coma Scale gives an easily recognizable estimation of the level of consciousness.

Pupils, eye movements, tone, and reflexes may be the only source of neurological localization.

- What are the different types of dysphasia? How would you distinguish between them?
- Compare dysarthria and dysphasia.
- How would you test for constructional apraxia? How would you test for neglect?
- Summarize the mini-mental state examination.
- Contrast cerebellar ataxia, sensory ataxia and Parkinson's disease in terms of their respective characteristic gaits.
- Describe a Romberg's test and what a positive result indicates.
- Discuss the components of the neurological examination of the eye.
- What is papilloedema? When might you see it?
- What is meant by the term nystagmus? Give some causes.
- How would you test trigeminal nerve function?
- How would you distinguish between an upper and lower motor neuron lesion of the facial nerve?
- What is Hallpike's manoeuvre?
- Contrast Weber's and Rinne's tests.
- What are the features of an upper motor neuron lesion in the lower limb?
- How would you test coordination in the upper limb? When might it be disturbed?
- What is reinforcement? Describe two manoeuvres you could ask the patient to perform.
- What modalities of sensation are routinely tested? How do their spinal cord terminations differ?
- What is the Glasgow Coma Scale? Name the three functions tested.
- Give your structured approach to the unconscious patient, beginning with resuscitation.

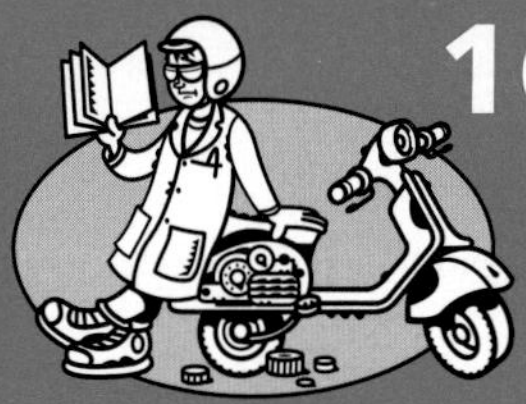

16. Further Investigations

In this chapter, you will learn about:
- Neurophysiological investigations.
- Routine investigations (blood tests, etc.) and how they relate to neurological problems.
- Imaging of the nervous system.

Neurophysiological investigations

Electroencephalography (EEG)

The EEG measures electrical potentials generated by the neurons lying underneath an electrode on the scalp, and compares this either with a reference electrode or a neighbouring electrode. The normal trace is symmetrical, and therefore asymmetries, as well as specific abnormalities, may indicate an underlying disorder. Interpretation of EEGs is complex, and you should not worry if you cannot pick up subtle abnormalities.

Before accurate brain imaging was possible, EEG was used to detect focal lesions. These are now more commonly picked up with computed tomography or magnetic resonance imaging, but EEG remains useful for detecting underlying abnormalities of cerebral function, and especially for:
- Epilepsy (see below).
- Diagnosis of encephalitis.
- In coma.
- Aid to diagnosis of Creutzfeldt–Jakob disease.
- Diagnosis of subacute sclerosing panencephalitis.

The main role of EEG is in the assessment of epilepsy. It can help in the following ways:
- Diagnosis of a seizure disorder.
- Classification of seizure type, which may optimize therapy.
- Assessment for surgical intervention.
- Diagnosis of pseudoseizures (especially with simultaneous video recording—telemetry).

'Invasive EEG monitoring' refers to electrodes inserted directly into the brain. This is undertaken before surgery (e.g. to remove an epileptic focus).

Different normal rhythms are characteristically found over different regions of the brain (Fig. 16.1).

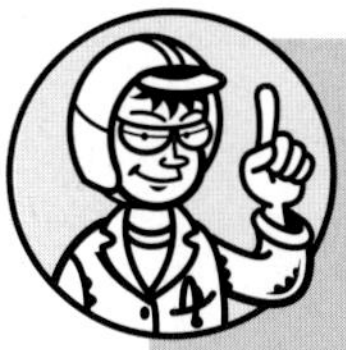

> The EEG may be normal in patients who have clearly had seizures. There is an increased likelihood of seeing an abnormality if a recording is made under conditions of sleep deprivation, hyperventilation or photic stimulation (flashing lights).

Other than these rhythmic activities, other abnormal activity may be generated in certain conditions (Figs 16.2 and 16.3).

Electromyography and nerve conduction studies

Usually performed together, these investigations examine the integrity of muscle, peripheral nerve and lower motor neurons. They are useful in:
- Determining the cause of weakness (e.g. neuropathy, myopathy, anterior horn cell disease).
- Determining the distribution of the abnormality (e.g. generalized/focal).
- Suggesting the type of myopathy (e.g. dystrophy or myositis) or neuropathy (e.g. axonal or demyelinating; motor, sensory or sensorimotor).
- Diagnosing myasthenia gravis.
- Assessing baseline deficits before surgery (e.g. carpal tunnel syndrome).
- Objectively assessing the response to medical therapies, especially new treatments in trials (e.g. human immunoglobulin in Guillain–Barré syndrome).

Normal muscle at rest is electrically silent (apart from actually during needle insertion), unless the needle is placed in the region of a motor end-plate (when miniature end-plate potentials can be recorded). During voluntary movement, individual motor unit potentials (recordings of the activity from the muscle fibres innervated by a single motor neuron) can be seen. Fig. 16.4 shows common abnormalities.

Normal EEG rhythms		
Rhythm	**Characteristics**	**Site and comments**
alpha	8–13 Hz (normal)	posterior; especially with eyes closed
beta	>13 Hz (normal)	anterior; increased with sedatives (e.g. barbiturates)
theta	4–7 Hz (normal)	normal in young and when drowsy
delta	<4 Hz (abnormal except in sleep)	slow rhythm generated over a structural lesion and in sleep

Fig.16.1 Normal EEG rhythms.

Some abnormal EEG activities	
Activity	**Interpretation**
generalized slow-wave activity	metabolic encephalopathy, drug overdose, encephalitis
focal slow-wave activity	underlying structural lesion
focal/generalized spikes or spike and slow wave activity	epilepsy
three-per-second (3/sec) bilateral, symmetrical spike-and-wave activity (Fig 13.4)	typical absence seizures (idiopathic generalized epilepsy)
periodic complexes (generalized sharp waves every 0.5–2.0 seconds)	CJD

Fig.16.2 Some abnormal electroencephalographic activities.

Fibrillations and fasciculations

Fibrillation potentials (up to 300 mV) are due to spontaneous contractions of individual muscle fibres after denervation, probably due to hypersensitivity of the muscle membrane to acetylcholine. They cannot be seen through the skin, but may be seen in the tongue in motor neuron disease.

Fasciculation potentials (up to 5 mV, usually every 3 or 4 seconds) are contractions of groups of muscle fibres after denervation, visible on both electromyography and through the skin as a twitch or ripple. They may be normal, especially in calf muscles, usually at a rate of 1/s.

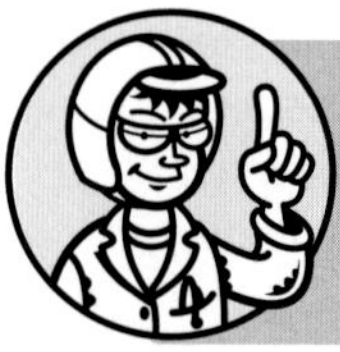

Fasciculations are a particular feature of motor neuron disease.

Other studies

These include:

- Magnetic brain stimulation.
- Evoked potentials (EPs):
  - Visual EPs.
  - Brainstem auditory EPs.
  - Somatosensory EPs.

Routine investigations

You should be aware of simple tests of neurological relevance. In this section, five areas of investigation are presented:

- Haematology (Fig. 16.5).
- Biochemistry (Fig. 16.6).
- Immunology (Fig. 16.7).
- Microbiology (Fig. 16.8).
- Cerebrospinal fluid findings (Fig. 16.9).

For each test, normal ranges are given, with neurological differential diagnoses for high and low

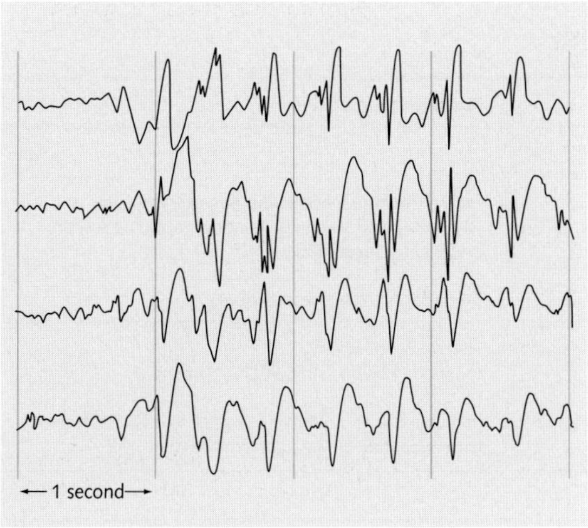

Fig.16.3 Three-per-second (3/s) spike-and-wave activity. Characteristic of absence seizures.

values. Cerebrospinal fluid protein levels are given in g/dL and serum levels are in g/L.

Imaging of the nervous system

Plain radiography

Skull radiography

Skull radiography has a limited role in current neurological practice. The main indication is head injury when more sophisticated imaging is not immediately indicated. The standard views are:

- Lateral.
- Postero-anterior.
- Towne's view (fronto-occipital).

Learn the normal skull radiographic markings (Figs 16.10 and 16.11) and the main abnormalities seen on skull radiographs (Fig. 16.12).

Spinal radiography

The standard views in spinal radiography are:

- Lateral.
- Postero-anterior.

Learn the main abnormalities seen on spinal radiographs (Fig. 16.13).

Computed tomography scanning

Using an X-ray source and a series of photon detectors housed in a gantry, computed tomography produces a series of consecutive two-dimensional axial brain digital images, which show the X-ray density of the brain tissue. The densities of different brain tissues vary according to their X-ray absorption properties, ranging between low (black: air, cerebrospinal fluid) to high (white: bone, fresh blood) (Figs 16.14 and 16.15).

The diagnostic yield of the computed tomography scan is increased by injecting iodine-containing contrast agents, which enhance the distinction between the different brain tissues and outline the areas of blood–brain barrier breakdown (around tumours or infarctions). Learn the main abnormalities seen on the computed tomography scan (Fig. 16.16).

Common abnormalities of the EMG and NCS	
Abnormality	**Change in electromyographic trace**
denervation	increased insertional activity; large amplitude, long duration, polyphasic MUPs, fibrillations; fasciculations
myopathy	small, short, polyphasic MUPs
myotonia	high-frequency bursts
myasthenia	abnormal decrement on repetitive stimulation; jitter with single-fibre studies (indicating variable neuromuscular transmission time)
Abnormality	**Change in nerve conduction**
axonal neuropathy	small action potential; normal nerve conduction velocity
demyelinating neuropathy	slow nerve conduction velocity; prolonged latency (time to travel from one point to the next); normal or slightly reduced action potential

Fig.16.4 Common abnormalities found with electromyography (EMG) and nerve conduction studies (NCS) (MUPs, motor unit potenials).

Haematology			
Test	**Normal range**	**Abnormality**	**Possible interpretation**
full blood count			
haemoglobin (Hb)	13.5–18.0 g/dL male; 11.5–16.0 g/dL female	low; anaemia	may cause non-specific neurological symptoms (e.g. dizziness, weakness, fainting); may suggest an underlying chronic illness
		high; polycythaemia	predisposes to stroke and chorea
mean cell volume (MCV)	76–96 fL	high; macrocytic anaemia	vitamin B_{12} deficiency (peripheral neuropathy, SCDC, dementia)
		low; microcytic anaemia	may indicate an underlying chronic illness; associated with idiopathic intracranial hypertension
white cell count (WBC)			
neutrophils	2–7.5 x 10^9	high; neutrophilia	meningitis or other infection
		low; neutropenia	leukaemia/lymphoma (infiltrative disease, space-occupying lesions, peripheral neuropathy) multiple myeloma (neuropathy, vertebral collapse, hyperviscosity syndrome)
lymphocytes	1.5–3.5 x 10^9	high; lymphocytosis	viral infection (transverse myelitis, Guillain–Barré syndrome)
		low; lymphopenia	leukaemia/lymphoma, as above
eosinophils	0.04–0.44 x 10^9	high; eosinophilia	hypereosinophilic syndrome (rare)
platelet count	150–400 x 10^9	high; thrombocythaemia	predisposes to stroke
		low; thrombocytopenia	intracranial bleeding
erythrocyte sedimentation rate (ESR)	<20 mm/h	high	vasculitis (e.g. PAN, SLE, giant cell arteritis) may cause cerebral, cranial, and peripheral nerve infarcts, confusion and fits)
coagulation tests			
activated partial thromboplastin time (APT or PTTK)	35–45 s	high	SLE; antiphospholipid syndrome
protein C, protein S	varies with laboratory	low; deficiency	inherited predisposition to thrombosis
factor 5 Leiden	varies with laboratory	present	mutation causes a single amino acid substitution in factor 5, which results in activated protein C resistance and predisposition to thrombosis
vitamin B_{12}	>150 ng/L	low; deficiency	peripheral neuropathy, SCDC, confusion/dementia
folate	2.1–2.8 mg/L	low; deficiency	peripheral neuropathy, dementia

Fig.16.5 Possible consequences of abnormalities in blood or serum levels of haematological indices. Individual laboratories may have different normal ranges (APT, activated partial thromboplastin; PAN, polyarteritis nodosa; PTTK, partial thromboplastin time; SCDC, subacute combined degeneration of the cord; SLE, systemic lupus erythematosus).

Magnetic resonance imaging

Nuclear magnetic resonance is the term that describes the interaction between the hydrogen protons in the different body structures and strong external magnetic fields. As the patient lies in the scanner, the naturally spinning hydrogen protons align with the strong magnetic field of the scanner. When a further external

Biochemistry			
Test	**Normal range**	**Abnormality**	**Interpretation**
urea and electrolytes (U and Es)			
sodium	135–145 mmol/L	high; hypernatraemia low; hyponatraemia	both may cause weakness, confusion, and fits
potassium	3.5–5.5 mmol/L	high; hyperkalaemia low; hypokalaemia	hyper/hypokalaemic periodic paralysis
urea	2.5–6.7 mmol/L	high; renal failure	confusion, peripheral neuropathy
creatinine	<150 mmol/L	high; renal failure	confusion, peripheral neuropathy
glucose (fasting)	4–6 mmol/L	high; diabetes low; hypoglycaemia	neuropathy, coma confusion, coma, focal signs
calcium	2.2–2.6 mmol/L	low; hypocalcaemia	tetany
liver function tests (LFTs) bilirubin and liver enzymes	bilirubin range: 3–17 μmol/L enzymes vary between laboratories	high	liver disease: confusion, tremor, neuropathy
creatine kinase	24–195 U/L	high	muscle disease: myositis, dystrophy
thyroid function tests thyroid stimulating hormone (TSH)	0.5–5 mU/L	low TSH; thyrotoxicosis high TSH; hypothyroidism	tremor, confusion, hyperreflexia apathy, confusion, hyporeflexia, neuropathy

Fig.16.6 Possible consequences of abnormalities in blood or serum levels of biochemical indices. Individual laboratories may have different normal ranges.

magnetic field (radiofrequency pulse) of a specific frequency is applied at a right angle, the protons 'flip' out of the main external magnetic field.

As the protons 'relax' back to their original position, they emit a radiofrequency signal that can be digitally analysed and displayed as an image. This 'relaxation' time has two components, known as T1 and T2, which determine the magnetic resonance parameters of the different brain tissues (Figs 16.14 and 16.15).

The paramagnetic agent gadolinium-labelled DTPA (diethylene triamine penta-acetic acid, or pentetic acid) is used as a contrast agent. Learn the main abnormalities seen on magnetic resonance imaging (Fig. 16.17).

Myelography

A water-soluble iodine-based medium is injected in the subarachnoid space through a lumbar or a cervical approach. This outlines the spinal canal and nerve root sheaths, allowing the assessment of the spinal canal and the nerve roots.

Cord compression caused by extra- or intramedullary lesions is identified as a compression or interruption of the column of contrast.

Postmyelographic computed tomography scanning allows further assessments to the nerve roots within the theca.

Angiography

Serial cranial radiographs are taken after the injection of an iodine-containing contrast agent into a large artery (aorta, carotid, vertebral) to allow the identification of cerebral vessels (Fig. 16.18). Simultaneous digital subtraction of the surrounding soft tissues and bony structures allows the use of more dilute contrast and shorter procedure time, although the spatial resolution of the images will be compromised.

Fig.16.7 Immunology.

Immunology	
Test	**Associated disorder**
antinuclear factor (ANA)	systemic lupus erythematosus (SLE): fits, confusion, neuropathy, aseptic meningitis, Sjögren's syndrome: gritty eyes, neuropathies, mixed connective tissue disease (MCTD)
anti-double-stranded DNA (dsDNA) antibodies	SLE
rheumatoid factor	rheumatoid arthritis: cervical spine subluxation, neuropathies, vasculitis
anti-Ro (SSA), anti-La (SSB) antibodies	Sjögren's syndrome
antiphospholipid antibodies (e.g. anticardiolipin)	antiphospholipid syndrome
anti-ribonucleoprotein (RNP) antibodies	MCTD; myositis, trigeminal nerve palsies
Jo-1 antibodies	polymyositis
antineutrophil cytoplasmic antibodies (ANCA)	pANCA (peripheral): polyarteritis nodosa cANCA (classical): Wegener's granulomatosis
antiacetylcholine receptor antibodies (AChR)	myasthenia gravis
anti-GM1 antibodies	multifocal motor neuropathy, Guillain–Barré syndrome
anti-GAD antibodies	stiff-man syndrome

Fig.16.8 Microbiology.

Microbiology	
Test	**Associated disorder**
VDRL (venereal disease reference laboratory)	primary syphilis; false positive in pregnancy, systemic lupus erythematosus, malaria
TPHA (*Treponema pallidum* haemagglutination assay)	syphilis; false positive with non-venereal treponemes (yaws, pinta)
hepatitis B surface antigen (HBsAg)	some cases of polyarteritis nodosa
HIV	AIDS

Fig.16.9 Cerebrospinal fluid findings.

CSF findings			
Disease	**Protein (g/dL)**	**Glucose**	**Cells**
normal	<0.5	>50% blood glucose	<5/mL lymphocytes, no polymorphs
bacterial meningitis	1.0–5.0	<50%	>1000/mL, polymorphs predominate
viral meningitis	0.5–1.0	normal	<1000/mL, lymphocytes predominate
tuberculous meningitis	1–10	<50%	<1000/mL, lymphocytes predominate

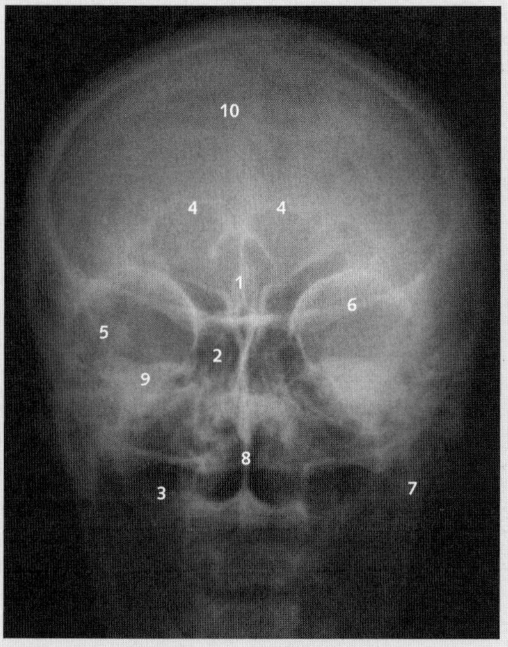

1 crista galli
2 ethmoidal air cells
3 floor of maxillary sinus (antrum)
4 frontal sinus
5 greater wing of sphenoid
6 lesser wing of sphenoid
7 mastoid process
8 nasal septum
9 petrous part of temporal bone
10 sagittal suture

Fig.16.10 Normal postero-anterior skull radiograph (courtesy of J. Weir and P. H. Abrahams).

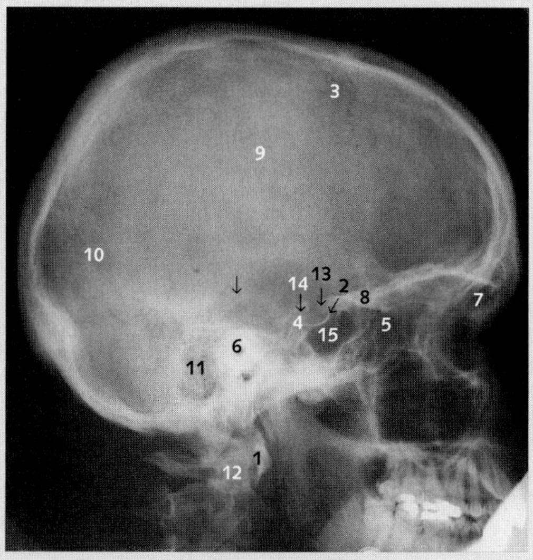

1 anterior arch of atlas (first cervical vertebral)
2 anterior clinoid process
3 coronal suture
4 dorsum sellae
5 ethmoidal air cells
6 external acoustic meatus
7 frontal sinus
8 greater wing of sphenoid
9 grooves for middle meningeal vessels
10 lambdoid suture
11 mastoid air cells
12 odontoid process (dens) of axis (second cervical vertebra)
13 pituitary fossa (sella turcica)
14 posterior clinoid process
15 sphenoidal sinus

Fig.16.11 Normal lateral skull radiograph (courtesy of J. Weir and P. H. Abrahams).

Venous digital subtraction angiography is possible, but the quality of the images obtained is distinctly inferior to those obtained through the arterial route.

The indications for angiography are:

- Extracranial atherosclerotic cerebrovascular disease (stenosis, particularly carotid), lumen irregularities or occlusions).
- Aneurysms and arteriovenous malformation.

Main abnormalities seen on skull X-ray	
Pathology	**Abnormality**
trauma	skull fractures, intracerebral haematomas (midline shift of a calcified pineal gland)
tumours	bone erosions (metastasis, multiple myeloma) or hyperostosis (meningiomas), calcifications (craniopharyngioma, glial tumours), enlargement/destruction of the pituitary fossa (pituitary tumours)
raised intracranial pressure	separation of the sutures (children), erosion of the posterior clinoids, thinning of the vault, and flattening of the pituitary fossa
developmental defects	craniostenosis, platybasia
inflammatory processes	opacification of the paranasal sinuses
vascular	calcified intracranial aneurysms and vascular malformations

Fig.16.12 Main abnormalities seen on skull radiograph.

Main abnormalities seen on spinal X-ray	
Pathology	**Abnormality**
trauma	fractures, fracture–dislocations, subluxations
tumours	erosion of the pedicles (long-standing tumours), erosions of the vertebral bodies (metastatic tumours)
degenerative disease	narrowing of disc spaces, calcification of the intervertebral discs, osteophyte formation

Fig.16.13 Main abnormalities seen on spinal radiograph.

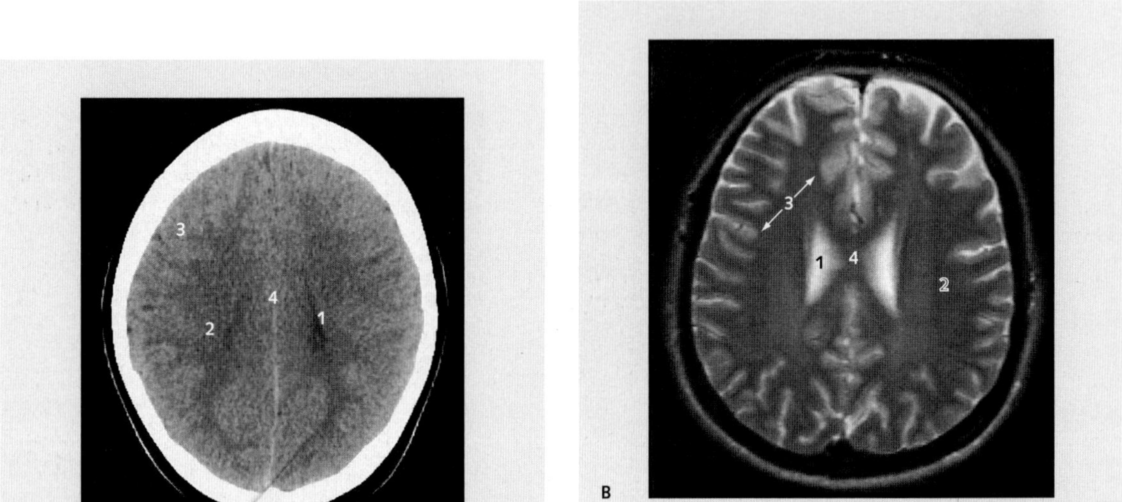

1 lateral ventricle
2 white matter
3 grey matter (arrows on MRI)
4 corpus callosum

Fig.16.14 (A) Computed tomography and (B) magnetic resonance imaging (T2-weighted image) showing the normal structure of the brain.

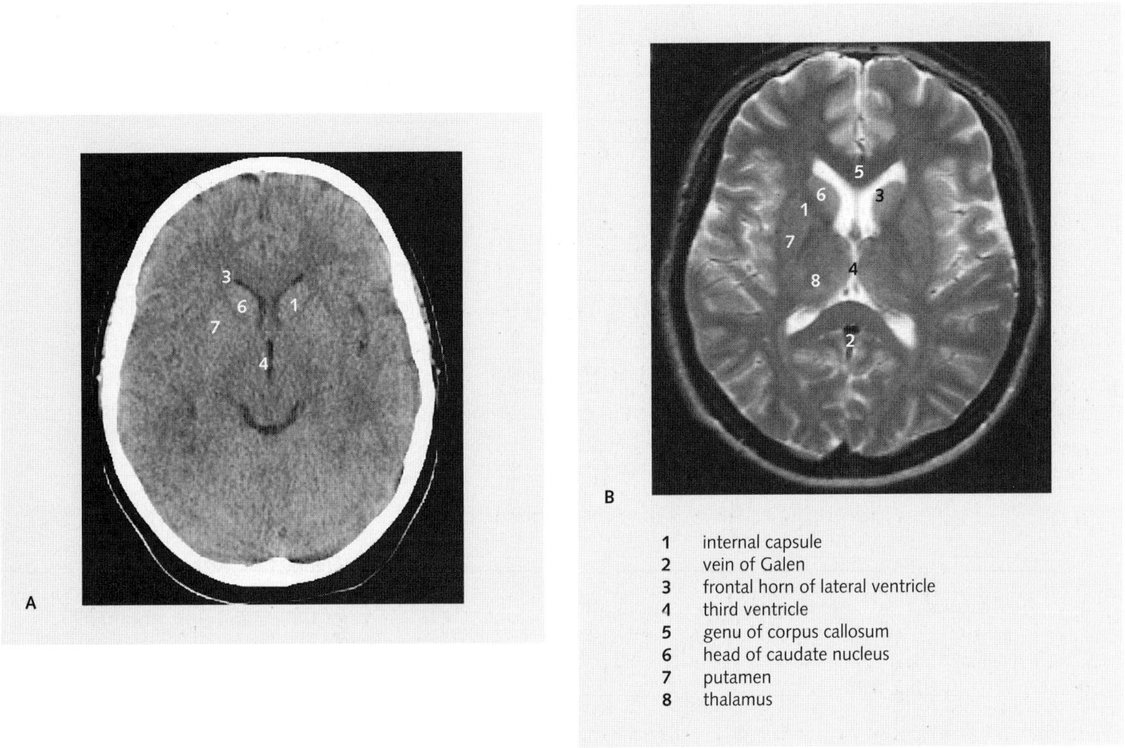

Fig.16.15 (A) Computed tomography and (B) magnetic resonance imaging (T2-weighted image) showing the normal structure of the brain.

Fig.16.16 Main abnormalities seen on computed tomography scanning (HD, high density; LD, low density).

Main abnormalities seen on CT scanning	
Pathlogy	**Abnormality**
trauma	extracerebral and intracerebral haematomas(HD), brain confusion (mixed HD and LD)
vascular lesions	infarction (LD), haemorrhage (HD), subarachnoid haemorrhage (HD) in the basal cisterns and sulcil, angiomos, and aneurysms (intensely enhancing lesions)
tumours	enhancing irregular lesions surrounded by LD (oedema)
degeneration	brain atrophy (ventricular enlargment, widening of the sulci, and flattening of the gyri)
hybrocephalus	ventricular enlargement whith no evidence of cortical atrophy
infections	abscesses(LD lesions surrounded by ring enhancement), focal encephalitis (LD)
spinal lesions	lesions of the vertebrae, the intervertebral discs, and the spinal canal

Main abnormalities seen on MRI	
Pathlogy	**Abnormality**
demyelinating disease	multiple sclerosis (periventricular white malter lesions)
tumours	lesions in the pituitary fossa, cerebellopontine angles, craniocervical junction, and the orbits (images are not affected by artefacts from the surrounding bony structures)
vascular diseases	large aneurysms and venous sinus thrombosis (magnetic resonance angiography (MRA))
infections	encephalitis, progressive multifocal leucoencephalopathy
spinal lesions	intramedullary lesions (syringomyelia, tumours, demyelination), extramedullary lesions (degenerative disease, tumours, abscesses)

Fig.16.17 Main abnormalities seen on magnetic resonance imaging.

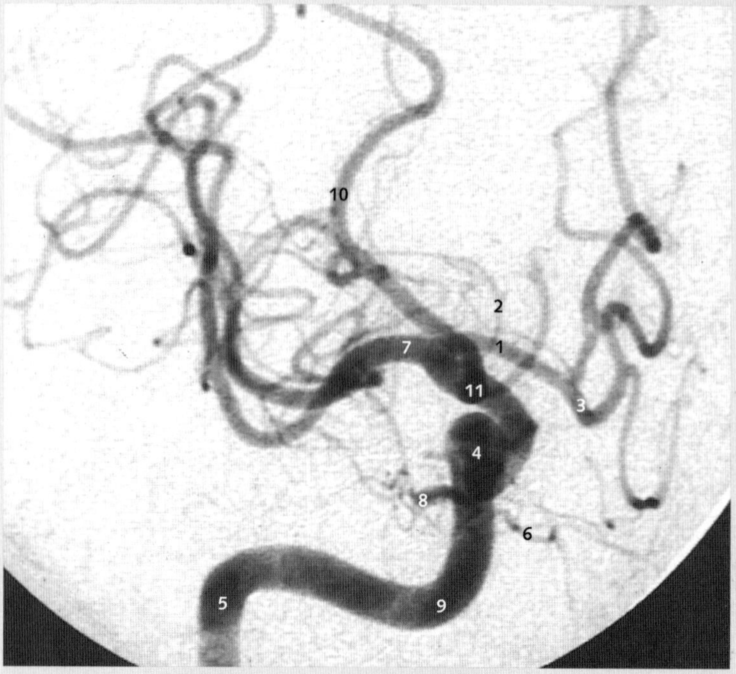

1 anterior cerebral artery
2 anterior choroidal artery
3 anterior communicating artery
4 cavernous portion of internal carotid artery
5 cervical portion of internal carotid artery
6 ethmoidal branch of ophthalmic artery
7 middle cerebral artery
8 ophthalmic artery
9 pertrous portion of internal carotid artery
10 posterior cerebral artery
11 posterior communicating artery

Fig.16.18 Arterial phase of a normal carotid angiogram (courtesy of J. Weir and P. H. Abrahams).

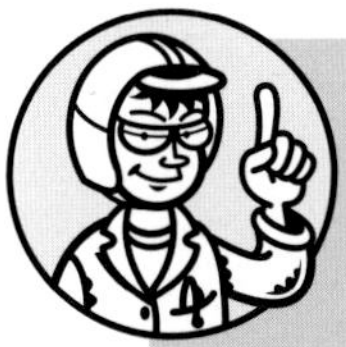

Advantages of magnetic resonance imaging:
- Absence of ionizing radiation.
- The ability to obtain images in coronal, sagittal, as well as axial plains.
- More sensitive to the pathological changes in the brain tissues.

Disadvantages:
- Cannot be used for patients with pacemakers (the magnetic field interferes with their function).
- Cannot be used for patients with ferromagnetic intracranial aneurysmal clips or implants (they distort the images and could be displaced by the strong magnetic field).
- Claustrophobia.

- Assessing cerebral vessel anatomy and tumour blood supply before neurosurgery.
- Interventional angiography: embolization of angiomas.

Duplex sonography

This technique offers a combination of real time and Doppler flow ultrasound scanning, allowing a non-invasive assessment of extracranial arteries. It is particularly helpful as a screening test for lesions at the carotid bifurcation which avoids the need for angiography in many patients. The quality of this technique is dependent on the experience and skill of the operator.

Cerebral ultrasonography

This technique is used in neonates, as other imaging requires sedation and/or high radiation doses. The ultrasound is performed through the sutures and fontanelles, which have not fused. It is particularly useful for detecting the presence of hydrocephalus and intraventricular haemorrhage in premature babies.

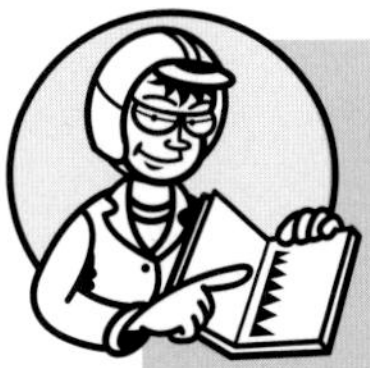

- What rhythms may normally be seen on an EEG? What is the role of the EEG in investigating patients?
- How might you investigate neuromuscular function in someone with myasthenia gravis? How would your findings differ from those in a patient with multiple sclerosis?
- How would you distinguish bacterial and viral meningitis on CSF culture?
- What are the basic differences between computed tomography and magnetic resonance imaging? Give examples of when each is appropriate.
- In what clinical situation might you order a cerebral angiogram? Describe the abnormality you would see.

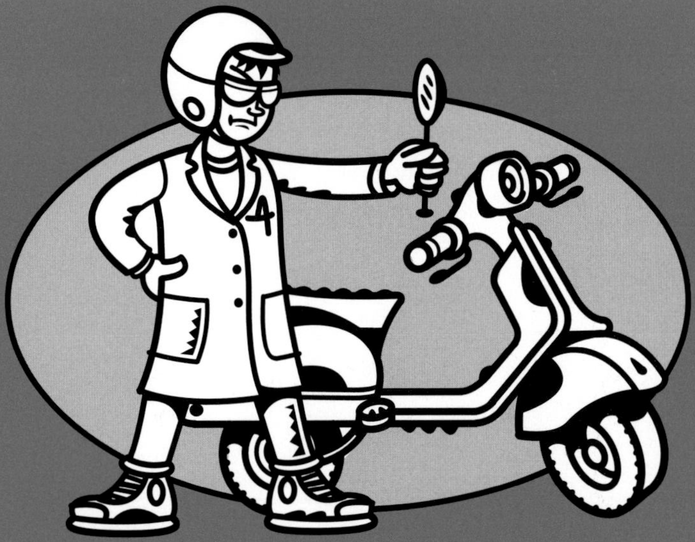

SELF-ASSESSMENT

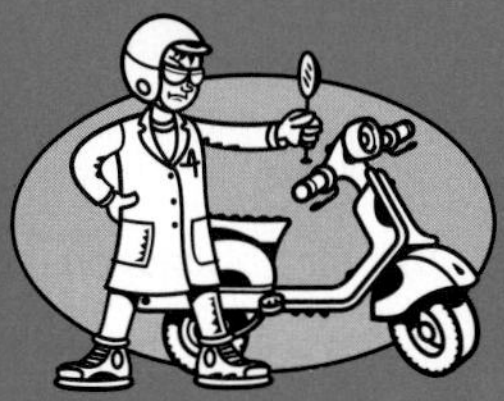

Multiple-choice Questions (MCQs)

Indicate whether each answer is true or false.

1. In the brain:

(a) The internal capsule is lateral to the lentiform nucleus.
(b) The amygdala lies in the frontal lobe.
(c) The frontal lobe is separated from the parietal lobe by the precentral sulcus.
(d) The hippocampus lies in the temporal lobe.
(e) The lateral sulcus lies between the parietal lobe and the occipital lobe.

2. In the development of the central nervous system:

(a) Cells of the neural tube form dorsal root ganglion cells.
(b) Cells of the neural tube form glia and neurons.
(c) The brain develops from three vesicles.
(d) Failure of neural tube closure can result in spinal and cranial defects.
(e) Basal plate cells develop into cells with sensory function.

3. In the ventricles:

(a) Cerebrospinal fluid is secreted by the choroid plexus.
(b) Blockage of the aqueduct causes a communicating hydrocephalus.
(c) The lateral ventricles drain directly into the fourth ventricle.
(d) The ventricular cavities are lined with pia mater.
(e) Cerebrospinal fluid has the same protein content as plasma.

4. Regarding the development of the brain:

(a) The retina emerges from the developing central nervous system.
(b) The mesencephalon refers to the pons and medulla.
(c) The hippocampal formation and amygdala are structures found in the diencephalons.
(d) The pituitary gland has an anterior part derived from the oral cavity.
(e) The tela choroidea is formed from two layers—dura mater and ependyma.

5. Regarding the central nervous system environment:

(a) There are roughly equal numbers of glial cells and neurons.
(b) Microglia are phagocytic.
(c) Astrocytes regulate interstitial calcium concentration.
(d) Schwann cells may myelinate several axons.
(e) L-glucose is preferentially transported across the blood–brain barrier.

6. Concerning the action potential:

(a) Inhibitory postsynaptic potentials are caused by increasing membrane permeability to cations (e.g. Na^+).
(b) Temporal summation occurs only when there is transmission at many synapses.
(c) There are few Na^+ channels at the axon hillock.
(d) Conduction velocity (m/s) in myelinated axons is six times the diameter (μm).
(e) After demyelination, axonal membranes can store more charge.

7. At the synapse:

(a) Neurotransmitters are released at all synapses.
(b) Axoaxonic synapses can inhibit action potential generation.
(c) Intracellular Na^+ is the signal for exocytosis.
(d) Dopamine synthesis is regulated by altering the activity of dopa decarboxylase.
(e) Neurotransmission can be terminated by uptake into the terminal bouton.

8. Regarding neurons:

(a) A high metabolic rate is required to maintain ion concentration difference across the membrane.
(b) Interneurons have long axons which influence cells in other parts of the nervous system.
(c) Their framework is supported by astrocyte glial processes.
(d) Electrical synapses may be bidirectional.
(e) Excitatory glutamatergic synapses typically have elliptical vesicles of neurotransmitter.

9. Regarding neurotransmission:

(a) There is a single receptor identified for glutamate.
(b) Muscarinic acetylcholine receptors are associated with a cation channel.
(c) Ionotrophic receptors are generally G-protein linked.
(d) An inhibitory postsynaptic potential is created by increasing the membrane permeability to chloride ions.
(e) Saltatory conduction is typically bidirectional.

10. Concerning the spinal cord:

(a) The spinothalamic tract carries ipsilateral sensory information.
(b) The dorsal columns carry ipsilateral sensory information.
(c) The lateral corticospinal tract carries crossed fibres.
(d) The tectospinal tract carries information to the midbrain.
(e) The dorsal columns carry information about pain and temperature.

11. Regarding the spinal cord:

(a) In adults, the cord ends at the level of L3.
(b) The dorsal column tract decussates in the cord.
(c) Tabes dorsalis leads to a loss of fine touch and proprioception.
(d) Hemisection of the cord leads to a contralateral sensory loss.
(e) The grey matter lies peripherally.

12. Concerning pain:

(a) Nociceptors have unencapsulated endings.
(b) Local circuits in the dorsal horn influence pain signal transmission.
(c) Opioids act only in the dorsal horn.
(d) In morphine overdose, the pupils are dilated.
(e) Naloxone is an antagonist at the μ receptor.

13. Concerning somatosensation:

(a) Rapidly adapting receptors continue firing while their stimulus is still present.
(b) Axons from proprioceptors are unmyelinated.
(c) The cell bodies of spinothalamic tract axons lie in dorsal root ganglia.
(d) The sensory homunculus has very small hands.
(e) The sensory cortex lies in the parietal lobe.

14. The following are likely complications of giving opioid drugs to patients in acute pain:

(a) Dependence.
(b) Emesis.
(c) Diuresis.
(d) Miosis.
(e) Sedation.

15. A patient requires analgesia for back pain:

(a) Conventional NSAIDs inhibit both COX-1 and COX-2.
(b) Selective COX-2 inhibitors are more effective than conventional NSAIDs.
(c) Ibuprofen 400 mg twice daily is a reasonable choice.
(d) Bed rest is the most appropriate non-drug therapy.
(e) In a patient with saddle anaesthesia and incontinence, urgent referral must be made.

16. Regarding analgesia:

(a) The body has an endogenous system of pain relief.
(b) Antidepressants may be effective in some types of pain.
(c) Opioids cause diarrhoea and vomiting as side effects.
(d) Naloxone has a similar duration of action to morphine.
(e) Non-steroidal anti-inflammatory drugs are selective COX-1 inhibitors.

17. Concerning the pyramidal tract:

(a) The pyramidal tract contains only axons originating in the primary motor cortex.
(b) The pyramidal tract passes through the posterior one-third of the internal capsule.
(c) The motor homunculus has large hands.
(d) Upper motor neuron lesions result in atrophy and fasciculation.
(e) The lateral corticospinal tract innervates distal limb muscles.

18. Concerning basal ganglia:

(a) The striatum has poor connections with the cortex.
(b) The substantia nigra sends a dopaminergic projection to the striatum.
(c) The indirect processing loop via the subthalamic nucleus excites the cortex.
(d) L-dopa is given to parkinsonian patients because it is metabolized by tyrosine hydroxylase.
(e) The basal ganglia are involved in the activation of motor programs.

19. Parkinson's disease:

(a) Is always an obvious diagnosis.
(b) Should be treated immediately with L-dopa.
(c) Is an upper motor neuron disorder, and therefore associated with increased tendon reflexes.
(d) Symptoms may respond to anticholinergic drugs.
(e) Is associated with depression.

20. In the cerebellum:

(a) Mossy fibres carry proprioceptive information.
(b) Purkinje cells send excitatory projections to the deep cerebellar nuclei.
(c) Cerebellar hemispheres process ipsilateral motor functions.
(d) Cerebellar lesions produce ataxia.
(e) Complex spikes recorded in granule cells signal error detection.

21. In the motor unit:

(a) Large innervation ratios give fine control over movement.
(b) Smaller motor neurons are recruited before larger ones.
(c) Fast fibres contain glycolytic enzymes.
(d) Fibre clumping occurs with diseases of the muscle fibres.
(e) Spontaneous muscle activity can occur in diseases of the motor neuron.

22. Concerning the vestibular system:

(a) The otolith organs detect head position.
(b) The vestibulospinal tracts influence antigravity muscles.
(c) The vestibular nuclei project to cranial nerve nuclei controlling eye position.
(d) The horizontal vestibulo-ocular reflex uses complementary information from both cranial nerves VIII.

(e) Proprioception is mediated only by sensations from the musculoskeletal system.

23. Parkinson's disease is characterized by:

(a) Loss of dopaminergic neurons in the pons.
(b) Tremor of 12 Hz or more.
(c) Rigidity.
(d) Macrographia.
(e) Bradykinesia.

24. Concerning the brainstem:

(a) The pyramidal tracts decussate at the top of the medulla.
(b) The trigeminal nucleus receives somatosensory information from cranial nerves other than the trigeminal.
(c) Cranial nerve X leaves the medulla lateral to the olivary nucleus.
(d) The nuclei of cranial nerves VI and VII are closely related.
(e) Cranial nerve III emerges between the cerebral peduncles.

25. In the autonomic nervous system:

(a) Preganglionic fibres are unmyelinated.
(b) All parasympathetic preganglionic neurons have their cell bodies in the brainstem.
(c) Muscarinic antagonists reduce heart rate.
(d) Acetylcholine is released at all ganglia.
(e) One preganglionic sympathetic neuron can synapse in several ganglia.

26. The following are true of Horner's syndrome:

(a) It may be caused by an underlying malignancy.
(b) Anhidrosis is always present.
(c) Carotid artery thrombosis may cause the pupil to constrict when adrenaline eye drops are given.
(d) It is a recognized complication of thyroid surgery.
(e) Vision is lost in the affected eye.

27. Regarding the sympathetic nervous system:

(a) It has positive chronotropic and inotropic effects on the heart.
(b) The coeliac ganglion supplies the colon.
(c) It acts to constrict the pupil.
(d) The interomediolateral column of cell bodies in the spinal cord runs from C5 to T1.
(e) It causes adrenaline and noradrenaline to be released by actions on the adrenal cortex.

28. A patient is brought into an Accident and Emergency Department unconscious and with neck stiffness:

(a) Lumbar puncture should be performed immediately.
(b) A purpuric rash is most suggestive of pneumococcal meningitis.
(c) Subarachnoid haemorrhage may be the underlying cause.
(d) Intracranial tumour is ruled out by neck stiffness.
(e) The patient should be observed for 30 minutes to see if helpful focal signs develop.

29. Regarding dementia:

(a) Patients with Pick's disease have a cortical dementia.
(b) Dementia is a rare clinical feature of Parkinson's disease.
(c) A mini-mental state score of 28 is suggestive of dementia, provided that the patient is not depressed or in an acute confusional state.
(d) EEG is very helpful in making the diagnosis.
(e) Alzheimer's disease is the cause of dementia in approximately 40% of cases.

30. Concerning anxiolytics and anticonvulsants:

(a) Benzodiazepines block GABA action by binding to the GABA receptor.
(b) Benzodiazepine action can be prolonged by active metabolites.
(c) Intravenous clonazepam is used to treat status epilepticus.
(d) Phenytoin toxicity is suggested by tremor, dysarthria and ataxia.
(e) Valproate has only one mechanism of action similar to phenytoin.

31. In cerebrovascular disease:

(a) Large anterior circulation strokes have a high early mortality rate.
(b) Lacunar infarctions can present with isolated dysphasia.
(c) Subarachnoid haemorrhage is usually caused by a rupture of a Charcot–Bouchard aneurysm.
(d) Lateral medullary syndrome is caused by acute occlusion of the posterior inferior cerebellar artery.
(e) Amaurosis fugax is suggestive of a contralateral carotid lesion.

32. A 60-year-old woman presents to an Accident and Emergency Department. She was found in the street 30 minutes previously and has been fitting since:

(a) A computed tomography brain scan is the first priority.
(b) She may respond to intravenous diazepam.
(c) If the fitting stops she can be discharged.
(d) The diagnosis is status epilepticus. Further investigation is not necessary.
(e) If the seizure continues, she should be transferred to a neurosurgical centre.

33. Regarding brain tumours:

(a) Glioblastoma multiformis is a tumour of childhood.
(b) Meningioma is the commonest benign primary brain tumour.
(c) Computed tomography scanning is the preferred method of investigating tumours of the pituitary fossa because, unlike magnetic resonance imaging, the

images will not be affected by artefacts from the surrounding bony structures.
(d) Calcified tumours are always benign.
(e) Bronchogenic carcinoma is the commonest primary systemic tumour.

34. Cerebral oedema:

(a) Vasogenic oedema is an intracellular oedema.
(b) Cytotoxic oedema affects both grey and white matter.
(c) Vasogenic oedema is usually responsive to treatment with steroids, mannitol and dehydration.
(d) Hydrocephalus may result in extracellular oedema.
(e) Hypoxic brain damage usually results in cytotoxic oedema.

35. Regarding developmental and associated disorders:

(a) Children with cerebral palsy have mental retardation.
(b) A patient in whom spina bifida is picked up on an incidental radiograph should be referred for a surgical opinion to prevent later deterioration.
(c) Hydrocephalus is diagnosed by ultrasonography in adults and children.
(d) Dementia with normal-pressure hydrocephalus may respond to surgery.
(e) Arnold–Chiari formation may cause headache.

36. Following one epileptic seizure in an adult:

(a) Driving is allowed but must stop if a second event occurs.
(b) A brain scan should be performed in most cases.
(c) Lumbar puncture is mandatory.
(d) EEG showing three-per-second spike-and-wave activity indicates a likely structural lesion.
(e) The probability of a second event within 3 years is 50%.

37. In central nervous system infections:

(a) *Neisseria meningitidis*, *Streptococcus pneumoniae* and *Haemophilus influenzae* are the commonest causative organisms of epidural spinal abscesses.
(b) Viral meningitis is a benign and self-limiting disease and no specific treatment is required.
(c) In meningitis, lumbar puncture should always be performed before initiating antibiotic treatment.
(d) Acyclovir is nephrotoxic and should be used only in confirmed cases of herpes simplex encephalitis.
(e) Toxoplasmosis is a common fungal infection in AIDS patients.

38. The following may precipitate seizures in susceptible individuals:

(a) Sleep.
(b) Sleep deprivation.
(c) Hyperventilation.
(d) Stress.
(e) Pneumonia.

39. In multiple sclerosis:

(a) Blurring of vision associated with orbital pain on eye movements is a typical presenting complaint.
(b) Flexing of the neck may produce 'electric shock'-like pains.
(c) Bence-Jones protein is seen on cerebrospinal fluid analysis.
(d) Signs may be seen on magnetic resonance imaging.
(e) Is usually fatal within 5 years of diagnosis.

40. A 79-year-old man presents with a left hemiparesis:

(a) If he is left handed, dysphasia is likely in a right hemisphere stroke.
(b) A posterior circulation stroke is likely.
(c) A carotid bruit may be heard.
(d) A haemorrhagic stroke is most likely.
(e) Rehabilitation in a specialist unit may be helpful.

41. The following are patients at high risk of stroke:

(a) A 55-year-old man presenting with amaurosis fugax.
(b) A 40-year-old woman with a long history of migraine.
(c) A 25-year-old man with polycystic kidney disease and hypertension.
(d) A 70-year-old smoker with hypertension.
(e) A 45-year-old man with a previous history of fully resolved bacterial meningitis.

42. The following are causes of cerebral palsy:

(a) Intrauterine infection.
(b) Maternal hypertension.
(c) Maternal hyperglycaemia.
(d) Birth trauma.
(e) Intraventricular haemorrhage.

43. Myotonic dystrophy:

(a) Is a cause of bilateral ptosis.
(b) Is a particular type of Duchenne's muscular dystrophy.
(c) Is associated with cardiac arrhythmias.
(d) Is inherited through either parent.
(e) Is associated with sustained muscle contractions.

44. Regarding muscular dystrophy:

(a) It is an X-linked inherited disorder.
(b) The genetic abnormality is similar for both Duchenne and Becker forms.
(c) Gower's sign may be present in children with the disorder.
(d) The weakness is primarily distal.
(e) The calf muscles are grossly enlarged.

45. Regarding neurofibromatosis:

(a) It is an autosomal recessive condition.
(b) Type 1, rather than type 2, presents with acoustic neuromas.

(c) Lisch nodules are areas of haemorrhage seen on the retina.
(d) Meningiomas are common complications of Type 2.
(e) Six or more café-au-lait spots > 5 mm may be suggestive of the diagnosis.

46. A 65-year-old smoker presents with fatigue and proximal muscle weakness:

(a) Lambert–Eaton myasthenic syndrome (LEMS) is a possible diagnosis.
(b) A normal chest X-ray excludes the presence of a small-cell lung cancer.
(c) The defect in LEMS is postsynaptic.
(d) Autonomic involvement is common.
(e) LEMS commonly affects trunk and proximal muscles.

47. The following are potential triggers of Guillain–Barré syndrome:

(a) Campylobacter infection.
(b) Influenza infection.
(c) MMR immunization.
(d) Chicken pox.
(e) Glandular fever.

48. In the eye:

(a) The cornea has no sensory innervation.
(b) Ganglion cell axons are unmyelinated inside the eye.
(c) The sclera is continuous with the arachnoid layer.
(d) The fovea contains only rods.
(e) Branches of the central retinal artery do not pass over the fovea.

49. Concerning central visual pathways:

(a) Fibres from the nasal half of the retina cross over in the chiasm.
(b) There are cells in the lateral geniculate nucleus that receive information from both eyes.
(c) Lesions of the optic tract affect both sides of the visual field.
(d) The primary visual cortex has a columnar organization.
(e) Most of the visual cortex is devoted to processing the peripheral visual field.

50. Regarding glaucoma:

(a) Intraocular pressure should be below 22 mmHg.
(b) Glaucoma is an uncommon cause of blindness.
(c) Acute open angle glaucoma is an ophthalmological emergency.
(d) Tropicamide dilating drops should be instilled into the eye to examine the extent of damage to the optic nerve.
(e) Glaucoma may be caused by blockage in the scleral sinus.

51. Regarding eye movements:

(a) The vestibulo-ocular reflex may be impaired in IIIrd nerve palsies.
(b) The frontal lobes have a role in saccadic eye movements.
(c) Smooth pursuit eye movements hold images steady on the optic disc.
(d) Vergence eye movements are important in accommodation.
(e) Saccadic and smooth pursuit eye movement may alternate.

52. Concerning the auditory system:

(a) The basilar membrane is of uniform width.
(b) Hair cells show different frequency sensitivities along the basilar membrane.
(c) Feedback from the brainstem travels in the olivocochlear bundle.
(d) Pathways from the cochlear nuclei travel only contralaterally up to the cortex.
(e) The primary auditory cortex is in the parietal lobe.

53. Regarding deafness:

(a) A positive Rinnes test excludes conductive deafness.
(b) In conductive hearing loss, sound will be heard loudest in the affected ear during Weber's test.
(c) Ménière's disease is a possible cause.
(d) Bone conduction is normally more important than air conduction for hearing.
(e) Cochlear implants are first-line treatment for sensorineural deafness.

54. Concerning taste and smell:

(a) Fungiform papillae are found on the anterior two-thirds of the tongue.
(b) The olfactory epithelium sends projections to the olfactory bulb.
(c) Taste afferents synapse in the solitary nucleus.
(d) Granule cells in the olfactory bulb project into the cortex.
(e) Afferents to the olfactory cortex synapse first in the thalamus.

55. In a 55-year-old woman with a brain tumour:

(a) In the presence of a dressing apraxia, the lesion is likely to be in the dominant parietal lobe.
(b) The presence of upper quadrant homonymous field defect suggests that the lesion is likely to be in the temporal lobe.
(c) Sensory inattention is suggestive of a dominant hemispheric lesion.
(d) Altered personality and loss of initiative suggests that the lesion is likely to be in the frontal lobe.
(e) The presence of dyscalculia suggests a temporal lobe lesion.

56. Concerning memory and the limbic system:

(a) Lesions of the hippocampus and surrounding area can produce amnesia.
(b) The parahippocampal gyrus is continuous with the cingulate gyrus.

(c) Primacy effects are caused by long-term memory.
(d) Procedural memory can be spared in amnesia.
(e) Working memory has a capacity of 7 ± 2 units of information.

57. Concerning the localization of cortical function:

(a) The cerebral hemispheres have similar processing functions.
(b) Frontal lobe lesions can result in disorders of object recognition.
(c) Planning deficits can result from frontal lobe lesions.
(d) Lesions to the motor cortex supplying the laryngeal muscles lead to copious production of nonsense sounds.
(e) Parietal lobe lesions can produce attentional disorders.

58. Concerning cognitive development and degeneration:

(a) The newborn child has no cognitive abilities.
(b) The sensorimotor stage is the first in Piaget's scheme of development.
(c) Successful ageing occurs without relative synaptogenesis.
(d) Glial cell numbers in the cortex increase with age.
(e) Social withdrawal in the elderly cannot be reversed.

59. Concerning brainstem-acting drugs:

(a) 5-HT_3 antagonists act only at the chemoreceptor trigger zone.
(b) Antihistamines reduce nausea caused by vestibular input to the vomiting centre.
(c) Dopamine agonists reduce nausea.
(d) The potency of an inhaled general anaesthetic agent is related to its blood : gas coefficient.
(e) General anaesthetic agents produce cardiovascular depression.

60. Regarding antidepressant treatment:

(a) Their use is never justified in bipolar disorders.
(b) Reactive depression has a clear precipitant.
(c) Tricyclic antidepressants are safe in overdose.
(d) Lithium toxicity may be indicated by a tremor.
(e) Antidepressants have their therapeutic effect 2 days after beginning treatment.

61. Regarding the limbic system:

(a) Wernicke–Korsakoff syndrome causes degeneration of the mammillary bodies.
(b) Herpes simplex encephalitis may be associated with memory impairment.
(c) The limbic system has strong connections with the hypothalamus.
(d) The amygdala lies on the border of the fourth ventricle.
(e) Long-term potentiation is a possible cellular mechanism for memory.

62. Localiziing signs to the temporal lobe may include:

(a) Olfactory hallucinations.
(b) Dysphasia.
(c) Hemiparesis.
(d) Psychotic symptoms.
(e) Emotional disturbance.

63. Localizing signs to the frontal lobe may include:

(a) Hemisensory loss.
(b) Neglect.
(c) Personality disturbance.
(d) Dysphasia.
(e) Intention tremor.

64. The following endocrine disorders may present with coma:

(a) Diabetes.
(b) Addison's disease.
(c) Thyroid dysfunction.
(d) Conn's syndrome.
(e) Cushing's disease.

65. The following are causes of cognitive impairment which have a degree of reversibility:

(a) Thyroid dysfunction.
(b) Subdural haematoma.
(c) Renal failure.
(d) Liver failure.
(e) Neurosyphilis.

66. Concerning nystagmus:

(a) Nystagmus is jerky, with the fast phase to the side of the lesion in unilateral vestibular lesions.
(b) Downbeating nystagmus is suggestive of a lesion at or around the superior colliculi.
(c) Pendular nystagmus is suggestive of long-standing impaired macular vision.
(d) Nystagmus is suggestive of a brainstem pathology if its direction varies with the direction of gaze.
(e) Nystagmus is generally symptomatic.

67. A 66-year-old patient presents with lower cranial nerve palsies:

(a) A wasted and fasciculating tongue is suggestive of pseudobulbar palsy.
(b) The jaw jerk is brisk in pseudobulbar palsy, but absent in bulbar palsy.
(c) Motor neuron disease causes features of both bulbar and pseudobulbar palsy.
(d) Speech is monotonous in bulbar palsy.
(e) Emotional lability is suggestive of pseudobulbar palsy.

68. Concerning dysphasia:

(a) Lesions of the angular gyrus cause a non-fluent dysphasia.

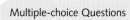

(b) Repetition is impaired in conductive dysphasia.
(c) Lesions at Broca's area cause fluent dysphasia.
(d) Dysphasias are caused by non-dominant hemispheric lesions.
(e) Cerebrovascular disease and brain tumours are the commonest causes of dysphasia.

69. The following are potential causes of a VIIth nerve palsy:

(a) Middle ear infection.
(b) Guillain–Barré syndrome.
(c) Stroke.
(d) Herpes zoster infection.
(e) Osler–Weber–Rendu syndrome.

70. Causes of ptosis include:

(a) VIth nerve palsy.
(b) Horner's syndrome.
(c) Congenital anomalies.
(d) Tabes dorsalis.
(e) Myopathies.

71. Regarding the examination of the cranial nerves:

(a) A defect of lateral gaze is generally due to a VIth nerve palsy.
(b) Sensory abnormalities over the left side of the forehead are likely to be due to a VIIth nerve lesion.
(c) The motor function of the VIIth nerve may be tested by getting the patient to raise their eyebrows.
(d) Hypoglossal nerve function is tested by looking at the elevation of the palate when saying 'ah'.
(e) Examination of the first cranial nerve is rarely performed.

72. Regarding gait disturbance:

(a) A high-stepping gait may be due to peripheral neuropathy.
(b) Parkinson's disease is characterized by the 'marche à la petit pas'.
(c) Heel–toe walking may be impaired in cerebellar disease.
(d) Injuries from falls rule out a hysterical gait disturbance.
(e) Romberg's test is positive if a patient is stable with their feet together and eyes open, and falls when they close their eyes.

73. On examination of the peripheral nerves:

(a) Power of muscle groups should be recorded in the standard format with a score out of 10.
(b) The presence of spasticity is indicative of an upper motor neuron lesion.
(c) Coordination need only be tested unilaterally.
(d) Vibration sense is tested with a 440 Hz tuning fork.
(e) Sensation should be tested routinely across all myotomes.

74. EEG:

(a) Is necessary for the diagnosis of brain death.
(b) May be used in the diagnosis of metabolic encephalopathy.
(c) If normal, makes epilepsy unlikely.
(d) Is normal following a stroke.
(e) May be abnormal in migraine.

75. The following are typical findings on cerebrospinal fluid analysis:

(a) Bacterial meningitis causes a high cerebrospinal fluid protein.
(b) Viral meningitis gives a low cerebrospinal fluid glucose level.
(c) The presence of neutrophils indicates a bacterial aetiology for infection.
(d) The normal glucose level is typically two-thirds the plasma level.
(e) Polymorphs may be found in normal cerebrospinal fluid.

76. A young man presents who, over the past 2 days, has developed weakness in his hands and feet. Since this morning, he has been unable to stand up and cannot lift his arms above his head:

(a) He may have a lumbosacral disc protrusion.
(b) A complaint of numb toes makes Guillain–Barré syndrome less likely.
(c) Increased reflexes and extensor plantar responses indicate a probable intracranial problem.
(d) A history of recent diarrhoea is unlikely to be important.
(e) Peak expiratory flow rate should be monitored.

77. A patient presents with central, crushing chest pain which radiates to the jaw and left arm:

(a) Referred pain is felt in superficial structures because the viscera have no pain receptors.
(b) The pain information is carried in Aδ and C fibres.
(c) If he subsequently suddenly loses consciousness, stroke is the most likely diagnosis.
(d) He may be at risk of cerebrovascular events.
(e) A recent stroke may change your management.

78. A known drug addict presents to an Accident and Emergency Department unconscious:

(a) The effects of cocaine overdose are similar to those of morphine overdose.
(b) Long-term psychiatric sequelae may result from addiction to psychotropic drugs.
(c) Tolerance rarely develops with LSD.
(d) Ecstasy may precipitate a dilutional hyponatraemia.
(e) Drug addicts should not be given opioid pain relief in the acute setting.

79. A 54-year-old patient collapses at home:

(a) Tongue biting confirms the diagnosis of a seizure.

(b) A tonic–clonic seizure confirms the diagnosis of epilepsy.
(c) A history of urination at the time of collapse may be important.
(d) Vertebrobasilar insufficiency is a cause if there is a history of neck extension.
(e) A drug-induced cause is possible if the patient is taking calcium channel blocking drugs.

80. The following are likely causes of coma in a known alcoholic:

(a) Hyperglycaemia.
(b) Intracranial haemorrhage.
(c) Drug overdose.
(d) Wernicke–Korsakoff syndrome.
(e) Subacute combined degeneration of the cord.

81. Choreiform movements may be seen in:

(a) Treated Parkinson's disease.
(b) Thyroid disease.
(c) Guillain–Barré syndrome.
(d) Motor neuron disease.
(e) Rheumatic fever.

82. Regarding the pituitary gland:

(a) Tumours in this region are generally adenomatous.
(b) It releases thyrotrophic releasing hormone.
(c) It receives hormones in a specialized circulation.
(d) Masses in the pituitary may cause a homonymous hemianopia.
(e) Deficiency of pituitary hormones (pan-hypopituitarism) may cause acromegaly.

83. A 64-year-old woman arrives in an Accident and Emergency Department unconscious:

(a) An immediate computed tomography scan is required.
(b) An ischaemic stroke is a likely diagnosis.
(c) A urine dipstick measurement may be relevant.
(d) She may have a Glasgow Coma Scale score of 2.
(e) Naloxone should be given if opioid overdose is a possibility.

84. When looking at the optic fundus:

(a) The optic disc is darker than the surrounding retina.
(b) If the margin of the disc is indistinct, then papilloedema is a possibility.
(c) Arteriovenous nipping is a sign of diabetic retinopathy.
(d) Optic atrophy can be caused by toxic insult.
(e) Pigmentation is always caused by a disease process.

85. A 25-year-old man is found by an ambulance crew after a road traffic accident:

(a) His motorcycle helmet should be removed.
(b) A Glasgow Coma Scale of zero implies death.
(c) Straw coloured fluid coming from the ears and nose may indicate serious head injury.
(d) Post-traumatic epilepsy is a risk.
(e) The most important thing is to maintain an airway and give adequate ventilation.

86. The following are consequences of an acoustic neuroma:

(a) Conductive deafness.
(b) Ipsilateral facial weakness.
(c) Nystagmus.
(d) Raised intracranial pressure.
(e) Distant metastases.

87. When clerking a patient, you find papilloedema. Your differential diagnosis might include:

(a) Intracranial tumour.
(b) Hypocapnoea.
(c) Guillain–Barré syndrome.
(d) Malignant hypotension.
(e) Optic neuritis.

88. In your approach to the unconscious patient:

(a) If the Glasgow Coma Scale is less than 8, an artificial airway is likely to be required.
(b) Cheyne–Stokes breathing is deep, sighing breathing, often seen in diabetic ketoacidosis.
(c) Signs of raised intracranial pressure include a rising blood pressure, with a slowing pulse.
(d) A head injury means a coexistent spinal injury until proven otherwise.
(e) Retinal haemorrhages may indicate an ischaemic stroke.

89. Regarding delirium:

(a) Systemic infection may present as an acute confusional state.
(b) Disorientation in terms of place is most marked.
(c) All patients should receive an antipsychotic drug.
(d) It commonly leads to permanent cognitive impairment.
(e) Occurs in 1% of hospital inpatients.

90. Mixed upper and lower motor neuron signs are seen in:

(a) Diabetic neuropathy.
(b) AIDS.
(c) Cervical spondylosis.
(d) Guillain–Barré syndrome.
(e) Motor neuron disease.

91. A patient presents with tremor:

(a) Overdose of nebulized β_2-antagonists is a cause.
(b) A fast tremor is unlikely to be a result of Parkinson's disease.
(c) In the presence of peripheral paraesthesiae and hyperventilation is an ominous sign.
(d) Lithium toxicity should be considered.
(e) It is a common sign of hypothyroidism.

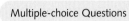

92. Regarding chronic alcohol abuse:

(a) A 'liver flap' is an early sign of liver impairment.
(b) Nutritional deficiencies are of little importance in Western countries.
(c) Korsakoff's syndrome is reversible, but Wernicke's syndrome has a poor prognosis.
(d) Confabulation is a feature of Korsakoff's syndrome.
(e) Delirium tremens develops 6–12 hours after stopping drinking.

93. A 54-year-old patient presents with diplopia:

(a) The presence of ptosis, and divergent squint is suggestive of a lesion of cranial nerve III.
(b) If diplopia is present when reading or looking down, then a lesion of cranial nerve VI is likely.
(c) The pupil is likely to be spared in diabetic lesions of cranial nerve III.
(d) Fluctuating diplopia is suggestive of myasthenia gravis.
(e) If caused by an acute palsy of cranial nerve III, and associated with an acute severe headache and signs of meningism, then a posterior communicating artery aneurysm should be excluded.

94. A 19-year-old man is referred by the orthopaedic surgeons before surgery for bilateral pes cavus:

(a) Spina bifida may be the cause.
(b) A chronic peripheral neuropathy, such as is seen with diabetes mellitus, may cause this picture.
(c) This could be caused by porphyria.
(d) The condition has probably developed in the past year.
(e) Nerve conduction studies may be abnormal.

95. Concerning antidepressants and antipsychotics:

(a) The cheese reaction occurs because of inhibition of cerebral monoamine oxidase by monoamine oxidase inhibitors.
(b) Tricyclics show an antimuscarinic and anti-adrenergic side-effect profile.
(c) Antipsychotic potency is proportional to D_4 blocking ability.
(d) The motor side effects of antipsychotics are due to effects on the pyramidal system.
(e) Clozapine blocks the D_2 receptor preferentially.

96. In a patient with bilateral wasting and weakness of the small hand muscles:

(a) The findings are explicable in terms of bilateral cerebral lesions.
(b) The findings could be caused by rheumatoid arthritis.
(c) Absence of the biceps jerk excludes cervical spondylosis as a cause.
(d) Extensor plantar responses exclude cervical spondylosis as a cause.
(e) Syringomyelia is one of the commonest causes.

97. A 25-year-old man presented to an Accident and Emergency Department with a head injury:

(a) Skull radiography is essential.
(b) The risk of chronic subdural haematoma is related to the severity of the head injury.
(c) He is said to have had a concussion if only minor macroscopic brain damage has occurred.
(d) Extradural haematoma is usually caused by a rupture of the sagittal or transverse sinuses.
(e) The risk of post-traumatic epilepsy is increased if he develops an epileptic seizure in the first 24 hours after injury.

98. Regarding numbness in the leg:

(a) A numb patch on the lateral surface of the thigh is often of ominous cause.
(b) Numbness on the sole of the foot should be associated with an absent knee jerk.
(c) If associated with a rash, may be caused by shingles.
(d) Bilateral proximal numbness is associated with diabetes mellitus.
(e) It is a common feature of motor neuron disease.

99. A 60-year-old man has a 5-year history of dizziness and sometimes faints when he stands up quickly:

(a) This sounds like epilepsy.
(b) A carotid bruit might be significant.
(c) If he also has impotence, unsteadiness and slurred speech, this could fit with multiple system atrophy.
(d) A drop of systolic blood pressure of 40 mmHg on standing might be incidental.
(e) The symptoms could be caused by cardiac disease.

100. Regarding metabolic and toxic diseases of the nervous system:

(a) Thiamine deficiency may result in neuropathy, dementia, or myelopathy (subacute combined degeneration of the cord).
(b) Abrupt alcohol withdrawal may result in delirium tremens which presents with tremor, hallucinations, seizures and autonomic overactivity.
(c) Lead poisoning causes chronic painful sensory neuropathy.
(d) Confusion, ataxia, and oculomotor disturbances are early features of Wernicke–Korsakoff syndrome.
(e) Carbon monoxide poisoning causes chronic encephalopathy with ataxia, dysarthria and tremor.

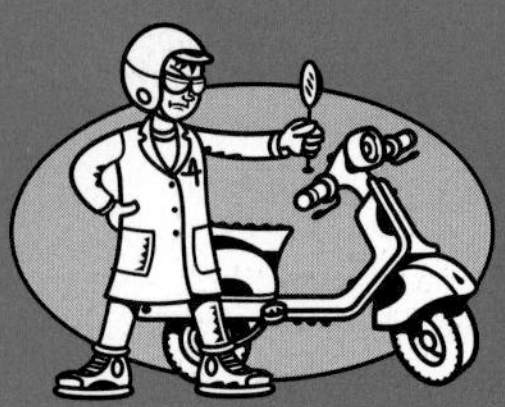

Short-answer Questions (SAQs)

1. Draw a cross-section through the spinal cord. Label the sensory tracts with the type of sensory information they carry.

2. A previously fit 25-year-old patient comes to outpatients with a short history of vertigo precipitated by head movements. Hallpike's manoeuvre was found to be positive.

   (a) How is Hallpike's manoeuvre carried out?
   (b) What are the clinical features of central and peripheral positional vertigo?

3. (a) What are the causes of tremor in a 60-year-old man?
   (b) Outline the features you would look for on examination to aid your diagnosis.

4. Why do parasympathetic signals reach their target organs more quickly than sympathetic signals?

5. A patient presents with the typical features of Guillain–Barré syndrome.

   (a) What are these?
   (b) What other diagnoses would you consider?

6. A 44-year-old woman presents with a traumatic cervical spinal injury following a road traffic accident. On examination, she is found to have paraparesis.

   (a) What are the possible pathological processes responsible for her neurological deficit?
   (b) Outline the management of this patient.

7. With a series of diagrams, describe the process of neurulation. What can happen if the neural tube fails to close?

8. (a) What are the three types of hydrocephalus?
   (b) Briefly outline the clinical features of hydrocephalus.

9. List the functions of glial cells.

10. A 38-year-old woman comes to outpatients with a history of two episodes of 'feeling funny', with an odd sensation in her right arm, followed by loss of consciousness.

    (a) What is the most likely diagnosis and how would you confirm this?
    (b) How would you treat the patient?

11. What does the jacksonian march tell us about the organization of the motor cortex?

12. Name two drugs that act on the brainstem to reduce vomiting and describe their different mechanisms of action.

13. With the aid of a diagram, show the activation cascade for light signal transduction in the photoreceptor.

14. A 60-year-old woman has tingling in her middle and index fingers, which is especially troublesome at night.

    (a) What is the most common cause of these symptoms?
    (b) What would you particularly look for in the history and examination?

15. A 32-year-old man complains that he has difficulty walking upstairs and getting up from a chair.

    (a) Where would you expect to find muscle weakness?
    (b) What are the possible diagnoses?

16. How do the contents of the middle ear transmit and amplify sound?

17. A 21-year-old woman with multiple sclerosis was admitted to hospital following a relapse.

    (a) Describe the possible clinical features of multiple sclerosis.
    (b) What investigations would have been used to confirm the diagnosis in this patient?

18. Why do we have loss of taste with a blocked-up nose?

19. Describe how we can distinguish between working memory and long-term memory.

20. A 55-year-old woman presents to outpatients with a 1-year history of difficulty in walking. On examination, she was found to be ataxic.

(a) Outline the clinical features of ataxic gait.
(b) How do you differentiate clinically between the two types of ataxic gait?

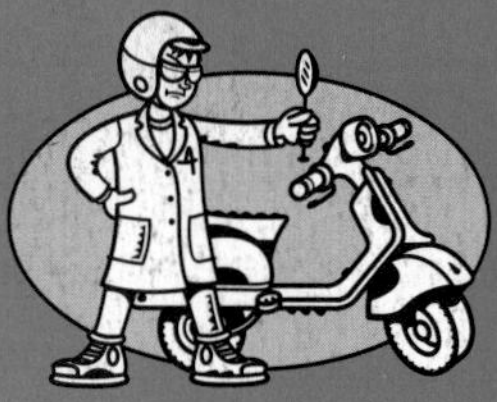

Essay Questions

1. Describe in outline how the various parts of the motor system contribute to motor processing.

2. A young man arrives in an Accident and Emergency Department at midnight when you are the house officer on duty. He is unconscious but breathing spontaneously. He is unaccompanied. Describe your management.

3. Discuss general medical disorders that may be associated with numbness of the hands and feet.

4. Discuss the clinical features of speech disorders.

5. What are the consequences of different types of damage to peripheral axons?

6. The mental state examination is an essential part of the neurological assessment. Discuss its different components.

7. Discuss the risk factors, the pathological mechanisms and the clinical features of stroke.

8. Describe the mechanism of opioid analgesia. What are the dangers of opioid overdose and how can they be treated?

9. Give an account of the central visual pathways with examples of how lesions can affect the visual field.

10. Give an account of the drug treatment of depression. Do you believe the monoamine theory?

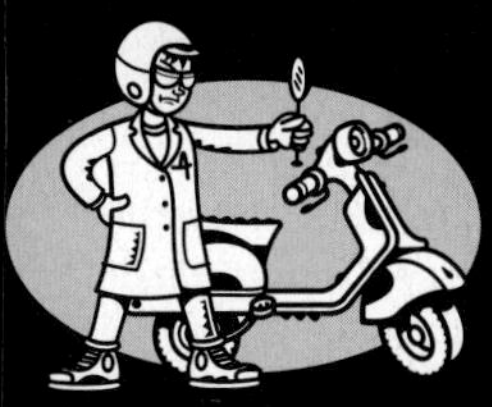

MCQ Answers

1. **The brain:**
   - (a) False—The internal capsule is medial to the lentiform nucleus.
   - (b) False—The amygdala lies in the medial temporal lobe.
   - (c) False—The frontal and parietal lobes are separated by the central sulcus.
   - (d) True—The hippocampus lies in the medial temporal lobe.
   - (e) False—The lateral sulcus divides the temporal lobe from the frontal and parietal lobes.

2. **Development of the central nervous system:**
   - (a) False—Cells of the neural crest form dorsal root ganglion cells.
   - (b) True—Glia and neurons originate from neural tube cells.
   - (c) True—These form the forebrain, midbrain and hindbrain structures.
   - (d) True—Spina bifida or anencephaly may result.
   - (e) False—Alar plate cells develop into sensory cells, basal plate into motor.

3. **The ventricles:**
   - (a) True—Cerebrospinal fluid is resorbed in the arachnoid granulations.
   - (b) False—This causes a non-communicating hydrocephalus.
   - (c) False—The lateral ventricles drain through the third ventricle.
   - (d) False—The ventricular cavities are lined with arachnoid mater.
   - (e) False—Cerebrospinal fluid has less protein than plasma under normal circumstances.

4. **Development of the brain:**
   - (a) True—The retina is a product of primitive forebrain development.
   - (b) False—Mesencephalon refers to the midbrain.
   - (c) False—They are part of the telencephalon.
   - (d) True—Rathke's pouch is an inward growth from the oral cavity, and forms the anterior pituitary.
   - (e) False—The tela choroidea comprises pia mater and the ependyma.

5. **CNS environment:**
   - (a) False—There are many more glia than neurons.
   - (b) True—Microglia are antigen-presenting cells which interact with the immune system.
   - (c) False—Astrocytes regulate interstitial potassium concentration.
   - (d) False—Schwann cells myelinate only one axon.
   - (e) False—D-glucose is the isomer transported across the blood–brain barrier.

6. **The action potential:**
   - (a) False—Cation entry causes depolarization and an excitatory postsynaptic potential.
   - (b) False—Spatial summation occurs with simultaneous transmission from many synapses.
   - (c) False—There is a high concentration of Na^+ channels at the axon hillock as this is where the action potential is generated.
   - (d) True—Large myelinated axons therefore have the fastest transmission.
   - (e) True—Axonal membranes have an increased capacitance.

7. **The synapse:**
   - (a) False—Electrical synapses have no transmitter.
   - (b) True—Axoaxonic synapses are often inhibitory.
   - (c) False—Intracellular Ca^{2+} is the signal for exocytosis.
   - (d) False—Dopamine synthesis is regulated by altering the activity of tyrosine hydroxylase.
   - (e) True—This is one mechanism for the termination of postsynaptic activation.

8. **Neurons:**
   - (a) True—The sodium–potassium ATPase consumes a lot of energy.
   - (b) False—Interneuron axons do not leave their cell group.
   - (c) True—Astrocytes also regulate insterstitial fluid potassium concentration and prevent the build-up of GABA.
   - (d) True—Electrical synapses may also be unidirectional.
   - (e) False—The vesicles are typically spherical.

9. **Neurotransmission:**
   - (a) False—There are several receptors, including NMDA, kainite and AMPA.
   - (b) False—Nicotinic receptors are associated with a cation channel.
   - (c) False—Metabotrophic receptors are generally G-protein linked.
   - (d) True—This hyperpolarizes the cell.
   - (e) False—Under physiological conditions, saltatory conduction is unidirectional.

10. The spinal cord:
- (a) False—The spinothalamic tract carries contralateral sensory information.
- (b) True—The dorsal columns have their decussation in the medulla.
- (c) True—These are motor fibres from the contralateral motor cortex.
- (d) False—The tectospinal tract carries information from the midbrain to the spinal cord.
- (e) False—The dorsal columns carry information predominantly about fine touch, vibration and position sense.

11. The spinal cord:
- (a) False—In adults, the cord generally ends at L1–L2.
- (b) False—The dorsal column tracts decussate in the medulla.
- (c) True—Tabes dorsalis is a bilateral lesion of the dorsal columns.
- (d) True—There are both ipsilateral (fine touch, proprioception) and contralateral (pain, temperature) losses in the Brown-Séquard syndrome.
- (e) False—The cell bodies (grey matter) lie centrally within the cord.

12. Pain:
- (a) True—Nociceptors have free nerve endings.
- (b) True—This is one of the sites of action for opioid analgesics.
- (c) False—Opioids also act on the brain and peripherally.
- (d) False—In morphine overdose, 'pin-prick' pupils are observed.
- (e) True—Naloxone is used in the treatment of opioid overdose.

13. Somatosensation:
- (a) False—Rapidly adapting receptors fire maximally at the beginning and end of a stimulus.
- (b) False—Axons from nociceptors are unmyelinated.
- (c) False—The cell bodies lie in the grey matter of the spinal cord.
- (d) False—Hands are important for exploration, and require dense sensory innervation.
- (e) True—The sensory cortex lies in the postcentral gyrus.

14. Giving opioid drugs to patients in acute pain:
- (a) False—Opioids given acutely for pain do not cause dependence.
- (b) True—Opioids should generally be prescribed with an antiemetic.
- (c) False—Urinary retention is a recognized complication.
- (d) True—Pupillary assessment (e.g. for brainstem lesions) will not be reliable.
- (e) True—The dose must be titrated to relieve the pain, but so as not to cause undue sedation or respiratory depression.

15. Analgesia for back pain:
- (a) True—NSAIDs are non-specific COX inhibitors.
- (b) False—There is no evidence to suggest that selective COX–2 inhibitors are more effective.
- (c) True—Ibuprofen is analgesic and anti-inflammatory, with a good side-effect profile.
- (d) False—Patients with back pain should generally be advised to carry out gentle exercise (ideally under the supervision of a physiotherapist).
- (e) True—This may represent a cauda equina syndrome produced by lumbar disc prolapse requiring urgent surgical intervention.

16. Analgesia:
- (a) True—This involves endorphins and enkephalins (opioids).
- (b) True—Some tricyclic antidepressants have been found to be effective in lower back pain.
- (c) False—The commonest side effects are constipation and nausea.
- (d) False—Naloxone has a much shorter duration of action.
- (e) False—Traditional NSAIDs inhibit both COX–1 and COX–2.

17. The pyramidal tract:
- (a) False—There are also fibres that regulate spinal reflexes from the sensory system.
- (b) True—The pyramidal tract passes through the posterior part of the internal capsule.
- (c) True—Hands need fine muscle control, and hence need dense motor innervation.
- (d) False—Lower motor neuron lesions lead to atrophy and fasciculation.
- (e) True—The medial corticospinal tract innervates the proximal.

18. Basal ganglia:
- (a) False—The striatum has connections with motor, sensory, association and limbic areas.
- (b) True—This pathway is deficient in Parkinson's disease.
- (c) False—The indirect loop inhibits the cortex.
- (d) False—L-dopa is metabolized by dopa decarboxylase.
- (e) True—The basal ganglia have a role in processing motor prorogrammes.

19. Parkinson's disease:
- (a) False—Signs may be very subtle.

(b) False—The longer the patient can manage without drugs the better, as tolerance to L-dopa soon develops.
(c) False—Motor neurons are not affected.
(d) True—Anticholinergics inhibit striatal output cells.
(e) True—Depression may aggravate symptoms.

20. The cerebellum:
(a) True—Mossy fibres carry proprioceptive inputs from the spinal cord.
(b) False—Purkinje cells send inhibitory inputs to deep cerebellar nuclei.
(c) True—In contrast to the cerebral cortex, which processes contralateral information.
(d) True—Typically ataxia manifests as a wide-based gait.
(e) False—Complex spikes in Purkinje cells may signal error detection.

21. The motor unit:
(a) False—If one neuron innervates many muscle fibres, coarse control of movement is produced.
(b) True—This is the case for both reflex and voluntary movements.
(c) True—Slow fibres have high levels of oxidative enzymes.
(d) False—Diseases of muscle fibres cause atrophy.
(e) True—Motor neuron disease causes fasciculations.

22. The vestibular system:
(a) True—The utricle and saccule detect head position and movement.
(b) True—This helps maintain posture.
(c) True—This is the mainstay of the vestibulo-ocular reflex.
(d) True—Inputs from both ears are integrated in the vestibular nuclei and have complementary effects on cranial nerves III and VI.
(e) False—Inputs from the motor system are also required.

23. Parkinson's disease:
(a) False—Loss of > 80% of dopaminergic neurons in the substantia nigra of the midbrain causes Parkinson's disease.
(b) False—The tremor is typically between 3–6 Hz.
(c) True—The rigidity is described as 'cog-wheeling'.
(d) False—Macrographia is small handwriting (micrographia), which is typical.
(e) True—Characterized by slow movements, paucity of facial expression and shuffling gait.

24. The brainstem:
(a) False—The pyramidal decussation is in the lower medulla.
(b) True—The trigeminal nucleus also receives inputs from cranial nerves VII, IX and X.
(c) True—This happens in the upper medulla.
(d) True—The VIth nerve nucleus lies slightly posterior, in the lower pons.
(e) True—Cranial nerve III leaves in the upper midbrain.

25. The autonomic nervous system:
(a) False—Postganglionic neurons are unmyelinated.
(b) False—There are also preganglionic parasympathetic cell bodies in the sacral region.
(c) False—Muscarinic antagonists release the heart from tonic parasympathetic inhibition.
(d) True—In both sympathetic and parasympathetic systems, acetylcholine is released.
(e) True—This coordinates the activation of ganglia at different spinal levels.

26. Horner's syndrome:
(a) True—Apical lung tumours, spinal cord tumours, neck tumours and brainstem tumours may all cause a Horner's syndrome.
(b) False—Anhidrosis is only a feature of central lesions.
(c) True—Central Horner's syndrome causes the pupil to react normally.
(d) True—Any surgical exploration of the neck may lead to damage to the sympathetic nerves to the face.
(e) False—Vision is retained, but acuity may be reduced and ptosis may be limiting.

27. The sympathetic nervous system:
(a) True—These effects are antagonistic to those of the parasympathetic nervous system.
(b) False—The coeliac ganglion supplies foregut structures.
(c) False—The sympathetic nervous system acts to dilate the pupil.
(d) False—The interomediolateral column runs from T1 to L2.
(e) False—Noradrenaline and adrenaline are released from the adrenal medulla.

28. Unconscious with neck stiffness:
(a) False—A computed tomography head scan should ideally be performed first.
(b) False—A purpuric rash is more typical of meningococcal disease.
(c) True—Blood irritates the meninges.
(d) False—Infiltrative tumours may cause neck stiffness.
(e) False—Urgent investigation is mandatory.

29. Dementia:
- (a) True—Pick's disease is a predominantly cortical dementia.
- (b) False—Dementia is a common feature of Parkinson's disease.
- (c) False—A mini-mental state score of 28 and above may be considered normal.
- (d) False—EEG is of no clinical relevance in dementia.
- (e) False—Alzheimer's disease is the cause of approximately 80% of dementia.

30. Anxiolytics and anticonvulsants:
- (a) False—Benzodiazepines facilitate GABA at the GABA receptor.
- (b) True—This may produce a prolonged sedative effect.
- (c) True—Although lorazepam is more often used.
- (d) True—There may also be nystagmus and diplopia.
- (e) False—Valproate also increases GABA content and action.

31. Cerebrovascular disease:
- (a) True—The mortality rate depends on the size and site of the infarct.
- (b) False—Lacunar infarctions involve predominantly sensory or motor tract, not higher functions.
- (c) False—Subarachnoid haemorrhage is usually caused by rupture of a berry aneurysm.
- (d) True—Symptoms include nystagmus, pain and temperature sensory loss and cerebellar signs.
- (e) False—Amaurosis fugax is suggestive of an ipsilateral carotid lesion.

32. Fitting in a 60-year-old woman:
- (a) False—Stopping the fit takes priority.
- (b) True—Diazepam or lorazepam can be used in status epilepticus.
- (c) False—A cause for the fit should be sought.
- (d) False—This is the correct diagnosis, but a cause must be sought.
- (e) False—If the seizure continues she should be transferred to the intensive care unit.

33. Brain tumours:
- (a) False—Tumours of glial cells are more commonly seen in adults.
- (b) True—Meningiomas comprise 20% of all brain tumours.
- (c) False—Magnetic resonance imaging is the investigation of choice for posterior fossa tumours.
- (d) False—Malignant tumours may also show calcification (e.g. oligodendroglioma).
- (e) True—Bronchogenic carcinoma accounts for nearly 50% of primary tumours which metastasize to the brain.

34. Cerebral oedema:
- (a) False—Vasogenic oedema is an intercellular oedema.
- (b) True—Cytotoxic oedema may affect grey or white matter.
- (c) True—Position (head up) may also help.
- (d) True—Hydrocephalus causes an extracellular oedema.
- (e) True—Toxic metabolites are released into the brain substance.

35. Developmental and associated disorders:
- (a) False—Intellectual function is often preserved.
- (b) False—Deterioration is unlikely.
- (c) False—Ultrasonography is only useful in infants.
- (d) True—This is a potentially treatable form of dementia.
- (e) True—Hydrocephalus may cause headache.

36. Epileptic seizure in an adult:
- (a) False—The patient is prevented from driving for 1 year.
- (b) True—An underlying cause should be sought.
- (c) False—A computed tomography scan may reveal a mass lesion which would make lumbar puncture dangerous.
- (d) False—Absence seizures are generally not due to an apparent structural abnormality.
- (e) True—The risk is highest in the first year.

37. Central nervous system infections:
- (a) False—These organisms are the commonest causes of meningitis.
- (b) True—In most cases.
- (c) False—Antibiotics should be given immediately if lumbar puncture is not available.
- (d) False—Acyclovir is a relatively safe drug and should be given whenever herpes simplex encephalitis is suspected.
- (e) False—Toxoplasmosis is caused by a protozoan parasite.

38. Seizures in susceptible individuals:
- (a) True—This is potentially a dangerous situation if the patient lives on their own, and slips into status epilepticus overnight.
- (b) True—This is one of the methods of inducing seizures used in EEG testing.
- (c) True—This is another method of inducing seizures.
- (d) True—Cases of seizures in high-stress situations have been reported.
- (e) True—Any intercurrent illness may precipitate a seizure.

39. Multiple sclerosis:
- (a) True—These are symptoms of optic neuritis.
- (b) True—This is known as Lhermitte's sign.

(c) False—Bence-Jones protein is an indicator for myeloma.
(d) True—Plaques of inflammation and demyelination may be seen.
(e) False—The average time from diagnosis to death is between 25 and 30 years.

40. A 79-year-old man with a left hemiparesis:
(a) False—The majority of left-handed people are still left hemisphere dominant.
(b) False—Anterior circulation stroke is more likely.
(c) True—However, its absence does not exclude a tight stenosis.
(d) False—Ischaemic stroke is more likely.
(e) True—Stroke units have been shown to reduce mortality significantly.

41. Patients at high risk of stroke:
(a) True—Amaurosis fugax can be thought of as a transient ischaemic attack of the retina, and commonly indicates carotid artery disease.
(b) False—However, migraine may cause a stroke-like picture, with focal neurological signs.
(c) True—There is an association between polycystic kidney disease and berry aneurysms which predispose to subarachnoid haemorrhage.
(d) True—Smoking and hypertension, along with old age, are all risk factors for cerebrovascular disease.
(e) False—A fully resolved meningitis does not predispose to intracerebral bleeds or ischaemia.

42. Causes of cerebral palsy:
(a) True—The 'TORCH' infections are the chief infective causes of cerebral palsy.
(b) True—Pre-eclampsia may lead to cerebral palsy, if not treated promptly.
(c) False—Hyperglycaemia commonly leads to large-for-dates babies.
(d) True—Although this is a minor cause of cerebral palsy (approximately 10% of cases).
(e) True—Any intracranial haemorrhage may lead to cerebral palsy.

43. Myotonic dystrophy:
(a) True—Myasthenia gravis is another cause.
(b) False—Muscular dystrophies are not associated with increased tone.
(c) True—Myotonic dystrophy causes a cardiomyopathy.
(d) True—Myotonic dystrophy is autosomal dominant in its inheritance.
(e) True—Myotonia means tonic spasm of the muscle.

44. Muscular dystrophy:
(a) True—Both Duchenne and Becker muscular dystrophies are X-linked.
(b) True—Both disorders are caused by mutations in the same gene.
(c) True—Boys with the disorder characteristically 'push up' off their thighs to reach a standing position.
(d) False—The weakness is primarily proximal, leading to the illusion of calf hypertrophy.
(e) False—The calf muscles are of normal bulk, but appear large (pseudohypertrophy) due to wasting of the thigh muscles.

45. Neurofibromatosis:
(a) False—Neurofibromatosis is an autosomal dominant ~~recessive~~ condition.
(b) False—Bilateral acoustic neuromas are a primary feature of type II neurofibromatosis.
(c) False—They are hamartomas of the iris, invisible to the naked eye.
(d) True—Gliomas and Schwannomas are also common.
(e) True—These findings are suggestive of type I neurofibromatosis.

46. Fatigue and proximal muscle weakness:
(a) True—LEMS is an important diagnosis to exclude as it is commonly seen in the presence of a malignancy.
(b) False—Repeated chest X-rays are important as symptoms may predate changes by up to 4 years.
(c) False—The presynaptic membrane which is affected in LEMS.
(d) True—In contrast to myasthenia gravis.
(e) True—Much less commonly, it affects the facial muscles (c.f. myasthenia gravis).

47. Potential triggers of Guillain–Barré syndrome:
(a) True—This is the commonest trigger for GBS.
(b) True—Influenza may trigger GBS.
(c) False—There are no reported cases of GBS following MMR.
(d) True—Herpes zoster is a recognized cause of GBS.
(e) True—Epstein–Barr virus may cause GBS.

48. The eye:
(a) False—The blink reflex relies on corneal innervation by the Vth nerve.
(b) True—This helps to maintain the transparency of the nerve fibres.
(c) False—The sclera is continuous with the dura mater.
(d) False—The fovea contains only cones.
(e) True—This would inhibit light reaching the area of highest cone density.

49. Central visual pathways:
(a) True—Temporal fibres remain on the ipsilateral side.

(b) False—Thalamic cells receive monocular input.
(c) False—Lesions of the optic tract affect one half of the visual field.
(d) True—The primary visual cortex is organized into ocular dominance columns.
(e) False—The fovea (central visual field) has proportionally greater representation in the cortex than does the peripheral field.

50. Glaucoma:
(a) True—The normal range is between 10–20 mmHg.
(b) False—Glaucoma is the third most common cause of blindness in the UK.
(c) False—Acute closed angle glaucoma is an ophthalmological emergency.
(d) False—Tropicamide drops dilate the pupil and may cause a catastrophic rise in intraocular pressure.
(e) True—The scleral sinus normally drains the aqueous humour, and a blockage causes a build-up of fluid.

51. Eye movements:
(a) True—The IIIrd and VIth nerves perform complementary functions in the vestibulo-ocular reflex.
(b) True—The frontal eye fields help to keep the fovea on a particular target.
(c) False—Smooth pursuit eye movements hold the image on the fovea — the optic disc corresponds to the blind spot.
(d) True—The eyes both look towards the midline when focussing on a near target.
(e) True—This is called optokinetic nystagmus and is used, for example, when looking out of a moving vehicle.

52. The auditory system:
(a) False—The basilar membrane is wider at the top than the bottom.
(b) True—Hair cells are grouped according to frequency selectivity.
(c) True—Fibres from the olivocochlear bundle provide feedback to the outer hair cells.
(d) False—The colliculi integrate information from both ears.
(e) False—The primary auditary cortex is in the temporal lobe.

53. Deafness:
(a) False—A positive Rinnes test indicates conductive deafness.
(b) True—It is as though the sensitivity of the nerve has been adjusted to compensate for the loss of air conduction.
(c) True—Vertigo is likely to be associated with the hearing loss in this case.
(d) False—Air conduction is more important than bone conduction under normal circumstances.
(e) False—Cochlear implants are only useful in selected cases. First-line treatment still comprises the use of hearing aids.

54. Taste and smell:
(a) True—Fungiform papillae comprise the majority of taste buds.
(b) True—The fibres gain access to the olfactory bulb through the cribriform plate.
(c) True—This relays information to the thalamus.
(d) False—Granule cells receive feedback from the anterior olfactory nucleus.
(e) False—There are direct projections from the olfactory bulb to the cortex.

55. A 55-year-old woman with a brain tumour:
(a) False—Constructional apraxias are localized to the non-dominant hemisphere.
(b) True—Temporal lobe damage causes visual field loss of the homonymous upper quadrant.
(c) False—Sensory inattention and neglect are characteristic of non-dominant hemisphere lesions.
(d) True—Personality changes are suggestive of frontal lobe damage.
(e) False—Dyscalculia suggests parietal damage.

56. Memory and the limbic system:
(a) True—These areas are involved in memory.
(b) True—The parahippocampal gyrus is the inferior continuation of the cingulate gyrus.
(c) True—The first items in a list are remembered first by activating long-term memory.
(d) True—Damage to the medial temporal lobe structures produces disruption of declarative memory, sparing procedural memory.
(e) True—There is a limited capacity for working memory.

57. The localization of cortical function:
(a) False—Different functions are localized to non-dominant and dominant hemispheres.
(b) False—These deficits occur with parietal lesions.
(c) True—Frontal lobe lesions can be accompanied by personality changes.
(d) False—Motor cortex lesions lead to pseudobulbar palsy.
(e) True—Neglect can result from parietal lesions of the non-dominant hemisphere.

58. Cognitive development and degeneration:
(a) False—Newborns have auditory capabilities and can respond to important stimuli such as faces.

(b) True—The sensorimotor stage comprises the first two years of life.
(c) False—Relative synaptogenesis compensates for the brain's inability to form new neurons.
(d) True—Although numbers of neurons decrease.
(e) False—Social withdrawal may be due to treatable causes (e.g. depression).

59. Brainstem-acting drugs:
(a) False—5-HT_3 antagonists also act on peripheral inputs.
(b) True—Antihistamines are useful in the treatment of vertigo.
(c) False—Dopamine antagonists are effective antiemetics.
(d) False—Potency is related to the oil : gas or oil : water partition coefficient.
(e) True—General anaesthetic agents also produce respiratory depression.

60. Antidepressant treatment:
(a) False—It may be required to control depressive symptoms, but close monitoring is needed.
(b) True—Although it may still require treatment if severe or prolonged.
(c) False—Tricyclic antidepressants are extremely dangerous — leading to cardiac arrhythmias and death in high doses.
(d) True—It is a fine tremor. Levels should be checked regularly.
(e) False—The antidepressant effect may not be seen for 2–3 weeks.

61. The limbic system:
(a) True—Wernicke–Korsakoff syndrome is secondary to chronic alcohol abuse and thiamine deficiency.
(b) True—Herpes simplex encephalitis commonly affects the temporal lobes.
(c) True—In this way, the hormonal processes can be influenced.
(d) False—The amygdala lies on the border of the third ventricle.
(e) True—This phenomenon has been demonstrated in hippocampal neurons.

62. Localizing signs to the temporal lobe:
(a) True—Temporal lobe epilepsy may produce olfactory hallucinations.
(b) True—A receptive dysphasia results from damage to Wernicke's area.
(c) False—Hemiparesis is a result of damage to the prefrontal gyrus.
(d) True—Temporal lobe epilepsy is often associated with psychotic symptoms.
(e) True—Emotional disturbance may go hand in hand with psychosis.

63. Localizing signs to the frontal lobe:
(a) False—The postcentral gyrus deals with sensory input.
(b) False—Neglect is a feature of parietal lobe damage.
(c) True—Typically, patients become more impulsive, aggressive and emotionally labile.
(d) True—Damage to Broca's area produces an expressive dysphasia.
(e) False—Intention tremor is a feature of cerebellar lesions.

64. Endocrine disorders presenting with coma:
(a) True—For example, diabetic ketoacidosis.
(b) True—Addisonian crisis may present in coma.
(c) True—Myxoedema (hypothyroidism) may cause confusional states and coma.
(d) False—Conn's syndrome presents with hypertension and electrolyte imbalance.
(e) False—Cushing's disease presents with the features of glucocorticoid excess.

65. Causes of cognitive impairment with a degree of reversibility:
(a) True—Hypothyroidism may cause a dementia-like picture.
(b) True—Drainage of the haematoma improves cognitive function.
(c) True—Dialysis may be required to reduce uraemia.
(d) True—Successful treatment may depend on a liver transplant.
(e) False—Penicillin treatment should be given to prevent further decline.

66. Nystagmus:
(a) False—Jerky nystagmus with the fast phase to the opposite side to the lesion is seen.
(b) False—Upbeating nystagmus suggests a lesion around the superior colliculi.
(c) True—Pendular nystagmus has normally been present since childhood.
(d) True—This may be mixed in form as well as direction.
(e) False—Nystagmus is usually asymptomatic.

67. A 66-year-old patient presenting with lower cranial nerve palsies:
(a) False—These symptoms are suggestive of a bulbar palsy.
(b) False—The gag reflex is absent in bulbar palsy.
(c) True—Wasting and fasciculation are common.
(d) False—Speech is nasal in quality.
(e) True—This is an indication of a central lesion.

68. Dysphasia:
(a) False—Lesions of Broca's area cause a non-fluent dysphasia.

(b) True—Content and fluency of speech is otherwise normal.
(c) False—Lesions of Broca's area cause a non-fluent dysphasia.
(d) False—The dominant hemisphere contains the language centre.
(e) True—Cerebrovascular disease is by far the commonest.

69. Potential causes of a VIIth nerve palsy:
(a) True—The VII nerve's course takes it close to middle ear structures.
(b) True—This causes a lower motor neuron weakness.
(c) True—This causes an upper motor neuron lesion.
(d) True—This is known as the Ramsay-Hunt syndrome, typically with herpetic vesicles visible within the ear.
(e) False—This is a type of hereditary haemorrhagic telangiectasia and has no association with VIIth nerve palsies.

70. Causes of ptosis:
(a) False—IIIrd nerve palsy may cause a ptosis.
(b) True—Horner's syndrome causes a partial ptosis.
(c) True—Most cases of ptosis in children are due to congenital anomalies.
(d) True—Syphilis is a rare cause of ptosis.
(e) True—Dystrophia myotonica may cause a bilateral partial ptosis.

71. Examination of the cranial nerves:
(a) True—The lateral rectus muscle is supplied by cranial nerve VI.
(b) False—The trigeminal nerve supplies sensation to the forehead.
(c) True—A defect suggests a lower motor neuron lesion.
(d) False—The hypoglossal nerve provides the motor supply to the tongue.
(e) True—If the patient reports disturbance of smell, it is most likely due to nasal congestion.

72. Gait disturbance:
(a) True—A unilateral lesion of the common peroneal nerve is another cause.
(b) False—Parkinson's disease causes a shuffling gait affecting all four limbs and the trunk.
(c) True—Individuals stagger to the affected side in unilateral lesions.
(d) False—They are unusual, but this depends on the degree of hysteria!
(e) True—A positive Romberg's test is indicative of proprioceptive sensory loss.

73. Examination of the peripheral nerves:
(a) False—The standard notation for power tests out of 5.
(b) True—Spasticity has the same meaning as increased tone.
(c) False—In unilateral cerebellar lesions, there may be a discrepancy between coordination on the left and right.
(d) False—Vibration is tested with a low frequency tuning fork (e.g. 128 Hz).
(e) False—Sensation should be tested across all dermatomes.

74. EEG:
(a) False—The UK guidelines do not require an EEG.
(b) True—Generalized slow-wave activity is seen.
(c) False—A normal resting EEG is found in approximately 50% of epileptic patients.
(d) False—There may be focal slow-wave activity.
(e) True—Although migraine is primarily a clinical diagnosis.

75. Typical findings on cerebrospinal fluid analysis:
(a) True—The protein level may be markedly raised.
(b) False—In viral meningitis, the glucose level is normal, or may be high.
(c) True—Lymphocytes are more typical of a viral aetiology.
(d) False—Normally, the glucose level is approximately 50% that of plasma.
(e) False—No polymorphs are seen, but a very small number of lymphocytes may be normal.

76. Weakness in the hands and feet in a young man:
(a) False—This does not explain the symptoms in his upper limbs.
(b) False—Numbness is a common complaint, but there may be no sensory signs.
(c) False—They indicate an upper motor neuron lesion.
(d) False—Campylobacter infection may be a precipitant for Guillain–Barré syndrome.
(e) False—The vital capacity should be measured.

77. Central, crushing chest pain, radiating to the jaw and left arm:
(a) False—There are nociceptors in the viscera, but their afferents synapse on the same pathway as superficial nociceptors, making the inputs indistinguishable to the brain.
(b) True—Aδ fibres are faster for sharp, stabbing pain. C fibres convey more dull, nagging pains.
(c) False—Cardiac arrhythmia is a more likely cause of syncope.
(d) True—Risk factors for ischaemic heart disease and cerebrovascular disease overlap.

(e) True—A haemorrhagic stroke would be a contraindication to thombolysis.

78. Unconscious drug addict:
(a) False—The effects of heroin overdose are similar to those of morphine (heroin = diamorphine).
(b) True—Long-term damage may lead to affective disorders and/or psychosis.
(c) False—Tolerance rapidly develops.
(d) True—This is made worse by hyperpyrexia, which encourages the patient to drink more water.
(e) False—Drug addicts also require pain relief, and may need higher doses as tolerance to opioids develops.

79. A 54-year old patient collapses at home:
(a) False—The tongue may have been bitten due to the patient's head banging on an object as they fell.
(b) False—A single seizure does not define epilepsy.
(c) True—Micturition syncope is commonest in elderly men.
(d) True—Patients typically give a history of hanging curtains, or reaching up to high shelves before collapsing.
(e) True—Postural hypotension is an important side effect of these drugs.

80. Causes of coma in a known alcoholic:
(a) False—Hypoglycaemia is a much more likely cause of coma.
(b) True—Head injuries are common in alcoholics and may lead to subdural haematomas.
(c) True—Alcoholism and drug addiction/suicide attempts commonly go hand in hand.
(d) True—Hepatic encephalopathy may cause drowsiness and coma.
(e) False—This is a complication of chronic alcohol abuse, but does not cause coma.

81. Choreiform movements:
(a) True—Long-term treatment with L-dopa may lead to the dose required being sufficient to cause chorea.
(b) True—Thyrotoxicosis may cause chorea.
(c) False—Chorea is caused by central problems.
(d) False—Motor neuron disease leads to paralysis.
(e) True—This is called Sydenham's chorea.

82. The pituitary gland:
(a) True—Microadenomas are the commonest pituitary tumours.
(b) False—Thyrotrophin releasing hormone is released by the hypothalamus, inducing the pituitary to release thyroid-stimulating hormone.
(c) True—The hypothalamic–pituitary axis has a specialized circulation.
(d) True—They do so by causing compression of the optic chiasm.
(e) False—Acromegaly is caused by excessive secretion of growth hormone in adulthood.

83. An unconscious 64-year-old woman:
(a) False—Resuscitation is the first priority.
(b) False—Stroke rarely causes loss of consciousness.
(c) True—The presence of ketones in the urine may lead to the suspicion of diabetic ketoacidosis as a diagnosis.
(d) False—Even a dead person scores 3 on the Glasgow Coma Scale.
(e) True—If there is not a rapid improvement, then the diagnosis should be reconsidered.

84. The optic fundus:
(a) False—The optic disc appears paler on fundoscopy.
(b) True—The disc margin should be crisp and distinct.
(c) False—Arteriovenous nipping is seen in hypertensive retinopathy.
(d) True—Methyl alcohol may cause optic atrophy and blindness.
(e) False—Pigmentation may be seen after laser treatment (e.g. for diabetic retinopathy).

85. A 25-year-old man after a road traffic accident:
(a) False—If possible, his helmet should be left in place until the cervical spine is cleared. However, if it is the only means of maintaining an airway, then it should be removed carefully.
(b) False—Even if dead, he will score 3/15 on the Glasgow Coma Scale.
(c) True—This may indicate cerebrospinal fluid leak from a basal skull fracture.
(d) True—Trauma is a common cause of adult-onset epilepsy.
(e) True—This takes priority, even over protection of the cervical spine.

86. Consequences of an acoustic neuroma:
(a) False—A sensorineural deafness results.
(b) True—The facial nerve runs in close proximity to the cerebellopontine angle.
(c) True—Nystagmus is a feature of VIIIth nerve lesions.
(d) True—Although this is a late sign.
(e) False—Acoustic neuromas are benign tumours of Schwann cell origin.

87. Papilloedema when clerking a patient:
- (a) True—Any space-occupying lesion can raise intracranial pressure sufficient to cause papilloedema.
- (b) False—Hypercapnoea causes papilloedema.
- (c) True—A high cerebrospinal fluid protein level may cause papilloedema.
- (d) False—Malignant hypertension is an important cause, which must not be missed.
- (e) True—This may represent the first presentation of multiple sclerosis in 50% of cases.

88. Approach to the unconscious patient:
- (a) True—The airway is unprotected at this level of coma.
- (b) False—The breathing described is known as Kussmaul breathing.
- (c) True—These are ominous signs.
- (d) True—The cervical spine should be cleared on X-ray whenever there is a suspicion of neck trauma.
- (e) False—Retinal haemorrhages may indicate a subarachnoid haemorrhage.

89. Delirium:
- (a) True—This is especially true in the elderly.
- (b) False—Disorientation in time is generally the most sensitive index.
- (c) False—The underlying cause must be sought and treated.
- (d) False—True delirium resolves completely on removal of the trigger.
- (e) False—Delerium occurs in up to 15% of patients on general medical and surgical wards.

90. Mixed upper and lower motor neuron signs:
- (a) False—Diabetic neuropathy is primarily a sensory and autonomic neuropathy.
- (b) True—HIV causes a wide range of neurological conditions, which vary in their presentation.
- (c) True—Lower motor neuron signs are seen at the level of the compression, with upper motor neuron signs below.
- (d) False—Guillain–Barré syndrome is a primarily motor neuropathy, so lower motor neuron signs only are seen.
- (e) True—The cardinal features of motor neuron disease are a mixed picture of upper and lower motor neuron lesions.

91. A patient presents with tremor:
- (a) False—Tremor is a common side effect of β_2-agonists.
- (b) True—The tremor of Parkinson's disease is typically 3–5 Hz.
- (c) False—These are all signs of a hyperventilatory state, which is rarely indicative of serious pathology.
- (d) True—Lithium toxicity causes a fine tremor.
- (e) False—Tremor is more common in hyperthyroidism.

92. Chronic alcohol abuse:
- (a) False—A liver flap indicates hepatic encephalopathy, which is a late sign of liver disease.
- (b) False—Deficiencies of thiamine, B_{12} and folate are common in Western societies.
- (c) False—Korsakoff's syndrome is the irreversible consequence of thiamine deficiency and alcohol abuse.
- (d) True—The patient confabulates to fill in gaps in his memory.
- (e) False—The dreaded 'DTs' develop 24–48 hours after the last drink.

93. A 54-year-old patient presents with diplopia:
- (a) True—There may also be pupil abnormalities.
- (b) False—These are the typical signs of a VIth nerve lesion.
- (c) True—In other IIIrd nerve lesions, the pupil is dilated and unreactive.
- (d) True—Diplopia may come on with fatigue (e.g. after looking at a computer screen all day).
- (e) True—A subarachnoid haemorrhage is likely.

94. A 19-year-old man before surgery for bilateral pes cavus:
- (a) True—Increased tone may be a consequence of spina bifida.
- (b) False—Pes cavus is caused by increased tone, which is not seen in diabetic neuropathy.
- (c) False—Porphyria causes a flaccid paralysis.
- (d) False—Chronic changes are needed to develop a permanent deformity.
- (e) True—Nerve conduction studies may be abnormal.

95. Antidepressants and antipsychotics:
- (a) False—The cheese reaction occurs due to inhibition of liver monoamine oxidase.
- (b) True—Side effects include dry mouth, constipation, urinary retention and postural hypotension.
- (c) False—Antipsychotic potency is proportional to D_2 receptor blocking activity.
- (d) False—They are extrapyramidal side effects.
- (e) False—Clonazepine acts preferentially on D_4 receptors.

96. Bilateral wasting and weakness of the small hand muscles:
- (a) False—Bilateral cerebral lesions would give bilateral upper motor neuron signs.

(b) True—Deformity may also be present.
(c) False—Cervical spondylosis causes compression of the C5 and C6 nerve roots, depressing the biceps reflex.
(d) False—Cervical spondylosis causes a progressive spastic quadriparesis with upper motor neuron signs in the legs.
(e) False—Syringomyelia is very rare.

97. A 25-year-old man with a head injury:
(a) False—A computed tomography scan or magnetic resonance imaging may be more appropriate for severe injury, mild injuries may not require investigation.
(b) False—Minor injuries can cause subdural haematomas.
(c) False—Concussion injuries show no macroscopic damage.
(d) False—Extradural haematoma is caused by tearing of the middle meningeal artery.
(e) True—There is an increased risk for the first week after head injury.

98. Numbness in the leg:
(a) False—Meralgia paraesthetica is a benign cause for these symptoms.
(b) False—The skin on the sole of the foot is supplied by S1, whereas the knee jerk is mediated by L3/L4.
(c) True—The rash will generally be dermatomal.
(d) False—Distal numbness in a glove and stocking distribution is typically associated with diabetic neuropathy.
(e) False—Sensory symptoms and signs are usually absent in motor neuron disease.

99. A 60-year-old man with a 5-year history of dizziness:
(a) False—There is no suggestion of a seizure.
(b) True—Impending stroke is a danger.
(c) True—Autonomic failure in the Shy–Drager syndrome may cause postural hypotension.
(d) False—A fall of > 20 mmHg on standing is significant.
(e) True—Cardiac arrhythmias may cause hypotension and light-headedness.

100. Metabolic and toxic diseases of the nervous system:
(a) False—Subacute combined degeneration of the cord is caused by vitamin B_{12} deficiency.
(b) True—Delirium tremens is an emergency, and reaches its peak 24–36 hours after stopping drinking.
(c) False—Lead poisoning causes chronic motor neuropathy, typically with wrist drop.
(e) True—Wernicke–Korsakoff syndrome is caused by thiamine deficiency.
(e) False—After an initial acute encephalopathy, chronic encephalopathy and parkinsonism develop.

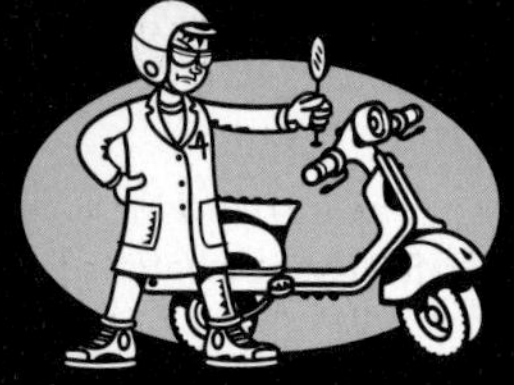

SAQ Answers

1. See Figs 3.4 and 3.5. Dorsal columns labelled with ipsilateral proprioceptive and fine touch information. Spinothalamic tract labelled with contralateral crude touch, pain and temperature information.

2. (a) Briefly describe how to perform this manoeuvre.
   (b) Positive Hallpike's manoeuvre can be due to a peripheral (semicircular canals) or central (brainstem) pathology (Fig. 15.24).

3. (a) (i) Part of a general illness; for example, thyrotoxicosis, alcohol dependence, hepatic failure. (ii) Owing to neurological disease [e.g. action tremor (drugs, essential), resting (parkinsonism), intention (cerebellar)]. Confused with tremor (e.g. pseudoathetosis).
   (b) Note: the question asked for examination, not history. (i) General (e.g. tachycardia, goitre, hepatomegaly). (ii) Specific [e.g. at rest, on action only, with intention, with eyes shut (pseudoathetosis), bradykinesia, rigidity, etc.] Is there a disturbance of eye movement?

4. Preganglionic fibres are myelinated and postganglionic fibres are unmyelinated. In the parasympathetic nervous system, the ganglia are close to their target organs, which means that most of the journey from the central nervous system to the target is along myelinated fibres. In the sympathetic nervous system, the ganglia are nearer to the cord (e.g. paravertebral chain and mesenteric ganglia). A greater fraction of the signal pathway in the sympathetic nervous system uses unmyelinated fibres.

5. (a) Days–weeks progressive, flaccid, hyporeflexic weakness, usually following a gastrointestinal or respiratory illness
   (b) See Chapter 15, p. 210

6. (a) Neurological damage may result from oedema, haemorrhage, compression of the cord by fractured or misaligned vertebrae, or transection of the cord by elements of the vertebral column.
   (b) The principles of management include immobilization to prevent further neural damage, preservation of skin integrity, preservation of bladder and bowel function, management of complications (respiratory, cardiovascular, gastrointestinal) and long-term rehabilitation.

7. Fig. 1.8. Neural tube defects can result in malformations of the vertebral column and skull. In the spine, these range from defects in the vertebral arch to complete exposure of the spinal cord. In the skull, failure of cranial neuropore closure can result in anencephaly, but less-severe malformations result in defects in the occipital bone.

8. (a) Obstructive, communicating, and compensatory hydrocephalus. Expand.
   (b) Clinical features depend on the age of the patient and on whether the hydrocephalus is acute or chronic (Fig. 11.6).

9. Astrocytes—support, nutrition, regulation of extracellular ion concentration, absorption of neurotransmitters, scar formation.
   Oligodendrocytes—myelination of central nervous system axons.
   Microglia—phagocytosis and antigen presentation.

10. (a) Epilepsy. History—from a witness, and from the patient (how exactly did she feel 'funny'? was she confused on waking? etc.). Examination—since episodes sound like focal seizures with secondary generalization, there may (but often are not) be focal signs.
    (b) Explain. Investigate (EEG, CT). Therapy. Advice (driving and avoid precipitants).

11. The jacksonian march is a seizure affecting the motor cortex, producing muscle movement that spreads over the body. As the disordered neuronal firing moves along the motor cortex, it produces action in different muscle groups, which implies that muscles within a group are represented in the same area of the cortex. The fact that movement spreads over the body indicates that the whole body is represented in the cortex in an orderly fashion. This is further evidence for the homuncular organization of the motor cortex.

12. Refer to Fig. 6.4.

13. Refer to Fig. 8.5.

14. (a) Carpal tunnel syndrome.
    (b) History: predisposing factors (e.g. occupation: cleaning windows and scrubbing floors can provoke, arthritis, not pregnancy at this age), relieving factors (shaking), history to suggest another cause? (e.g. neck pains, numb feet). Examination: evidence of median nerve compression, no evidence of generalized neuropathy.

15. (a) Proximally.
    (b) Inherited (e.g. Becker's or limb girdle muscular dystrophy, metabolic myopathy, not Duchenne's at this age). Acquired (e.g. polymyositis, myasthenia gravis, endocrine disease, neoplastic).

16. The ossicles transmit vibrations from the tympanic membrane to the oval window. The base plate of the stapes has a much smaller surface area than the tympanic membrane so that pressure changes due to

sound waves are amplified in the perilymph by movement of the stapes.

17. (a) The symptoms and signs depend on the anatomical location of the plaques (optic nerve: optic neuritis with reduced visual acuity, central scotoma, afferent pupillary defect and pale optic disc; brainstem: abnormal eye movements, limb ataxia, dysarthria and vertigo; spinal cord: sensory symptoms and signs with occasional sensory levels, spastic weakness, sphincter disturbance). Other features include dementia, euphoria, facial pain and painful tonic spasms.
(b) Multiple sclerosis is a clinical diagnosis. Magnetic resonance imaging is the most helpful investigation and is abnormal in almost all cases. Cerebrospinal fluid shows oligoclonal bands in 90% of cases. Evoked potentials may be prolonged.

18. We sense a loss of taste because olfaction contributes much more than taste receptors to our perceived sense of taste. In a blocked-up nose, olfactory stimuli have difficulty reaching the olfactory epithelium in the roof of the nasal cavity and so we rely on the poorer information from taste buds.

19. Primacy and recency effects, amnesic patients with preserved long-term memory and poor working memory, the coding system used for information storage and capacity for information storage.

20. (a) The clinical features of sensory and cerebellar ataxic gaits should be discussed.
(b) Romberg's test would help to differentiate between these two types of ataxia. Expand.

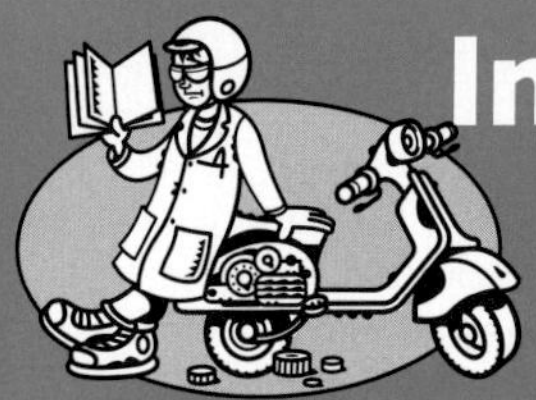

Index